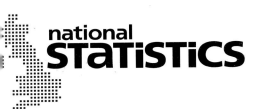

national
STATISTICS

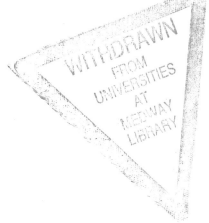
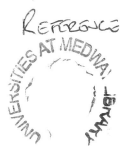
FOCUS ON Health

2006 edition

Editors: Madhavi Bajekal, Velda Osborne, Mohammed Yar and Howard Meltzer

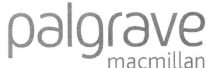
palgrave
macmillan

First published 2006 by
PALGRAVE MACMILLAN
Houndmills, Basingstoke, Hampshire RG21 6XS and
175 Fifth Avenue, New York, NY 10010
Companies and representatives throughout the world.

PALGRAVE MACMILLAN is the global academic imprint of the Palgrave Macmillan division of St. Martin's Press, LLC and of Palgrave Macmillan Ltd. Macmillan® is a registered trademark in the United States, United Kingdom and other countries. Palgrave is a registered trademark in the European Union and other countries.

ISBN 1-4039-9325-4

This book is printed on paper suitable for recycling and made from fully managed and sustained forest sources.

A catalogue record for this book is available from the British Library.

10   9   8   7   6   5   4   3   2   1
15   14   13   12   11   10   09   08   07   06

Printed and bound in Great Britain by
William Clowes Ltd, Beccles, Suffolk.

A National Statistics publication

National Statistics are produced to high professional standards as set out in the National Statistics Code of Practice. They are produced free from political influence.

About the Office for National Statistics

The Office for National Statistics (ONS) is the government agency responsible for compiling, analysing and disseminating economic, social and demographic statistics about the United Kingdom. It also administers the statutory registration of births, marriages and deaths in England and Wales.

The Director of ONS is also the National Statistician and the Registrar General for England and Wales.

For enquiries about this publication, contact:
E-mail: focuson.health@ons.gov.uk

For general enquiries, contact the National Statistics Customer Contact Centre.
Tel: 0845 601 3034 (minicom: 01633 812399)
E-mail: info@statistics.gsi.gov.uk
Fax: 01633 652747
Post: Room 1015, Government Buildings,
          Cardiff Road, Newport NP10 8XG

You can also find National Statistics on the internet at www.statistics.gov.uk

Contents

List of figures, maps and tables

4:   Smoking, drinking and drug use

8: Cancer

Appendices

9: Mental health

Page

11: Use of services

12: Caring and carers

Symbols and conventions

Rounding of figures. In tables where figures have been rounded to the nearest final digit, there may be an apparent discrepancy between the sum of the constituent items and the total as shown.

Non-calendar years:
Financial year – e.g. 1 April 2001 to 31 March 2002 would be shown as 2001/02
Academic year – e.g. September 2000/July 2001 would be shown as 2000/01
Combined years – e.g. 2000–02 shows data for more than one year that have been combined, illustrated in footnotes to tables and figures
Data covering more than one year – e.g. 1998, 1999 and 2000 would be shown as 1998–2000

Symbols. The following symbols have been used throughout the report:

..   not available
-    not applicable
0   nil or less than one

Adults and children:
The general convention followed in this report is:

- Children (boys/girls) for those aged 0–15
- Adults (men/women) for those aged 16 and over
- People (males/females) for all ages or ages spanning children and adults (e.g. 11–18).

The exceptions are Chapters 8 (*Cancer*) and 13 (*Mortality*) where 'adults' are defined as those aged 15 and over.

List of contributors

Authors:	Madhavi Bajekal
	Paul Bebbington
	Claudia Breakwell
	Anita Brock
	Claudia Cooper
	Nicola Cooper
	Melissa Coulthard
	David Dix
	Peter Goldblatt
	Clare Griffiths
	Velda Osborne
	Mike Quinn
	Steve Rowan
	Emmanuel Stamatakis
	Susan Westlake
	Levin Wheller
	Helen Wood
	Mohammed Yar
Production Manager:	Sini Dominy
Production Team:	Alan Herve
	Aidan Steer
	Steve Whyman
Design and layout:	Desktop Publications
	Michelle Franco

Acknowledgements

The editors wish to thank all their colleagues in the Office for National Statistics (ONS) who have helped in the preparation of this report. Special thanks go to our colleagues in the ONS Health and Care Division, and the `Focus on´ team in ONS.

We have received valuable advice from our independent referees: Lorna Booth (Department of Health), Adrienne Cullum (NICE), Sue Davies (ONS), Maria Evandrou (Southampton University), Douglas Fleming (RCGP), Rachael Harker (ONS), Mike Hope (DWP), Lesz Lancucki (NHS Health and Social Care Information Centre), Azeem Majeed (Imperial College), Jane Pearson-Moore (Department of Health), Steve Smallwood (ONS), Diane Stockton (ISD Scotland), Angus Walls (Newcastle University), and Joanne White (Health Protection Agency).

We are grateful also to our colleagues from the following Departments and devolved administrations: Department of Health; Scottish Executive; General Register Office for Scotland; Northern Ireland Statistics and Research Agency; National Assembly for Wales; Department for Work and Pensions; Office of the Deputy Prime Minister; Home Office; the National Institute for Clinical Excellence (NICE), Health Protection Agency; NHS Health and Social Care Information Centre.

Introduction

Madhavi Bajekal and Peter Goldblatt

Chapter 1

Background

Focus on Health is part of the 'Focus on' series of publications from the Office for National Statistics (ONS). The series combines data from the 2001 Census and other sources to illustrate various topics, and provides links to further information. Other reports in the 'Focus on' series cover social inequalities, older people, people and migration, ethnicity and identity, gender, families and religion. 'Focus on' reports consist of a short overview of the topic, followed by a full report containing more comprehensive analysis. *Focus on Health* is the fourth of the full reports in the series to be published. The overviews and full reports can be viewed or downloaded from the National Statistics website: www.statistics.gov.uk/focuson

This report builds on a long tradition of reporting on health issues by ONS and its predecessor organisations. The earliest of these, the Registrar General's Annual Reports initially focused on mortality and fertility,[1] fulfilling a legal obligation to report on the statistics derived from vital registration. Subsequently, the range of reporting was extended to make use, as in this volume, of census information. This was achieved through the decennial supplement series, with its comparisons of information recorded at census and death on topics such as occupation,[2] area of residence,[3] and through the collection of health-related information in the census itself, such as activity restriction and disability.[4] More recently, a number of multiple source reports have been produced to make use of the wider range of information available from surveys, disease notification registers and administrative sources such as healthcare records.[5]

Focus on Health draws on a similar range of sources, describing some of the key issues and trends in present day health in the UK. In such a wide field it is impossible to be comprehensive; so choices have been made about what to include. In general, information on each topic area is drawn from the preferred source for that topic with references to other data sources or publications which might supplement this report. While the aim is to present information for the UK as a whole, we include details for parts of the UK where available and trends are highlighted throughout.

The report is aimed at a general audience and presents clear analyses supported by charts, maps and tables that are easy to understand. The report brings together statistics in a number of broad topic areas and will provide a resource for all those with an interest in health issues, including policy makers, researchers, students and members of the general public. We welcome feedback and suggestions for future reports in the 'Focus on' series: please email focuson.health@ons.gov.uk.

Key concepts

The conceptual basis for this report lies in the framework for health and care statistics, which is intended to underpin the production and development of National Statistics on this topic.[6] Fellegi and Wolfson[7] describe a framework for social statistics as a "structured, meaningful description of the state of society and social activity .... based on a defensible understanding of dynamic relationships among the main factors or variables." The primary reason for having a framework is to ensure that the statistical system is comprehensive, integrated and coherent and meets user needs. While this report does not set out to provide a comprehensive or encyclopaedic account of the health domain, it does aim to illustrate, by example, the key elements of an integrated and coherent framework.

Health

Health is a positive concept, involving the whole person in the context of their situation. It is a state of physical, mental and social well being, not simply the absence of disease and disability.[8] Consequently it relates to both the health status of individuals and the care they receive from health and social services and elsewhere. As health information systems need to be capable of supporting national strategies for achieving health improvement, such systems need to provide reliable statistics for the planning, monitoring and evaluation of health development and services; the assessment of national and local progress in improving health; and the dissemination of this information to professionals, researchers and, most importantly, the public. In this context, the report provides information on population health status as well as specific issues relating to current health targets and service delivery.

The framework

A model of health developed for the World Health Organisation (WHO) in the early 1990s represents the determinants of health as layers of influence, one over another.[9] This model emphasises that individuals are endowed with age, sex and constitutional factors (such as genetics and other aspects of family background) which influence their health potential, but which are fixed. Surrounding the individuals are layers of influence that, in theory, could be modified. These range from personal behaviours and way of life, to social and community influences in interactions with friends, family and neighbours, to wider determinants on a person's ability to maintain health, such as living and working conditions and access to essential goods and services, and finally to the overall economic, cultural and environmental conditions prevailing in a society. These different layers of determinants do not operate in isolation, but interact in complex relationships.

To draw out the policy relevance of measuring these determinants of health, it is necessary to include in the statistical framework the actions and policies that impact on individuals and on the determinants.

Figure 1.1 (see overleaf) illustrates the statistical framework of domains that need to be measured to paint a picture of health status, identify the impact of individual actions and traits, society and organisations on health, and to monitor change over time.

This framework identifies a model in which health status depends on the determinants of health and the mechanisms that influence these. Both the determinants and influences may operate at a micro level, affecting the individual directly, or at a macro level, operating through society or institutions. Some will have an immediate and direct effect and others will largely act through the influence of wider determinants of health – such as poverty, education and employment – and the actions of governments and other players aimed at maintaining and improving the population's state of health. All actions and determinants impact on health status through the individual's life course.

The most immediate determinants of health that the individual experiences are lifestyle, behaviour and stress (micro-level determinants). These include, for example, behaviours harmful to health such as cigarette smoking, stressful life events and work stress. These are all influenced by life chances and opportunities –gender and ethnicity, educational and occupational opportunities, genetic make-up, etc. The individual-level determinants are however influenced by wider determinants (the macro level). The most immediate of these are the hazards which members of society face in their everyday lives – from road traffic, infections, air and water quality. These are, in turn influenced by the wider social and cultural environment (work, neighbourhood in which you live).

In terms of policies and actions that impact on health, individuals are affected most immediately by the service that they obtain from the health system. This is most directly influenced by the organisation of health services in their area, the resources available to the service and by its accessibility, responsiveness and quality. It is also increasingly acknowledged that much health care takes place within the family and that private and alternative sources of health care have an important role in the prevention and treatment of illness. At the macro level, health system provision is influenced by policies and external societal pressures that act upon service delivers. These in turn are influenced by wider social attitudes and the affordability of a particular level of health care expenditure.

As important to health are policies and actions that have a broader impact on the social determinants of health (poverty, employment conditions, environmental controls, road and food safety policies, social isolation, housing, etc.). Thus there is a synergy between each of the quadrants shown in Figure 1.1. What the figure does not show, because they are many and complex, are the inter-relationships between the various sectors and segments. These are however an essential element of the overall framework.

Contents and structure of the report

The chapters in this report are organised to cover five broad themes: self-assessed health status and activity limitations (2, 3); health-related behaviours (4, 5, 6); diagnosed disease and morbidity (7, 8, 9); preventive and curative healthcare services and informal and formal long-term health and social care (10, 11, 12); and lastly, mortality (13). Thus, we begin by first taking stock of the current health status of the population. We then sequentially examine the pathway to mortality over the life-course: starting with the patterning of health-damaging behaviours (or, the 'proximal' causes of disease), the prevalence of ill-health and disease, the provision of health services and social care and lastly, the main causes of mortality in the population.

Health status

The increasing importance of self-reported health has its roots in the WHO definition of health, which maintains that health encompasses mental and social wellbeing and should not simply be equated with the absence of disease. The value of self-reported health can best be understood as the operationalisation of the WHO definition of health and the recognition that subjective assessments by individuals are a valid measure of both overall population health status and the impact of functional limitations on daily life.

Chapters 2 (General health) and 3 (Limiting long-term illness) of this report analyse self-assessed or perceived general health and reported limitations in daily activities due to a long-term illness, health problem or disability. Questions on both topics have been long used in a variety of specialist health and general purpose surveys of the population and were also included in the UK Census in 2001. Both chapters present analyses of differences in health status by factors such as social position, material deprivation, education, employment, living arrangements and ethnicity. Regional and local variations in population health status are also discussed.

Overall, both chapters show that people who were disadvantaged in terms of their educational, employment and socio-economic background had higher rates of reported poor

Figure **1.1**

Framework for Health and Care Statistics

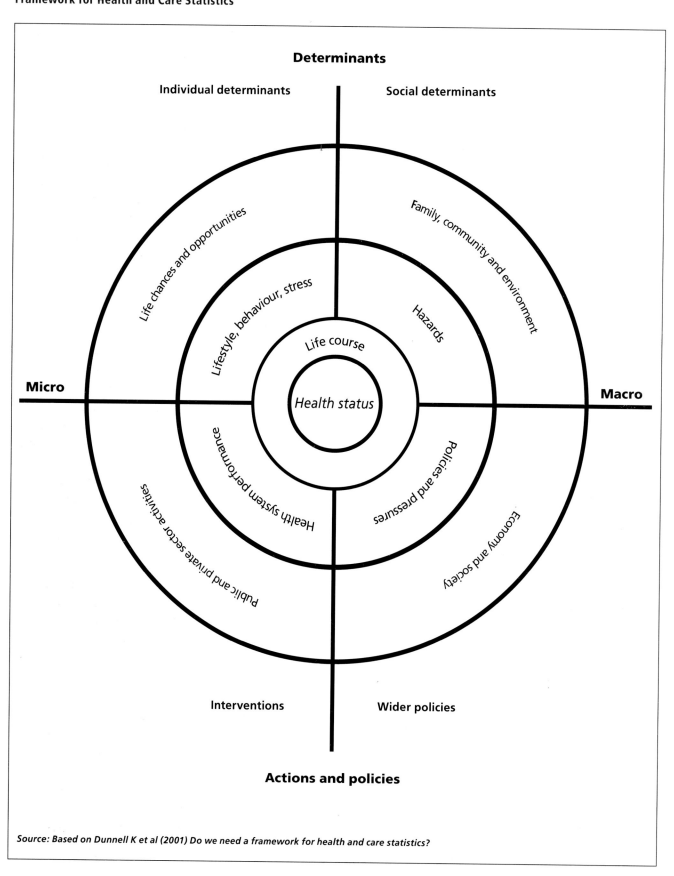

health and activity limitations. Of the four countries of the UK, on average the population of England had better reported health than the others; but within England, the enduring 'north south' divide persisted, with higher rates of poor health in the north of the country compared with the south.

Health-related behaviours

Lifestyle and behavioural risk factors such as smoking, diet and lack of physical activity have long been recognised as harmful to health and as contributing to the major burdens on the health service and society as a whole. Since the *Black Report*,[10] persistent differences between social groups in risky health behaviours have provided an important explanation for social inequalities in health. Reduction in behavioural risk factors has formed a key element of public health strategies in the UK since the early 1990s, and particularly since *Our Healthier Nation*[11] in 1999 signalled a shift in focus to both improving health and reducing inequalities in health.

Chapter 4 *(Smoking, drinking and drug use)* presents the most recent statistics on age, gender and socio-economic differences in levels of smoking, heavy drinking and drug-taking and trends over time in the prevalence of these risk factors. Among adults (aged 16 and over) the overall prevalence of smoking, drinking and drug-taking was higher for men than women in all age groups. In contrast, among children (aged 11–15), the prevalence of smoking was higher in girls, whilst the prevalence of drinking and drug-taking were about the same in boys and girls.

The proportion of adults who smoked cigarettes fell substantially in the 1970s and the early 1980s and continued to decline, but more gradually, into the early 1990s, since when it has levelled out at about 27 per cent. In the 1970s men were far more likely than women to be smokers. During the 1970s and 1980s the gap between men and women narrowed: it has still not disappeared completely but had fallen to four percentage points in 2003. Recent trends in drinking and drug-taking suggest that the prevalence of these has remained relatively stable, but there are differences between sexes, age groups and occupational classes.

Chapter 5 (*Obesity, eating and physical activity*) summarises the available evidence on socio-economic patterns and trends in obesity, eating, and physical activity and discusses the links between these. Physical activity and diet are the behaviours most closely linked to the development and maintenance of obesity, which is an important disease risk factor in its own right. The prevalence of obesity has increased markedly among adults and children since the 1990s and there is no sign that the upward trend is easing. Over the same period there has

been a decline in levels of physical activity in the population. While there is no evidence of change in total calorific intake, there have been changes in patterns of eating such as increased consumption of alcohol, energy-dense foods and reliance on ready-meals. The available evidence does not give clear answers as to whether it is changes in diet or physical activity that are primarily responsible for the marked increase in obesity.

Chapter 6 (*Sexual behaviour and health*) describes trends in sexual behaviour and some of the health consequences of these behaviours. There has been a change in sexual behaviour, and attitudes towards sex and sexuality, over the last thirty years. The chapter presents evidence on the growth in risky behaviour and the increase in almost all sexually transmitted diseases, particularly chlamydia. There were an increasing number of people living with HIV, with new diagnoses tripling over the last 15 years. From 1995 onwards, the number of cases of heterosexually transmitted HIV increased rapidly, with this becoming the predominant source of transmission.

Morbidity

Unlike mortality, morbidity in the population is notoriously difficult to measure. This is mainly because there is no clear dividing line between health and ill-health and rates of diagnosed conditions may depend on many factors including individuals' illness behaviour, or attitude to seeking advice and treatment from a healthcare professional, and the supply and availability of appropriate screening, diagnostic and treatment services. There are several potential measures of morbidity in the population – such as sickness absence rates, doctor consultation and hospital admission rates, and disease registers – with each providing a different, albeit incomplete, measure of the underlying morbidity in the population.

A key measure of population morbidity includes conditions diagnosed when patients present significant health problems (i.e. those that are not self-limiting, are serious, potentially disabling or life-threatening) to their general practitioner. Chapter 7 (*Morbidity*) looks at the prevalence of eleven chronic diseases which are either major causes of preventable ill-health in the populations (such as coronary heart disease, hypertension and diabetes) or are common conditions which significantly impair the quality of life of those who suffer from them (such as arthritis, back problems, hay fever and migraine). The chapter makes use of latest available data both from patient records maintained by general practitioners and self-reported diseases in population health interview surveys to examine variation in prevalence of specific diseases and overall morbidity by socio-economic status and ethnicity.

Chapter 8 (*Cancer*) focuses on one of the most common fatal diseases – cancer – analysing information available on incidence and mortality in England and Wales, and survival in England. The chapter provides trends in the incidence of all malignant cancers (combined) over the period 1971–2001, and mortality from all cancers over the period 1950–2003. Trends in the incidence, survival and mortality of some of the most common cancers are then discussed in detail along with associated possible causes and risk factors. Survival from many cancers has improved substantially over time (e.g. colorectal and breast cancers). Around a third of people develop cancer at some point in their lives and it accounts for a quarter of all deaths.

Chapter 9 (*Mental health*) presents data on the prevalence and treatment of mental health disorders. About a tenth of adults worldwide, an estimated 450 million people, are affected by mental disorders at any one time,[12] and depression, schizophrenia, alcohol-related disorders and bipolar affective disorder are among the ten disorders accounting for most years lived with disability.[13] In Great Britain, one in six adults has a neurotic disorder, and one in seven has considered suicide at some point in their lives. Psychosis is less common, but causes considerable distress and disability in those affected. Rates of mental illness in the community have not changed significantly in recent years, and more people are being treated with medication. However, it is estimated that about half of people with neurotic disorders, and a quarter of people with psychosis are not in regular contact with health services, including many likely to benefit from treatment.

Healthcare

Three chapters focus on the provision and use of healthcare services: from health protection and disease prevention services through to primary and secondary health services and, lastly, health and social care provided in the community and in long-stay institutions.

Chapter 10 (*Preventive healthcare*) focuses on intervention programmes at the population level aimed at health protection and early detection of diseases (such as immunisation and screening) and some health promotion activities (for example, breastfeeding and dental care) directed at individuals to maximise positive health outcomes. Some of the major public health intervention programmes have existed in some form for a long enough time to demonstrate a considerable, and ongoing, impact on health. The success of vaccination in reducing childhood mortality is an important example. Other UK-wide programmes, such as screening for breast and cervical cancers, have developed more recently but have in turn had a significant effect on survival. The decrease in drinking among pregnant women, and the improvements in oral health among

adults and to some extent among children, are indicative of the impact of health promotion activities in raising awareness of the importance of healthy lifestyles.

Chapter 11 (*Use of services*) provides an overview of the use of primary and secondary health services by the population. Primary healthcare is often described as those health services which provide the first (or primary) point of contact for patients, in contrast to secondary (or referral) services. In the UK, most contacts within the National Health Service (NHS) take place in general practice with GPs performing a 'gate-keeper' role to refer patients to specialist hospital services for treatment. Over the years there have been important changes to the way NHS services are delivered. NHS Direct and Walk-in Centres have been set up to complement GP services and these appear to be gaining in popularity. All the indicators of healthcare utilisation analysed in this chapter – such as GP consultations, prescription items dispensed, day case and hospital inpatient admissions – show an upward trend.

While the NHS provides treatment for health problems, individuals may also need other forms of health and social care because of long-term physical or mental illness, disability or frailty associated with old age. Chapter 12 (*Caring and carers*) describes the available statistics on care provided for those in need of support and assistance in living their daily lives, whether informally by family and friends or formally through community services or institutions such as residential and nursing homes. The inclusion of a question on the provision of informal, or unpaid care, in the 2001 Census for the first time has provided a unique opportunity to analyse the social, economic, and health characteristics of carers in the UK. Most adult carers were middle-aged, female and married, caring for members of their family not living in the same household and providing practical help with tasks such as preparing meals, shopping and doing laundry. Though the overall proportion of people providing care does not vary greatly by social position or household tenure, a higher proportion of carers in lower socio-economic groups and in social housing provided the most intensive levels of care. In terms of formal care, the proportion of the population living in medical and care institutions has remained relatively stable since 1991. However, there has been an increase in the provision of community-based home care services in the last decade with an increasing proportion of services being provided by the independent sector.

Mortality

Information on mortality plays a key role in identifying health needs and allocating resources, planning health services and assessing health system performance. Chapter 13 (*Mortality*), examines trends in mortality in the 25 years between 1979 and 2003. Over this period the age distribution of the population of the UK has changed: the elderly population (aged 85 and over) has almost doubled. As the population structure changes the major causes of death also change. This chapter therefore analyses the most common causes of death by age group starting with infants, moving onto children aged under 15, young adults aged 15–44, older adults aged 45–64 and 65–84, and finally the elderly. Over the last 25 years, mortality rates at all younger ages, except among men aged 15–44, have fallen in the UK resulting in more people living longer and an increasing proportion of deaths occurring in older ages. Over this period, the decline in death rates from circulatory disease that began in the early 1950s has continued; while rates of cancer mortality began to fall only from the 1990s.

Downloadable data and glossary

All the data underlying the statistics presented in this report are available as downloadable excel files on the ONS website, with one file for each chapter. The glossary provides explanations and definitions of key concepts and terms used.

References

1. Registrar General (1839) *First Annual Report of the Registrar General of Births, Deaths and Marriages: 1837*, HMSO: London.

2. Drever F (ed.) (1995) *Occupational Health Decennial Supplement.* Series DS No 16, HMSO: London.

3. Griffiths C and Fitzpatrick J (eds.) (2001) *Geographic variations in health.* Series DS No 16, TSO: London.

4. Drever F and Whitehead M (eds.) (1997) *Health Inequalities.* Series DS No 15, TSO: London.

5. Charton J and Murphy M (eds.) (1997) *The Health of Adult Britain.* Series DS No 12, 13, TSO: London.

6. Dunnell K, Allin P and Goldblatt P (2001) *Do we need a framework for health and care statistics?* Proceedings, Statistics Users' Annual Conference, November 2001, Imac Research.

7. Fellegi I and Wolfson M (1999) Towards systems of social statistics – some principles and their application in Statistics Canada. *Journal of Official Statistics* **15**, 3, 373–393.

8. Preamble to the Constitution of the World Health Organisation as adopted by the International Health Conference, New York, 1946.

9. Dahlgren G and Whitehead M (1991) *Policies and strategies to promote social equity in health*, Institute of Futures Studies: Stockholm.

10. Townsend P, Davidson N and Whitehead M (1988) *Inequalities in Health: The Black Report and The Health Divide*, Penguin Books.

11. Department of Health (1999) *Saving Lives: Our Healthier Nation.*

12. Thornicroft G and Maingay S (2002) The global response to mental illness. *BMJ* **325**, 608–609.

13. World Health Organization (2001) *World Health Report 2001*, WHO: Geneva.
www.who.int/whr/2001

General health

Claudia Breakwell

Chapter 2

Introduction

Questions on self-assessed general health have been widely used in both specialised health surveys and general surveys of the population. In 2001 for the first time a question on self-assessed general health was included in the UK Census. Each person in a household was asked to rate their health over the last 12 months. The possible responses were 'good', 'fairly good' or 'not good'.

Poor self-assessed health has been found to be a powerful predictor of admission to hospital, disability and subsequent mortality.[1, 2] The increased risk associated with poor self-assessed health was found to be greater than that associated with objective health status (measured by clinical assessments, laboratory or functional tests), poor life satisfaction and low income.[3, 4]

Self-assessed health draws together an individual's perception of all aspects of their health and wellbeing.[5] While self-assessed health status is recognised as a good measure of health-related quality of life, concerns remain about the reliability of subjective assessments. These are known to vary systematically across population sub-groups (by ethnicity and social class) and over time. They reflect difference in illness, health seeking behaviour, expectations and cultural norms for health.

Unlike simple indicators based on the presence or absence of disease, an important property of the general health status indicator is that it includes the entire spectrum of health states ranging from 'good' to 'not good' health. It therefore provides information on the distribution and the sociodemographic profile of those in 'good' and 'not good' health. In this chapter, the commentary is focused mainly on the prevalence of 'good' and 'not good' health, with the intermediate 'fairly good' health category discussed only where relevant.

Distribution of health status by age and sex

In the 2001 Census, 40.3 million people living in the UK rated their general health as 'good' and a further 13 million rated it as 'fairly good'. These 53.3 million people represent over 90 per cent of the total UK population while just 9 per cent (or 5.5 million people) rated their health over the last year as 'not good'. Children (aged 0–15) had the highest rate of 'good' general health at over 91 per cent, with an additional 8 per cent with general health rated 'fairly good'.[6]

Rates of 'good' health decrease steadily with age with corresponding increases in rates of 'fairly good' and 'not good' health (Figure 2.1). The 'not good' health rate reaches its peak

in the oldest age band whereas the 'fairly good' health rate drops slightly for those aged 85 and over. While individuals aged over 65 account for just 16 per cent of the population, they represent 40 per cent of all those with health rated as 'not good'.

Figure **2.1**

Self-assessed general health: by age, 2001

United Kingdom

Percentages

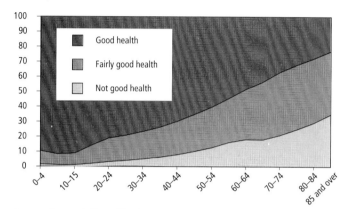

Source: Census 2001, Office for National Statistics; Census 2001, General Register Office for Scotland; Census 2001, Northern Ireland Statistics and Research Agency

The age-related pattern in rates of general health was similar for males and females. Overall, rates of 'good' health were lower for women than men (aged 16 and over), but there was little difference in rates between girls and boys. The difference in the rates of 'good' health between men and women ranged from six percentage points for 20- to 24-year-olds (84 versus 78 per cent respectively) to nothing for 60- to 64-year-olds (48 per cent). The most substantial difference between the rates for 'fairly good' health also occurred in the 20–24 age group where women reported higher rates of 'fairly good' health than men (18 versus 13 per cent).

The 'not good' health rates show a different pattern with the rates for males slightly higher than for females among children and those aged between 55 and 69 years old. Rates of 'not good' health for women over pensionable age increased sharply and women over 85 had the highest rate of 'not good' health, nearly four percentage points higher than the rate for men in the same age band.

Overall the age-standardised rates of 'good' health were 73 per cent for males, compared to 70 per cent for females in 2001 (Figure 2.2). A further 19 per cent of males, compared to 22 per cent of females, rated their general health as 'fairly good'. Thus, there was no overall difference between the male and female 'not good' health rates once the age distribution of the population was taken into account. The main difference between the sexes occurs in the positive answers for general health with more men than women rating their self-assessed general health as 'good'.

Figure **2.2**

Self-assessed general health (age-standardised): by sex, 2001

United Kingdom
Percentages

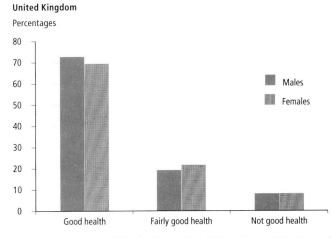

Source: Census 2001, Office for National Statistics; Census 2001, General Register Office for Scotland; Census 2001, Northern Ireland Statistics and Research Agency

In 2001 the life expectancy at birth for females was 80 years compared to 76 years for males.[7] Healthy life expectancy is defined as the number of years a person can expect to live in 'good' or 'fairly good' health. The difference between life expectancy and healthy life expectancy can be regarded as an estimate of the number of years a person can expect to live in 'not good' health. In 2001, females at birth could expect to live 12 years in 'not good' health compared to nine years for males.[8] Hence, although women live longer than men, on average they also spend a larger number of years and a greater proportion of their life in 'not good' health compared to men.[9]

Health status of residents in communal establishments

In 2001 over one million people in the UK (just under 2 per cent of the population) were living in some form of communal establishment. Over a fifth (22 per cent) of these individuals, compared to less than a tenth (9 per cent) of the total UK population, rated their general health as 'not good'. Half of residents in communal establishments (51 per cent) rated their health as 'good' compared with nearly three-quarters (69 per cent) of the whole population.

Data from the 2001 Census shows that, among residents of communal establishments, rates of 'good' health gradually decreased with age from 84 per cent in children to 14 per cent in 70- to 74-year-olds. Rates then increased slightly and

reached 22 per cent for residents aged 85 and over. While both the rates of 'fairly good' and 'not good' health increase with age, the 'not good' health rate increases faster than the 'fairly good' health rate. Thus, for individuals aged over 65 the rate of 'not good' health is actually higher than the rate of 'fairly good' health, but this difference then drops to just over one percentage point for those aged 85 and over.

There were marked differences between the rates of self-assessed health by sex. Females in communal establishments had a 'good' health rate (43 per cent) markedly lower than among males (60 per cent). Consequently, both the 'fairly good' and 'not good' health rates were lower for male residents in communal establishments than for females (males: 24 and 16 per cent; females: 31 and 26 per cent respectively). These differences can largely be explained by the fact that the age profile of women resident in communal establishments was much older than that of men. One in five men (22 per cent) resident in communal establishments were aged 65 and over, compared to over half (57 per cent) of all women. Many of the factors covered below are inappropriate for residents of communal establishments (for example; housing tenure, housing deprivation and living arrangements). Therefore all further analysis in this chapter refers solely to the population of private households, and excludes the population resident in communal establishments.

Socio-economic variation

Social position

Age-standardised rates of 'good' self-assessed general health decreased with declining social position in 2001 (Figure 2.3 – see overleaf). The rate among people in higher managerial and professional occupations was 82 per cent, decreasing to 77 per cent in lower managerial and professional groups and 74 per cent for those in intermediate occupations. Small employers and own account workers had a 'good' health rate of 74 per cent, whereas 71 per cent of people in lower supervisory and technical occupations and semi-routine occupations rated their general health in the past year as 'good'. The lowest rate of 'good' general health (66 per cent) for any occupational group was found among those employed in routine occupations. The National Statistics Socio-Economic Classification (NS-SEC) also includes those who had never worked or were long-term unemployed. This group had by far the lowest rate of 'good' general health, which at 50 per cent was over 30 percentage points lower than the higher managerial and professional occupations.

Within the same occupation group males consistently reported higher age-standardised rates of 'good' health compared with females, the difference between the sexes being greatest, at

Figure **2.3**

Self-assessed general health[1] (age-standardised): by NS-SEC,[2] 2001

United Kingdom

Percentages

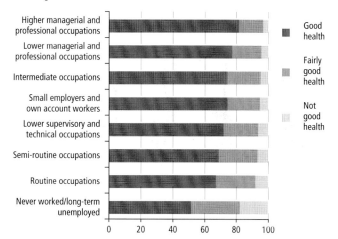

1 Excluding residents of communal establishments.
2 For persons aged 16–64.

Source: Census 2001, Office for National Statistics; Census 2001, General Register Office for Scotland; Census 2001, Northern Ireland Statistics and Research Agency

seven percentage points, in the lower supervisory and technical occupations and the routine occupations groups. There was little difference in the 'not good' health rates by social position between males and females.[10] Consequently, the variation in the 'fairly good' rates by social position and gender was the converse of that observed for 'good' health: females reported higher rates of 'fairly good' health than males, with the largest difference (six and five percentage points) between the sexes for those in routine or lower supervisory and technical occupations.

Economic activity

In 2001, of the 37 million people aged 16–64 who were asked about their economic activity, 28 million (74 per cent) were economically active while 9 million (26 per cent) were economically inactive. Three-quarters (76 per cent) of the economically active group reported their self-assessed health as 'good' compared with only half (51 per cent) of the economically inactive group. This large difference can partly be explained by the inclusion in the economically inactive group of those who were permanently sick or disabled and those who were retired who are likely to report lower rates of 'good' health.

Among the economically active group, rates of 'good' health also vary by employment status (e.g. full-and part-time workers). Full-time workers were more likely to rate their general health as 'good' compared with those working part-

time (77 and 73 per cent respectively). Further, those who are self-employed also had a higher rate of 'good' health (78 per cent) than employees (76 per cent). Three in five unemployed people reported their health as 'good' (62 per cent), a rate 14 percentage points lower than the average for the economically active group.

The rates of general health varied much more within the economically inactive group (Figure 2.4). As expected those classified as permanently disabled or sick had the lowest rates of 'good' health (11 per cent) and the highest rate of 'not good' health (63 per cent). The highest rate of 'good' general health in the economically inactive was among those classified as looking after home/family (61 per cent), this group also had the lowest rate of 'not good' health (8 per cent).

Figure **2.4**

Self-assessed general health[1] (age-standardised): by economic activity,[2,3] 2001

United Kingdom

Percentages

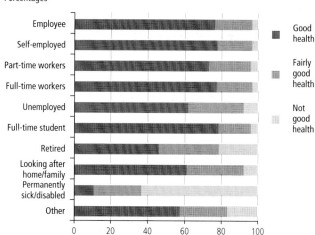

1 Excluding residents of communal establishments.
2 For people aged 16–64.
3 Those working 31 or more hours per week are classified as full-time, those working 30 or less hours per week as part-time.

Source: Census 2001, Office for National Statistics; Census 2001, General Register Office for Scotland; Census 2001, Northern Ireland Statistics and Research Agency

Overall, economically active men reported higher rates of 'good' health than women (77 per cent compared with 74 per cent), and this difference persists across all the economically active groups except among part-time workers, where both sexes had a similar rate (72 per cent for males and 73 per cent for females).

Gender differentials were reversed in the economically inactive group where women reported a higher rate of 'good' health (54 per cent) than men (43 per cent). A third (33 per cent) of all economically inactive males rated their health as 'not good' compared with just a fifth (19 per cent) of females in the same group.

Educational qualifications

Twenty per cent of the population aged 16–74 in the UK in 2001 had been educated to degree level or higher, a further 44 per cent had obtained lower qualifications while 36 per cent had no qualifications or qualifications of an unknown level. Over three-quarters (76 per cent) of those with a degree or higher level qualification reported their general health as 'good' after age-standardisation compared with just three-fifths (58 per cent) of people with no or unknown qualifications (Figure 2.5). People who had lower qualifications had a 'good' health rate the same as that for the UK population (71 per cent).

Figure **2.5**

Self-assessed general health[1] (age-standardised): by highest level of qualification,[2] 2001

United Kingdom

Percentages

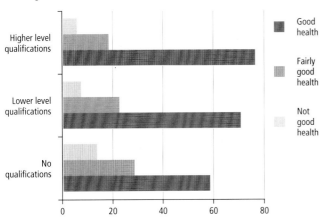

1   *Excluding residents of communal establishments.*
2   *For persons aged 16–74.*

Source: Census 2001, Office for National Statistics; Census 2001, General Register Office for Scotland; Census 2001, Northern Ireland Statistics and Research Agency

As we would expect, the gradient for 'not good' health rates is reversed. People with no qualifications were twice as likely as those who had obtained a higher level education to report 'not good' health (13 versus 6 per cent). Similar patterns of variation in health status by level of educational attainment were found for males and females. However, in all qualification groups women reported higher rates of 'fairly good' and 'not good' health than men and conversely, men reported the higher rates of 'good' health.

Housing tenure

In 2001, 71 per cent of the total population of Great Britain owned their homes.[11] A further 18 per cent were living in social housing, 9 per cent in privately rented accommodation and just 2 per cent were living rent free.

Figure **2.6**

Self-assessed general health[1] (age-standardised): by housing tenure, 2001

Great Britain[2]

Percentages

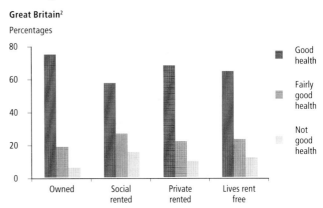

1   *Excluding residents of communal establishments.*
2   *Data are only provided for Great Britain because Northern Ireland uses a different coding system to the rest of the UK to describe tenure.*

Source: Census 2001, Office for National Statistics; Census 2001, General Register Office for Scotland; Census 2001, Northern Ireland Statistics

Individuals living in social housing reported the lowest rates of 'good' health (57 per cent). Occupants of privately rented accommodation and those who live rent-free fared better with rates of 'good' health at 68 and 64 per cent respectively; while owner-occupiers had the highest rate of 'good' health at 75 per cent (Figure 2.6).

The gradient of 'not good' health rates by tenure group was the opposite to that observed for 'good' health: rates for those living in socially rented housing (16 per cent) were ten percentage points higher than for those in owner-occupied homes (6 per cent). Males and females showed patterns across housing tenure that were very similar.

Age-specific rates of general health allow a closer look at the difference between individuals living in social housing and those who own their homes. In every age group owners reported higher rates of 'good' health than those who live in socially rented homes. This difference is widest in the 50–54 age group where two in five (37 per cent) of those living in socially rented housing report being in 'good' health compared with two in three (65 per cent) of owner-occupiers. Children (aged under 16) living in social housing report a rate of 'not good' health twice that of children living in owned housing (2 per cent compared with 1 per cent).

Housing deprivation

Housing deprivation is a derived variable from the Census that takes into account whether a household is overcrowded, is a shared dwelling, does not have sole use of a bath/shower or toilet or does not have central heating. In 2001, 8.6 million people lived in a household that was classified as deprived in at least one of these four dimensions, representing 15 per cent of the population in Great Britain.[12]

People living in households classified as not deprived in the housing dimension had a rate of 'good' general health seven percentage points higher, at 72 per cent, than those living in deprived housing (65 per cent). The differentials in 'good' health rates by housing deprivation were particularly marked for those aged 30–74 years when compared to the younger or older age bands (Figure 2.7). The difference in age-specific rates of 'good' health for those living in non-deprived versus deprived households increased from three percentage points in the 0–15 age group to a high of 12 percentage points for adults aged between 45 and 59 years old, and then declined to three percentage points for those aged 75 and over.

Figure **2.7**

Rate of 'good' general health:[1] by age and housing deprivation, 2001

Great Britain[2]

Percentages

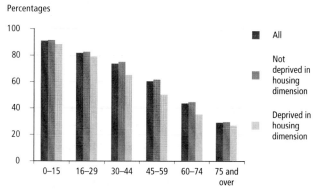

1 *Excluding residents of communal establishments.*
2 *Data is only provided for Great Britain because Northern Ireland uses a different coding system to the rest of the UK to describe housing deprivation.*

Source: Census 2001, Office for National Statistics; Census 2001, General Register Office for Scotland; Census 2001, Northern Ireland Statistics and Research Agency

The impact of deprived housing on health is well documented and also strongly linked to income.[13] Vulnerable groups such as the elderly, very young and those suffering from limiting long-term illness are at particular risk due to lengthy periods spent indoors. The social and physical characteristics of the surrounding area are also vital in maintaining good health. The fact that poor quality accommodation is often situated in impoverished surroundings with few local amenities contributes further to making vulnerable individuals housebound.

Marital status

The 2001 Census allows categorisation of marital status for those aged 16 and over into five distinct groups: single, married, separated (but still legally married), divorced and

widowed. Self-assessed general health varied considerably between marital groups (Figure 2.8). Rates of 'good' general health ranged from 66 per cent among those who were married to 51 per cent for those who were widowed; with intermediate values for those who were single (63 per cent), divorced (56 per cent) and separated (55 per cent).

Figure **2.8**

Self-assessed general health[1] (age-standardised): by marital status, 2001

United Kingdom

Percentages

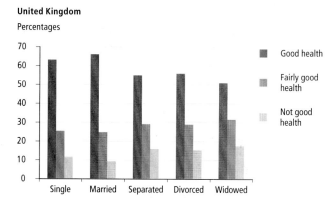

1 *Excluding residents of communal establishments.*

Source: Census 2001, Office for National Statistics; Census 2001, General Register Office for Scotland; Census 2001, Northern Ireland Statistics and Research Agency

The widowed population reported the highest rate of 'not good' health at 17 per cent while those who were married reported a rate eight percentage points lower (9 per cent). Those who were separated or divorced had 'not good' health rates of 16 and 15 per cent respectively; this rate drops to 12 per cent for the single population.

General patterns in reported health by marital status were very similar: rates of 'not good' health were virtually the same for both sexes whereas for 'good' health males reported slightly higher rates than females regardless of martial status. Separated males and females show the largest difference in 'good' health rates, with men reporting a 'good' health rate of 59 per cent compared with 53 per cent for women.

Living arrangements

While the previous section categorised people in terms of their legal marital status, analysis by family status provides an alternative measure based on living arrangements. A family comprises a group of people consisting of a married or cohabiting couple with or without children or a lone parent with children. People were categorised into 'couple families', 'lone parent families' or 'not in a family'. Further distinctions are also drawn between adults, dependent children and non-dependent children.[14]

Age-standardised rates of general health show members of couple families, whether adults or children have higher rates of 'good' health than lone parent families by between four and five percentage points (Figure 2.9). Of all respondents classified as part of a family, both male and female lone parents had the lowest rates of 'good' health (67 and 62 per cent respectively). Dependent children, both girls and boys, in couple families were the healthiest of all with 92 per cent reporting their self-assessed general health as 'good'.

Figure **2.9**

Self-assessed general health[1] (age-standardised): by family status of individual in household, 2001

United Kingdom
Percentages

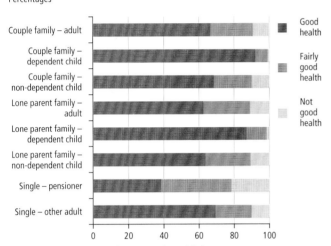

1 *Excluding residents of communal establishments.*

Source: Census 2001, Office for National Statistics; Census 2001, General Register Office for Scotland; Census 2001, Northern Ireland Statistics and Research Agency

Lone pensioners reported the lowest rate of 'good' health and conversely the highest rates of 'fairly good' and 'not good' health. Over a fifth (22 per cent) of lone pensioners rated their general health as 'not good' and a further 40 per cent rated it as 'fairly good'. Age-standardising the population over 65 allows comparison between pensioners in couple families and lone pensioners. Pensioners in a couple family reported rates of 'good' health four percentage points higher than lone pensioners (42 per cent compared with 38 per cent).

Ethnic variation

Information on ethnic background collected in the 2001 Census allows analysis of self-assessed general health in the UK by ethnic group after controlling for differences in age profile. Age-standardised rates of general health show that the White population in the UK, which accounts for over 92 per cent of the population, had the highest reported rates of 'good' health at 72 per cent (Figure 2.10). Asians, who comprised 4 per cent

of the population, had rates eight percentage points lower at 64 per cent. The 'fairly good' health rates mirrored this pattern but the variation between ethnic groups with the lowest and highest rates was much smaller at four percentage points.

Figure

Self-assessed general health[1] (age-standardised): by ethnic group, 2001

United Kingdom
Percentages

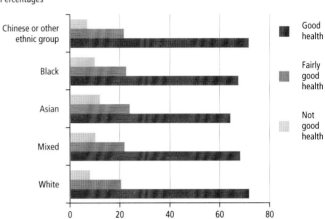

1 *Excluding residents of communal establishments.*

Source: Census 2001, Office for National Statistics; Census 2001, General Register Office for Scotland; Census 2001, Northern Ireland Statistics and Research Agency

Over one in 10 Asian people (12 per cent) reported their general health to be 'not good' making this the ethnic group with the highest rate of 'not good' health. The Black and the Mixed race populations, which represent 2 and 1 per cent of people in the UK respectively, reported rates of 'not good' general health at 10 per cent. Among all ethnic groups the lowest rates of 'not good' health were found in the 'Chinese and other' group at just 7 per cent, one percentage point lower than the rate of the White population (8 per cent).[15]

Females consistently reported lower rates of 'good' health than males for all ethnic groups (Table 2.11 – see overleaf). Gender differences in rates of 'good' health were most pronounced in the Asian and Black populations where the reported rate for women was over six percentage points lower than the rate for men (61 versus 67 per cent and 64 versus 71 per cent respectively). Conversely, there were no gender differences in the age-standardised rates of 'not good' health for the White, Mixed and 'Chinese and other' groups (8, 10 and 7 per cent respectively). However, Black and Asian females had higher overall 'not good' health rates than their male counterparts. Asian females had a rate of 13 per cent compared with 10 per cent for Asian males while Black females had a rate of 11 per cent compared with 9 per cent for Black males.

Table 2.11

Self-assessed general health[1] (age-standardised): by sex and ethnic group, 2001

United Kingdom   Percentages

	Males			Females		
	Good health	Fairly good health	Not good health	Good health	Fairly good health	Not good health
All	72.85	19.18	7.97	69.76	21.99	8.25
White	73.13	18.98	7.89	70.18	21.73	8.09
Mixed	70.17	20.10	9.73	66.18	23.39	10.42
Asian	67.34	22.27	10.39	60.81	25.70	13.49
Black	70.76	20.32	8.92	64.50	24.43	11.07
Chinese or other ethnic group	72.88	20.39	6.73	70.35	22.54	7.11

1 Excluding residents of communal establishments.

Source: Census 2001, Office for National Statistics; Census 2001, General Register Office for Scotland; Census 2001, Northern Ireland Statistics and Research Agency

Geographic variation

There is considerable variation in the age distributions of regional populations in the UK (Table 2.12). In order to make geographical comparisons it is necessary to use age-standardised rates of general health. The age-standardised rate of 'good' general health for the UK was 71 per cent. A further 21 per cent of people rated their general health as 'fairly good' leaving just 8 per cent of the population who rated their own health as 'not good'.

Within the UK, England and Scotland had the highest age-standardised rates of 'good' health, at 71 per cent, compared to 69 per cent in Wales and 70 per cent in Northern Ireland. Conversely, rates of 'not good' health were 8, 9, 11 and 10 per cent respectively.

There were also substantial variations between the various English Government Office Regions (GORs), where a clear north south divide is apparent in the rates of 'not good' health. The GORs with the lowest rates of 'not good' health were the South East and the East (6 per cent). Rates in the South West (7 per cent), London, East Midlands and West Midlands (all 8 per cent) were just under or the same as the UK.

The North East and North West had the next highest rates (10 per cent), followed by Yorkshire and Humber (9 per cent) with an overall rate just one percentage point higher than the UK.

The difference in the percentage of people reporting 'good' health in the local authority (LA) with the highest (79 per cent) and the lowest rates (61 per cent) was 17 percentage points compared to six percentage points at regional level. Map 2.13

Table 2.12

Self-assessed general health[1] (age-standardised): by region, 2001

United Kingdom   Percentages

	Good health	Fairly good health	Not good health
United Kingdom	71.26	20.62	8.12
North East	67.73	21.90	10.36
North West	69.72	20.70	9.58
Yorkshire and the Humber	69.84	21.25	8.91
East Midlands	70.65	21.56	7.79
West Midlands	69.96	21.62	8.42
East	73.39	20.24	6.37
London	71.04	20.77	8.19
South East	74.41	19.65	5.93
South West	73.06	20.18	6.76
England	71.47	20.71	7.82
Scotland	70.86	20.27	8.88
Northern Ireland	70.42	19.01	10.49
Wales	68.82	20.64	10.55

1 Excluding residents of communal establishments.

Source: Census 2001, Office for National Statistics; Census 2001, General Register Office for Scotland; Census 2001, Northern Ireland Statistics and Research Agency shows the proportion of people in each LA with self-assessed general health over the past 12 months rated as 'good' grouped into quintiles. Areas with higher than average 'good' health rates appear in a darker colour and can be seen to be predominantly in the south east of the country. Of the 87 LAs in the top quintile of 'good' health rates, 80 were in England (representing 23 per cent of all English LAs) and seven in Scotland (22 per cent of Scottish LAs). Both Wales and Northern Ireland had no LAs in the top quintile. The highest ranked LAs in Northern Ireland – North Down and Ballymena – and in Wales – Gwynedd, were all in the second quintile with a 'good' health rate of 74 per cent.

Map 2.14 (see overleaf) shows the proportion of people in LAs who rated their health as 'not good', grouped into quintiles. In this case the highest rates occur in inner city London, Northern Ireland, South Wales and the North of England. In total, 12 out of the 87 LAs categorised as having the highest rates of 'not

good' general health are in Wales, representing 55 per cent of all Welsh LAs. Local authorities in Northern Ireland are also over-represented with 12, or 46 per cent of all LAs in Northern Ireland, in the highest 'not good' health quintile. Twenty-two per cent of LAs in Scotland appear in the highest quintile compared with just 16 per cent of LAs in England.

All 10 LAs with the highest rates of 'good' health were found in England (Table 2.15 – see overleaf). The 10 LAs with the highest rates of 'not good' health were dispersed with one in England (Easington), five in Wales (Merthyr Tydfil, Blaenau Gwent, Rhondda Cynon Taff, Neath Port Talbot and Caerphilly), one in Scotland (Glasgow City), and three in Northern Ireland (Belfast, Derry and Strabane). Nine of the 10 LAs with the highest rates of 'good' health also appear in the list of 10 LAs with the lowest rates of 'not good' health.

Caution must be exercised when interpreting results that show

Map **2.13**

Rates of 'good' general health[1] (age-standardised): by local authority,[2] 2001

United Kingdom

All people

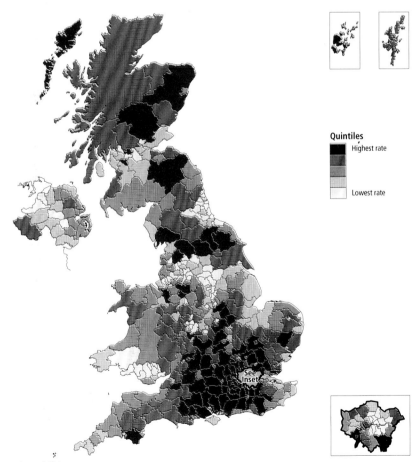

Quintiles
Highest rate

Lowest rate

1   Excluding residents of communal establishments.
2   Local authorities ranked from highest to lowest and then divided into five groups.

Source: Census 2001, Office for National Statistics; Census 2001, General Register Office for Scotland; Census 2001, Northern Ireland Statistics and Research Agency

© Crown copyright. All rights reserved (ONS.GD272183.2005).

Map **2.14**

Rates of 'not good' general health[1] (age-standardised): by local authority,[2] 2001

United Kingdom

All people

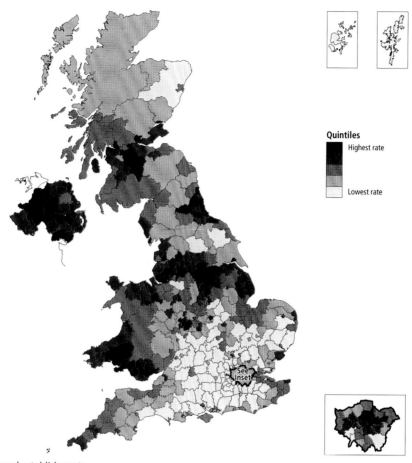

Quintiles

Highest rate

Lowest rate

1   *Excluding residents of communal establishments.*
2   *Local authorities ranked from highest to lowest and then divided into five groups.*

Source: Census 2001, Office for National Statistics; Census 2001, General Register Office for Scotland; Census 2001, Northern Ireland Statistics and Research Agency

© *Crown copyright. All rights reserved (ONS.GD272183.2005).*

geographical variation as previous studies have shown that when considering other confounding factors, such as socio-economic status, geographical site can account for just one per cent of the variation.[16] However, a northwest-southeast divide in social class inequalities existed in Great Britain during 2001, with each of the seven social classes having higher rates of poor health in Wales, the North East and North West regions of England than elsewhere.[17]

Trends

The 2001 Census was the first to include a question on general health. Therefore in order to analyse trends over time in general health survey data needs to be used. The General Household Survey (GHS) is a nationally representative interview survey of private households in Great Britain. Information is collected on a wide range of topics, including on self-assessed

general health status using a question with exactly the same wording as in the 2001 Census.[18]

Data from the GHS only covers Great Britain but Northern Ireland carries out an equivalent survey, the Continuous Household Survey (CHS).[19] This survey is modelled on the GHS using similar sampling, weighting and stratifying techniques, and asks exactly the same questions of health, and in the same sequence. Data from the CHS and GHS have been combined after weighting, to ensure correct proportions of the population are represented, and then age-standardised to produce combined UK figures from 1990 to 2003.

Survey-based estimates will not be directly comparable to the 2001 Census estimates due to differences in methodology between the two types of sources. One person on behalf of all household members generally completes the Census form,

Table 2.15

Local authorities with the highest and lowest age-standardised rates of 'good' and 'not good' general health,[1] 2001

United Kingdom　　　　　　　　　　　　　　　　　　　　　　　　　　　　　　　　　　　Percentages

Top 10 'Good health'		Top 10 'Not good health'	
Elmbridge	79.27	Merthyr Tydfil	16.25
Chiltern	79.21	Easington	15.43
South Bucks	79.09	Glasgow City	14.70
Hart	78.82	Blaenau Gwent	14.37
Surrey Heath	78.70	Belfast	14.20
Wokingham UA	78.64	Rhondda; Cynon; Taff	13.85
Mole Valley	78.46	Neath Port Talbot	13.62
Winchester	78.33	Derry	13.60
Richmond upon Thames	78.21	Caerphilly	13.48
Waverley	78.19	Strabane	13.37
Bottom 10 'Good health'		**Bottom 10 'Not good health'**	
Easington	61.40	Chiltern	4.20
Merthyr Tydfil	61.68	Hart	4.23
Glasgow City	62.25	Wokingham UA	4.27
Blaenau Gwent	62.97	Elmbridge	4.44
Tower Hamlets	63.16	Surrey Heath	4.49
Manchester	63.57	Mole Valley	4.50
Newham	63.95	Winchester	4.53
Rhondda; Cynon; Taff	64.17	South Bucks	4.55
Caerphilly	64.19	Horsham	4.58
Bolsover	64.23	Waverley	4.60

1　Excluding residents of communal establishments.

Source: Census 2001, Office for National Statistics; Census 2001, General Register Office for Scotland; Census 2001, Northern Ireland Statistics and Research Agency

while both the GHS and CHS are face-to-face interview surveys. Furthermore, the Census estimates include people living in communal establishments while the surveys exclude the population living in institutions.

The proportion of males in the UK reporting that their health over the last 12 months was 'good' rose by four percentage points between 1990 and 2003 to 64 per cent, the highest it has been since 1998 (Figure 2.16 – see overleaf). The 'not good' health rate for males has remained constant at 12 per cent over the time period with the exception of years 1994 and 1995. In these two years the 'not good' health rate rose by two percentage points to reach its highest value of 14 per cent. In contrast both the 'good' and 'fairly good' health rates show a greater degree of variability over the same period. While the cumulative proportion of males rating their health as 'good' or 'fairly good' remained constant at over 85 per cent, the variability in male health status over time occurs in the distribution between the two positive health states.

The proportion of women reporting their general health as 'good' remained fairly constant at approximately 60 per cent between 1990 and 2003 (Figure 2.16 – see overleaf). Rates of 'fairly good' health dropped by two percentage points, from 29 to 27 per cent, while the 'not good' health rate increased by one percentage point from 12 to 13 per cent.

Both men and women experienced similar trends over time in health status. Fewer women than men rated their health as 'good' whereas fewer men than women rated their health as 'not good' corroborating the similar pattern seen in the 2001 Census data.

Figure 2.16

Trends in general health: by sex, 1990–2003[1]

United Kingdom

Percentages

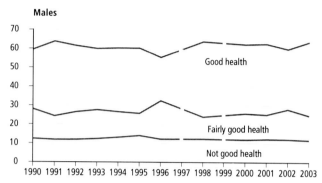

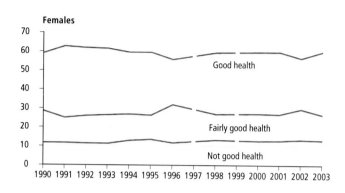

1   Data not available for 1997 and 1999.

Source: General Household Survey, Office for National Statistics; Continuous Household Survey, Northern Ireland Statistics and Research Agency

Conclusion

A total of 40.2 million residents of the UK in 2001 rated their general health over the past 12 months as 'good', a further 13 million rated it as 'fairly good', with the remaining 5.5 million people reporting health as 'not good'. Rates of 'good' health decreased with age, whilst the rates of 'fairly good' and 'not good' health increased. Adult females consistently reported lower rates of 'good' health and higher rates of 'fairly good' and 'not good' health than adult males.

Substantial variation between the various regions has shown an apparent north-south divide in the rates of 'not good' general health. The South East, East, South West, London, East Midlands and West Midlands reported rates of 'not good' health lower than the UK average while in Wales, the North West, North East, Yorkshire and Humber and Scotland rates were higher than average.

Economic factors are also seen to have a strong association with self-assessed general health status and have been shown previously to have an adverse impact on health.[20] Those who were economically active had 'good' health rates 50 per cent higher than the economically inactive while people with higher managerial and professional occupations reported rates of 'good' health 25 per cent higher than those in routine occupations. Variation in general health has long been associated with levels of educational qualification, with those who had higher level qualifications reporting higher rates.

Social variations between populations have known implications for self-assessed health, which are also echoed in these results.[21] Married respondents and people in couple families reported lower rates of 'not good' health than those who were not married or were lone parents while most minority ethnic groups reported higher rates of 'not good' health than the White population.

Notes and references

1.   Idler E and Benyamini Y (1997) Self rated health and mortality: a review of twenty seven community studies. *J Health Soc Behaviour* **38**, 21–37.

2.   Burstrom B and Fredlund P (2001) Self rated health: is a good predictor of subsequent mortality among adults in higher social classes? *J Epidemiol Community Health* **55**, 836–840.

3.   Mossey J M and Shapiro E (1982) Self-rated health: a predictor of mortality among the elderly. *AM J Public Health* **72**, 800–808.

4.   Sadana R, Mathers C D, Lopez A D, Murray C J L and Iburg K M (2002) Comparative analysis of more than 50 household surveys on health status, in Murray C J L, Saloman J A, Mathers C D and Lopez A D (eds.) *Summary Measures of Population Health*, WHO:Geneva, 369–371.

5.   Kaplan G and Baron-Epel O (2003) What lies behind the subjective evaluation of health status? *Social Science and Medicine* **56**, 1669–1676.

6.   As is standard practice in household surveys we can assume that the form filler answered the question on behalf of young children living in the household.

7.   Healthy Life Expectancy at birth and at 65 in Great Britain and England, 1981–2001: at www.statistics.gov.uk/statbase

8. Life Expectancy at birth and at 65 in Great Britain and England, 1981–2001: at www.statistics.gov.uk/statbase

9. Robine J M, Romieu I and Michel J P (2003) Trends in Health Expectancies, in Robine J M, Jagger C, Mathers C D, Crimmins E M and Suzman R M (eds.), *Determining Health Expecancies*, Wiley, 76–93.

10. Drever F, Doran T and Whitehead M (2004) Exploring the relation between class, gender, and self-rated general health using the new socioeconomic classification. A study using data from the 2001 Census. *J Epidemiol Community Health* **58**, 590–596. This study reported a substantial gender gap in the rates of 'not good' health for the 'Higher managerial and professional occupations' NS-SEC group (3.5 per cent for males and 4.4 per cent for females). However the analysis was restricted to data for ages 25–64 in Great Britain, excluding the long-term unemployed.

11. Data are only provided for Great Britain because Northern Ireland uses a different coding system to the rest of the UK to describe tenure.

12. Data are only provided for Great Britain because Northern Ireland uses different deprivation indicators.

13. *Housing and Health: building for the future (2003)* British Medical Association, Board of Science and Social education.

14. A dependent child is a person aged 0–15 in a household, or aged 16–18, in full-time education living in a family with his or her parents.

15. The category 'Chinese and other' has to be used in order to provide UK data on ethnicity. In Northern Ireland, the ethnic minority population is too small for the Chinese population and people from other ethnic groups to be split. This creates a disclosivity issue, meaning the two categories must be combined.

16. Au D M, McDonnell M B, Martin D C and Fihn C (2001) Regional variations in Health Status. *Medical Care* **39(8)**, 879–888.

17. Doran T, Drever F and Whitehead M (2004) Is there a north-south divide in social class inequalities in health in Great Britain? Cross sectional study using data from the 2001 Census. *BMJ* **328**, 1043–1045.

18. For more information on the GHS see www.statistics.gov.uk/LIB2002

19. For more information on the CHS see www.esds.ac.uk/government/nichs

20. Kennedy B, Kawachi I, Glass R and Prothrow-Stith D (1998) Income distribution, socioeconomic status, and self-rated health in the United States: multilevel analysis. *BMJ* **317**, 917–921.

21. Browning C R, Cagney K A and Wen M (2003) Explaining variation in health status across space and time: implications for racial and ethnic disparities in self-rated health. *Social Science and Medicine* **57**, 1221–1235.

Limiting long-term illness

Levin Wheller

Chapter 3

Background

Most of us suffer periods of ill health in our lives, but these are usually acute illnesses, short-lived problems that do not have a substantial limiting effect on our day to day activities. However a large number of people in the UK suffer with chronic, or long-term illnesses which limit the activities they can perform in their daily lives.

Individuals with long-term illnesses, health problems or disabilities can face restrictions in the type or amount of work they can do and difficulties performing everyday tasks that most of us take for granted. For these and other reasons, long-term illness and disability are important social issues that have been included in numerous national surveys since the 1970s and, more recently, in the 1991 and 2001 Censuses.

A question on limiting long-term illness (LLTI) was introduced into the 1991 Census,[1] and repeated in 2001 in a revised form. Because of the different wording of the LLTI question in 1991 and 2001, the results from these two years are not directly comparable. The LLTI question in the 2001 Census asks 'Do you have any long-term illness, health problem or disability which limits your daily activity or the work you can do?' Respondents are instructed to include problems due to old age. Since 1971, questions on long-standing and acute illness have been included in the General Household Survey (GHS). However, unlike the Census, the sample size of the GHS is too small to provide reliable estimates for small areas or minority population groups.

Limitations covered by LLTI may include difficulties in walking, reaching, stretching and bending down, as well as sight, hearing and communication problems. Limitations may result from health problems as varied as asthma, diabetes, cancer and depression.

Prevalence of limiting long-term illness

A large number of people in the UK reported having an LLTI in 2001: 10.3 million people living in private households, along with a further 530,000 people in communal establishments. In total 18 per cent of the UK population had an LLTI (Table 3.1). The 10.3 million individuals with an LLTI in private households comprised 4.8 million males and 5.5 million females. Over half of people with an LLTI living in private households (5.4 million individuals) were aged 60 and over. Although people aged 60 and over make up 20 per cent of the UK population in private households, they represent 53 per cent of all people with an LLTI.

People reporting an LLTI may not always consider themselves as being in poor health. For example, someone with diabetes, whose condition is well controlled, may say they are in good health, even though the illness may restrict their activities. Of the 10.3 million people in private households who reported having an LLTI, 1.6 million (16 per cent) reported being in 'good health', with 4.2 million in 'fairly good health' (41 per cent) and 4.5 million (43 per cent) in 'not good health'.

Table 3.1

Limiting long-term illness: by age and type of residential establishment, 2001

United Kingdom

Numbers and percentages

	All	0–15	16–29	30–44	45–59	60–74	75 and over
All people in private households	57,742,457	11,807,188	9,924,336	13,177,326	11,055,653	7,746,138	4,031,816
with limiting long-term illness	10,325,083	514,331	619,515	1,381,669	2,344,997	3,046,687	2,417,884
percentage with limiting long-term illness	17.88	4.36	6.24	10.49	21.21	39.33	59.97
All people in communal establishments	1,045,766	51,690	398,068	93,204	59,824	70,138	372,842
with limiting long-term illness	530,381	4,265	33,632	40,762	40,151	60,635	350,936
percentage with limiting long-term illness	50.72	8.25	8.45	43.73	67.12	86.45	94.12
All people	58,788,223	11,858,878	10,322,404	13,270,530	11,115,477	7,816,276	4,404,658
with limiting long-term illness	10,855,464	518,596	653,147	1,422,431	2,385,148	3,107,322	2,768,820
percentage with limiting long-term illness	18.47	4.37	6.33	10.72	21.46	39.75	62.86

Source: Census 2001, Office for National Statistics; Census 2001, General Register Office for Scotland; Census 2001, Northern Ireland Statistics and Research Agency

The 2001 Census showed a steady increase in rates of LLTI with age for both males and females resident in private households (Figure 3.2). While less than 5 per cent of males and females aged 0–4 had an LLTI, just over 10 per cent of males and females in the 35–39 age group had an LLTI. Rates doubled again with around 20 per cent of men and women aged 50–54 reporting an LLTI. This upward trend continued beyond pensionable ages, where the highest rates of LLTI were found. In the 65–69 age group, 41 per cent of males and 38 per cent of females had an LLTI or disability, with these rates gradually rising to 69 per cent for males and 78 per cent for females aged 90 and over.

Figure **3.2**

Limiting long-term illness:[1] by age and sex, 2001

United Kingdom

Percentages

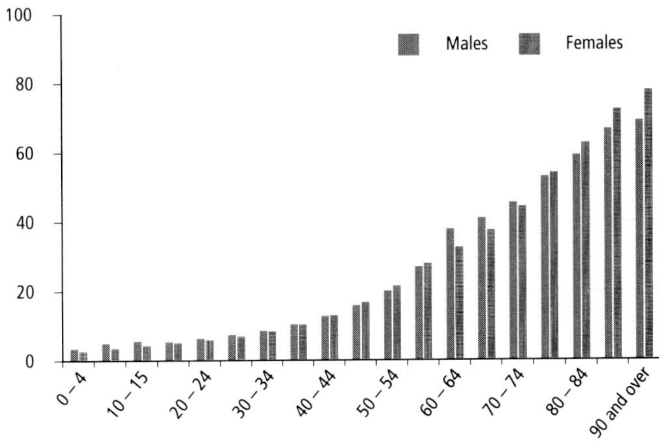

1 *Excluding residents of communal establishments.*

Source: Census 2001, Office for National Statistics; Census 2001, General Register Office for Scotland; Census 2001, Northern Ireland Statistics and Research Agency

Differences in rates of LLTI between males and females are small (around one percentage point) in all age groups up to 59 years. However some substantial differences are found between the sexes in persons aged 60 and over. In the 60–74 age group, males have a higher prevalence of LLTI than females (41 and 38 per cent respectively). This trend is reversed for those aged 75 and over with more women (62 per cent) than men (57 per cent) reporting an LLTI.

Overall, 17 per cent of males, compared to 19 per cent of females, had an LLTI in 2001 (18 per cent of all people in private households). Much of this difference can be explained by the fact that women tend to live longer than men. The latest estimate of expected life free from LLTI (healthy life expectancy)[2] shows that in 2001, women aged 65 could expect to live for another 19 years, with 10 years of this time free from LLTI, compared with 16 and nine years respectively for men.

The different age distributions of males and females in the UK means that once these populations are age-standardised, the differential in LLTI rates between males and females is reversed. Age-standardised rates of LLTI were 17 per cent for males and 16 per cent for females, compared with unstandardised rates of 17 and 19 per cent respectively.

Limiting long-term illness in communal establishments

In addition to the population of private households, there were a further one million people in the UK living in communal establishments in 2001. Just over half (51 per cent) of all people resident in institutions had an LLTI. Rates of illness increased more rapidly with age in establishments than in private households. Only 8 per cent of people aged 0–15 resident in establishments had an LLTI. This rose to 44 per cent of people aged 30–44 and to 94 per cent of people aged 75 and over.

The overall rate of LLTI in all types of establishment was 62 per cent for females and 38 per cent for males, a difference of 24 percentage points. This difference is largely explained by the fact that the female population of communal establishments is much older than the male population. Although there were 290,000 females aged 75 and over in all communal establishments in 2001, there were only 80,000 male residents in the same age group. All further analysis in this chapter refers solely to the population of private households, and excludes the population resident in communal establishments.

Types of illnesses and limitations

Though the Census identifies people with an LLTI, it does not ask what types of illness people have, or in what way people are limited by their illnesses. Other surveys do cover these issues. The GHS looks at the types of illnesses people suffer from, and the Family Resources Survey (FRS) examines the ways in which people are limited by their long-term illnesses. Both surveys only consider residents of private households aged 16 and over.

In 2002–03, the FRS asked people who had an LLTI to specify their limitations within eight categories. The most common types of limitation or disability among both males and females were with mobility; lifting, carrying or moving objects; and manual dexterity (Figure 3.3 – see overleaf). Over 60 per cent of males and females aged 16 and over with an LLTI had mobility problems, with similar percentages of both sexes having problems lifting, carrying or moving objects. Around one in five males (23 per cent) and one in four females (27 per cent) with an LLTI had problems with manual dexterity (e.g. holding a mug/ turning a tap with either/ both hands).[3]

Figure **3.3**

Disabilities among adults[1] with a limiting long-term illness: by sex, 2002/03

Great Britain

Percentages

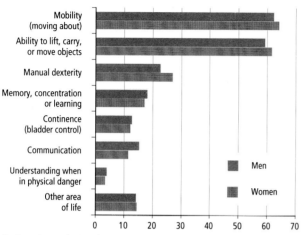

1 *People aged 16 and over in private households.*

Source: Family Resources Survey, Department for Work and Pensions

Figure **3.4**

Conditions affecting adults[1] with a limiting long-term illness: by sex, 2002

Great Britain

Percentages

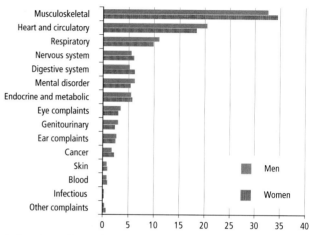

1 *People aged 16 and over in private households.*

Source: General Household Survey, Office for National Statistics

Problems with continence; communication; and memory, concentration and learning were less prevalent, with higher percentages of males than females suffering from these types of limitation, especially communication.

In the GHS, respondents with an a limiting long-standing illness (the GHS uses the term limiting long-standing illness rather than the term limiting long-term used in the Census), are asked 'what is the matter with you?' and responses are coded into the International Classification of Diseases (ICD). The GHS data can be used to estimate the relative prevalence of different chronic health problems among people with limiting long-standing illnesses.

The most common type of health problem affecting people with an LLTI was musculoskeletal complaints. Problems in this category, including arthritis and back pain, affected about a third of men (33 per cent) and women (35 per cent) (Figure 3.4). The FRS showed that the most commonly reported limitations concern mobility; lifting, carrying or moving objects; and manual dexterity – all of which are related to musculoskeletal diseases, and conditions affecting muscles, joints and bones.

The next most common condition reported by people with an LLTI were heart and circulatory diseases, where complaints include chronic heart disease and hypertension (20 per cent of males and 18 per cent of females). Respiratory diseases such as asthma and bronchitis affected 11 per cent of males and 10 per cent of females. Illnesses such as diabetes, thyroid disorders

and obesity (endocrine and metabolic diseases) affected 6 per cent of females and 5 per cent of males, whereas 6 per cent of males and 5 per cent of females reported mental disorders such as dementia, anxiety, depression and phobias.

Geographical variation

There is considerable variation in the age distributions of regional populations of the UK. In order to make equitable geographical comparisons it is necessary to use age-standardised rates of LLTI. The age-standardised rate of LLTI among residents of private households was 16 per cent for the UK, according to the 2001 Census.

In the UK, England had the lowest age-standardised prevalence of LLTI, at 15 per cent. This compares to rates of 17 per cent for Scotland, and 19 per cent for both Wales and Northern Ireland. There were also substantial variations between the various English Government Office Regions (GORs), where a clear north-south divide is apparent.

The GORs with the lowest prevalence of LLTI in England were the South East and the East, which both had a rate of 13 per cent (Table 3.5). The South West (14 per cent), London (15 per cent) and the East Midlands (15 per cent) all had rates lower than the UK as a whole. The North East had the highest rate of LLTI for any English GOR, sharing a prevalence of 19 per cent with both Wales and Northern Ireland. The North West (18 per cent) had the next highest rate within England, while Yorkshire and the Humber (17 per cent), and the West Midlands (16 per cent) had successively lower rates.

Table 3.5

Limiting long-term illness[1] (age-standardised): by Region, 2001

United Kingdom	Percentages
South East	12.6
East	13.3
South West	14.0
London	15.1
England	15.2
East Midlands	15.4
UK	15.7
West Midlands	16.0
Yorkshire and the Humber	16.6
Scotland	17.3
North West	17.8
North East	19.4
Wales	19.4
Northern Ireland	19.5

1 *Excluding residents of communal establishments.*

Source: Census 2001, Office for National Statistics; Census 2001, General Register Office for Scotland; Census 2001, Northern Ireland Statistics and Research Agency

Overall, the analysis of geographical differences at local authority (LA) level, reveals even greater disparities than at GOR level. Map 3.6 (see overleaf) shows the proportion of people in each LA with an LLTI, illustrating that high rates were recorded in Wales and the North East, as well as in most LAs in Northern Ireland and inner city London. In contrast, lower rates were found in suburban areas to the south and west of London, as well as along the coast in the South East of England.

The difference between the best and worst GORs in terms of the prevalence of LLTI is around six percentage points (South East 13 per cent, Northern Ireland 19 per cent). However, at LA level, the gap between the lowest rate (Elmbridge, South East) of 10 per cent and the highest rate (Easington, North East) of 27 per cent is almost three times as large, at 17 percentage points.

All 10 LAs with the lowest rates of LLTI are found in the South East of England (Table 3.7 – see overleaf). Of the 10 LAs with the highest rates of LLTI only two are found in England, with five in Wales, one in Scotland, and two in Northern Ireland.

The LA with the lowest rate of LLTI outside England is Aberdeenshire (Scotland), with a rate of 13 per cent, three percentage points more than the lowest rate in England. In Wales, Monmouthshire has the lowest prevalence of LLTI at 15 per cent, while in Northern Ireland, the lowest rate is also 15 per cent in North Down.

Ethnicity

The 2001 Census shows the different ethnic groups in the UK to have varied rates of age-standardised LLTI (Figure 3.8 – see overleaf). One in five Asians had an LLTI, making this the ethnic group with the highest rate of LLTI (20 per cent). Rates of LLTI among the Mixed (18 per cent) and Black (17 per cent) populations were higher than among the White population (16 per cent). People of Chinese and other ethnic backgrounds had the lowest overall rate of LLTI at 13 per cent, three percentage points lower than the White population.

Black and Asian females had higher overall rates of LLTI than their male counterparts. The largest difference was found between Asian females and males, with rates of 22 and 19 per cent respectively. Black females had a rate of 18 per cent compared with 16 per cent for Black males. White males (16 per cent) and females (15 per cent) had very similar rates, whereas males and females in Mixed and Chinese and other groups had the same rates of LLTI, at 18 and 13 per cent respectively.

Socio-economic variation

Educational attainment

In 2001, there were over 15 million people aged 16–74 in the UK who had 'no qualifications', or qualifications of an 'unknown level'. LLTI was most prevalent in this group, affecting 24 per cent of males, and 23 per cent of females.

Of the 18.9 million people with lower level qualifications, 14 per cent of both males and females had an LLTI. The group with higher level qualifications (8.3 million people) had a lower rate still, with 11 per cent of males and 12 per cent of females suffering from an LLTI (Figure 3.9 – see overleaf). Rates of LLTI among men with the highest qualifications were less than half the rate of those with unknown or no qualifications, whereas for females, the rate was just over half.

Economic activity

In 2001, 27.6 million people in the UK aged 16–64 were economically active, and a further 9.5 million people were economically inactive, with 2.1 million of this group classified as 'permanently sick or disabled'.

Age-standardised rates of LLTI varied by working status (e.g. full- and part-time workers) and whether people were economically active or inactive. The rate of LLTI among economically inactive males was 52 per cent, more than seven times higher than the rate among economically active males (7 per cent). Economically inactive females had a rate of LLTI of 29

Map **3.6**

Limiting long-term illness[1] (age-standardised): by local authority,[2] 2001

United Kingdom

All people

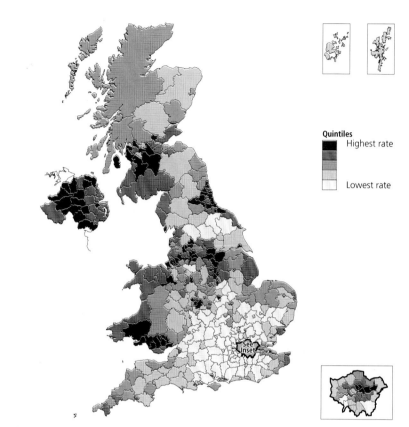

Quintiles
Highest rate

Lowest rate

1 Excluding residents of communal establishments.
2 Local authorities ranked from highest to lowest and then divided into five groups.

Source: Office for National Statistics; Census 2001, General Register Office for Scotland; Census 2001, Northern Ireland Statistics and Research Agency

Table **3.7**

Local authorities with the highest and lowest rates of limiting long-term illness (age-standardised),[1] 2001

United Kingdom

Percentages

Rank	Local Authority	Region	%	Rank	Local Authority	Region	%
1	Elmbridge	South East	9.6	425	Knowsley	North West	23.1
2	South Bucks	South East	9.8	426	Caerphilly	Wales	23.5
3	Chiltern	South East	9.8	427	Derry	Northern Ireland	23.7
4	Hart	South East	9.9	428	Rhondda; Cynon; Taff	Wales	23.9
5	Wokingham	South East	10.0	429	Glasgow City	Scotland	24.1
6	Surrey Heath	South East	10.0	430	Strabane	Northern Ireland	24.2
7	Windsor and Maidenhead	South East	10.3	431	Blaenau Gwent	Wales	24.3
8	Mid Sussex	South East	10.4	432	Neath Port Talbot	Wales	24.4
9	Waverley	South East	10.4	433	Merthyr Tydfil	Wales	26.7
10	Horsham	South East	10.4	434	Easington	North East	26.9

1 Excluding residents of communal establishments.

Source: Census 2001, Office for National Statistics; Census 2001, General Register Office for Scotland; Census 2001, Northern Ireland Statistics and Research Agency

Figure **3.8**

Limiting long-term illness[1] (age-standardised): by sex and ethnic group,[2] 2001

United Kingdom

Percentages

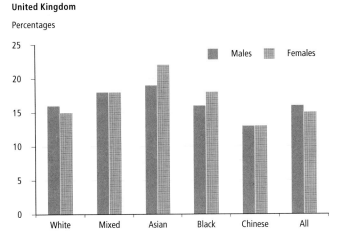

1 Excluding residents of communal establishments.
2 Chinese includes 'other ethnic group' catgegory.

Source: Census 2001, Office for National Statistics; Census 2001, General Register Office for Scotland; Census 2001, Northern Ireland Statistics and Research Agency

Figure **3.9**

Limiting long-term illness[1] (age-standardised): by sex and highest level of qualification, 2001

United Kingdom

Percentages

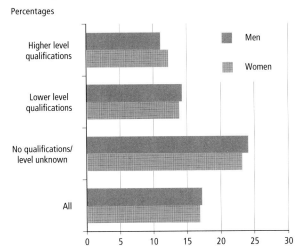

1 People aged 16–74 living in private households.

Source: Census 2001, Office for National Statistics; Census 2001, General Register Office for Scotland; Census 2001, Northern Ireland Statistics and Research Agency

per cent, 23 percentage points lower than inactive males, and more than four times higher than the rate for economically active women (7 per cent) (Table 3.10).

Of all economically active groups, the rate of LLTI was highest among the unemployed, where 17 per cent of males and 14 per cent of females had an LLTI. For both males and females, these rates were more than twice those found among male

Table **3.10**

Limiting long-term illness[1] (age-standardised): by sex and economic activity,[2] 2001

United Kingdom   Percentages

	All	Men	Women
Economically active	*7.21*	*7.46*	*6.86*
Employee	6.67	6.83	6.48
part-time	8.12	13.29	7.44
full-time	6.27	6.46	5.86
Self-employed	7.27	7.15	7.66
part-time	10.13	12.24	8.68
full-time	6.76	6.40	6.82
Unemployed	15.81	16.60	14.42
Full-time student	8.24	9.02	7.49
All part-time	8.41	12.91	7.54
All full-time	6.31	6.45	5.97
Economically inactive	**35.87**	**51.74**	**29.29**
Retired	43.49	46.52	40.43
Looking after home/family	14.82	22.22	14.19
Permanently sick/disabled	94.56	95.15	93.86
Other (incl. part-time students)	26.72	30.43	24.11
All	**14.35**	**14.46**	**14.25**

1 People aged 16–64 living in private households.
2 Those working 31 or more hours per week are classified as full-time, those working 30 or less hours per week as part-time.

Source: Census 2001, Office for National Statistics; Census 2001, General Register Office for Scotland; Census 2001, Northern Ireland Statistics and Research Agency

and female employees (7 and 6 per cent respectively). There was little difference between the rates of LLTI for employees and those who were self-employed (around 7 per cent of males and females in both groups). Full-time students had rates of LLTI of 9 per cent for males and 7 per cent for females.

Differences in rates of LLTI between those who work full-time and part-time were more pronounced among males than females. Males working part-time had a rate of LLTI at 13 per cent, compared with 6 per cent for those working full-time, representing a gap of seven percentage points. Among females there was a difference of only two percentage points, with 8 per cent of females working part-time having an LLTI, compared with 6 per cent of those working full-time.

Not unexpectedly, among the economically inactive groups, those who were classed as permanently sick or disabled had the highest rates of LLTI: 95 per cent for males and 94 per cent for females. The next highest rates were found among those who had retired (47 per cent males, 40 per cent females) and 'other' economically inactive people (30 per cent of males, 24 per cent of females with an LLTI). The lowest rates of LLTI among economically inactive individuals were found among people looking after the home or family (males 22 per cent and females 14 per cent).

Census data shows clear differences in economic activity status between those who have and those who do not have an LLTI. Among those of working age (16–64), around three in five people with an LLTI were economically inactive compared with only one in five of those without an LLTI. As shown by recent research,[4] among adults of working age there was a large overlap between people who say they are work restricted and those reporting limitation in daily activities. This overlap is likely to be reinforced in the 2001 Census because of the explicit inclusion of work restriction (limitation in the *work you can do*) in the Census question on LLTI.

Work capacity and economic activity therefore capture distinct though related constructs. This may in part explain why people with an LLTI are less likely to report working part-time (60 per cent compared with 70 per cent), or being unemployed (12 per cent compared with 5 per cent) than people who do not have an LLTI.

Social position

Age-standardised rates of LLTI were lowest among those in higher managerial and professional occupations (7 per cent), increasing to 9 per cent in lower managerial and professional groups; 10 per cent in intermediate occupations; 11 per cent among small employers and own account workers and 12 per cent in lower supervisory and technical groups and 13 per cent in semi-routine occupations (Figure 3.11). The highest rate of LLTI (15 per cent) for any occupational group was found among those employed in routine occupations.

The National Statistics Socio-Economic Classification (NS-SEC) also includes those who had never worked or were long-term unemployed. This group had by far the highest rate of LLTI, which at 37 per cent was more than double the highest rate in any other occupational group. In most categories, there was little difference between rates for males and females. However males have notably higher rates of LLTI than females in the 'never worked and long-term unemployed' groups (41 and 34 per cent respectively).

Figure **3.11**

Limiting long-term illness (age-standardised): by sex and NS-SEC,[1] 2001

United Kingdom

Percentages

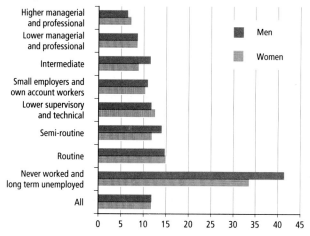

1   People aged 16–64 living in private households.

Source: Census 2001, Office for National Statistics; Census 2001, General Register Office for Scotland; Census 2001, Northern Ireland Statistics and Research Agency

Marital status

Rates of LLTI varied between the different marital status categories, but were fairly similar between males and females within each marital status group (Figure 3.12). Age-standardised rates of LLTI were highest among those who were widowed (29 per cent) followed by those who were divorced or separated (25 per cent), then those who were single (23 per cent). Married people had the lowest rate of LLTI at 18 per cent.

Figure **3.12**

Limiting long-term illness (age-standardised): by marital status,[1] 2001

United Kingdom

Percentages

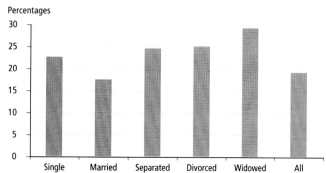

1   People aged 16 and over living in private households.

Source: Census 2001, Office for National Statistics; Census 2001, General Register Office for Scotland; Census 2001, Northern Ireland Statistics and Research Agency

Family status

In addition to marital status, the Census allows us to explore differences in rates of LLTI by the family status of an individual. Both male and female lone parents had a rate of LLTI at 20 per cent, compared with a rate of 15 per cent for males and females who were part of a two-parent (couple) family (Figure 3.13). Among dependent children, rates of LLTI were significantly higher in lone parent families (7 per cent of boys, 5 per cent of girls) than in couple families (4 per cent of boys and 3 per cent of girls had an LLTI). The highest age-standardised rates of LLTI were found among single pensioners who were not part of a family; 52 per cent of males and 46 per cent of females had an LLTI.

Figure 3.13

Limiting long-term illness[1] (age-standardised): by sex and family status, 2001

United Kingdom

Percentages

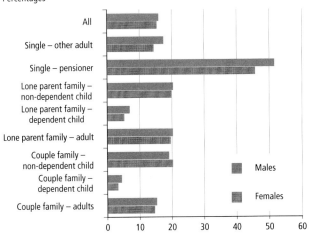

All
Single – other adult
Single – pensioner
Lone parent family – non-dependent child
Lone parent family – dependent child
Lone parent family – adult
Couple family – non-dependent child
Couple family – dependent child
Couple family – adults
Males
Females
0
10
20
30
40
50
60

1 *Excluding residents of communal establishments.*

Source: Census 2001, Office for National Statistics; Census 2001, General Register Office for Scotland; Census 2001, Northern Ireland Statistics and Research Agency

By age-standardising the population over 65, rates of LLTI between single pensioners and pensioners in couple families can be directly compared. Males and females aged 65 and over who were living alone had rates of LLTI of 52 and 49 per cent respectively. The corresponding rates among pensioners who were in a family were 47 and 46 per cent. Lone pensioners therefore display rates of LLTI five percentage points higher among males and three points higher among females.

Housing tenure

Data from the Census on household tenure in Great Britain reveals that age-standardised rates of LLTI were highest for both males and females living in social housing, at 30 and 27 per cent respectively (Figure 3.14). In 2001, 9.5 million people in Great Britain lived in social housing, with 2.9 million of them having an LLTI.

Figure 3.14

Limiting long-term illness[1] (age-standardised): by sex and housing tenure, 2001

Great Britain[2]

Percentages

35
30
25
20
15
10
5
0
Males
Females
Owned
Social housing
Private rented
Rent free
All

1 *Excluding residents of communal establishments.*
2 *Data are only provided for Great Britain because Northern Ireland uses a different coding system to the rest of the UK to describe tenure.*

Source: Census 2001, Office for National Statistics; Census 2001, General Register Office for Scotland; Census 2001, Northern Ireland Statistics and Research Agency

People owning their own accommodation had the lowest rate of LLTI after age-standardisation, at 13 per cent for both males and females, whereas 18 per cent of males and 17 per cent of females who were renting privately had an LLTI. Rates of LLTI among social housing tenants were more than double that of people who owned their accommodation.

Age-specific rates of LLTI also showed a marked difference between residents of social housing and owner-occupiers. The prevalence of LLTI among those living in social housing was at least double that of those living in owned accommodation in all groups up to age 59.

This marked contrast in LLTI rates results in children aged 0–15 living in social housing having rates of LLTI equal to owner-occupiers aged 30–44 (Figure 3.15 – see overleaf).

Proportionately, the greatest difference in the prevalence of LLTI between owner-occupiers and residents of social housing was in the 30–44 age group. In this age group, social housing tenants had a rate of LLTI over three times higher (25 per cent) than people who own their own homes (7 per cent). Though the size of this difference decreased in the oldest age groups (60–74, 75 and over), the proportion of social housing tenants with an LLTI remained 66 per cent higher than owner-occupiers in the 60–74 age group, and 20 per cent higher among those aged 75 and over.

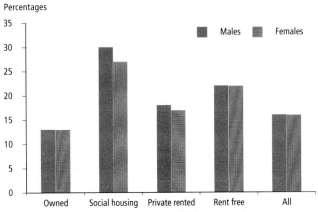

Figure **3.15**

Limiting long-term illness:[1] by age and housing tenure, 2001

Great Britain[2]

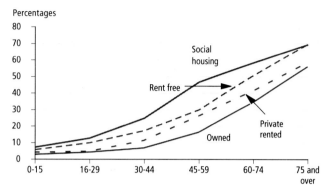

1 Excluding residents of communal establishments.
2 Data are only provided for Great Britain because Northern Ireland uses a different coding system to the rest of the UK to describe tenure.

Source: Census 2001, Office for National Statistics; Census 2001, General

Housing deprivation

Housing deprivation is another census variable that allows us to analyse the relationship between an individual's conditions and their health. A household is defined as deprived if it is either overcrowded, in a shared dwelling, does not have sole use of a bath or shower, or has no central heating.

In 2001, 8.6 million people in Great Britain lived in homes that were deprived, representing 16 per cent of the population after age-standardisation. Men and women living in deprived housing had a higher rate of LLTI after age-standardisation (20 per cent) than people living in non-deprived households (15 per cent).

Conclusion

The 2001 Census shows that in 2001, 10.3 million people, or 18 per cent of the UK population resident in private households were suffering from a limiting long-term illness (16 per cent after age-standardisation). Rates of LLTI increased with age for both males and females. The 2002/2003 FRS revealed that the most common limitations among both males and females with an LLTI were difficulties with mobility; lifting, carrying or moving objects; and manual dexterity. The 2002 GHS showed that musculoskeletal conditions were the most common forms of LLTI, a finding in line with the functional limitations highlighted by the FRS.

Rates of LLTI were highest in Wales, Northern Ireland and the North of England, while the East, South East and South West had the lowest rates. Data on education and employment show there was an association between higher levels of

qualifications and full-time economic activity (whether as an employee or self-employed) and low rates of long-term illness. Economically inactive people tended to have much higher rates of LLTI.

Overall, people who were disadvantaged in terms of their educational, employment and socio-economic background appeared to have higher rates of LLTI. Minority ethnic groups (excluding 'Chinese and other') had raised rate of LLTI compared to the White population, while people living in deprived and social rented housing also had higher rates of LLTI. Socially, there was a relationship between closer family composition and lower rates of illness, with married males and females displaying the lowest rates of LLTI, and children in couple families having lower rates of illness than those in lone parent families.

References

1. Charlton J and Wallace M (1994) Long-term illness: Results from the 1991 Census. *Population Trends* **75**, 18–25.

2. Healthy Life Expectancy at birth and at 65 in Great Britain and England, 1981–2001 at: www.statistics.gov.uk/statbase/ssdataset. asp?vlnk=8486

3. Martin *et al* (1988) *The prevalence of disability among adults*, HMSO: London.

4. Bajekal M, Harris T, Breman R and Woodfield K (2004) DWP In-house reports 128: *Review of Disability Estimates and Definitions*, DWP: London, p47, 62.

Smoking, drinking and drug use

Susan Westlake and Mohammed Yar

Chapter 4

Introduction

Behaviours such as smoking, heavy drinking and drug-taking have long been recognised as harmful to health. The 2004 White Paper *Choosing Health: Making Healthy Choices Easier,*[1] was specifically aimed at supporting action to reduce the number of people who smoke; encourage and support sensible drinking, and reduce the harm caused by illegal drugs. Various strategies exist to alleviate problems. For example, smoking cessation clinics support people who wish to give up, and guidelines for sensible drinking have been produced.

It is generally recognised that smoking is the largest single preventable cause of premature mortality and one of the main underlying determinants of health inequalities.[2, 3] It is estimated that in each year between 1998 and 2002, over 106,000 deaths in the UK, around a sixth of the total, were from smoking-related causes and smoking was the direct cause of about three in five of all cancers.[4]

Drinking excessively causes many problems for individuals and society, ranging from road traffic accidents and anti-social behaviour to ill-health. Long-term alcohol misuse increases the likelihood of diseases such as cirrhosis of the liver, cancer and haemorrhagic stroke.[5] *The Alcohol Harm Reduction Strategy for England*[5] was published in 2004. Scotland, Wales and Northern Ireland have produced similar initiatives.

For each of the three behaviours – smoking, drinking and drug-taking – this chapter presents the latest data on patterns of prevalence and trends and associated morbidity and mortality. Wherever available, separate data for children (aged less than 16) and adults (aged 16 and over) is presented.

Smoking

Smoking among adults

The Department of Health's *Public Service Agreement 2005–2008* (PSA)[6] contains a target of reducing adult smoking rates in England to 21 per cent or less by 2010; with a reduction in prevalence among routine and manual occupational groups to 26 per cent or less. Data from the 2003 General Household Survey (GHS) show that in Great Britain around a quarter (26 per cent) of adults, aged 16 and over smoked cigarettes. More men (28 per cent) than women (24 per cent) were smokers. Cigarette smoking is more common among adults aged 20–34 than other age groups. In 2003, 36 per cent of adults aged 20–24 and 34 per cent of adults aged 25–34 were smokers compared with 15 per cent of those aged 60 and over.[7]

The proportion of adults who smoked cigarettes fell substantially in the 1970s and the early 1980s – from 45 per cent in 1974 to 35 per cent in 1982. After 1982 it declined

gradually until the early 1990s, since when it has levelled out at 26 to 28 per cent.

In the 1970s men were far more likely than women to be smokers. In 1974, 51 per cent of men and 41 per cent of women smoked cigarettes (Figure 4.1). During the 1970s and 1980s the gap between men and women narrowed. It has still not disappeared completely but had fallen to four percentage points in 2003.[7] Men are more likely than women to stop smoking.[8]

Figure **4.1**

Cigarette smoking prevalence:[1] by sex, 1974–2002[2]

Great Britain

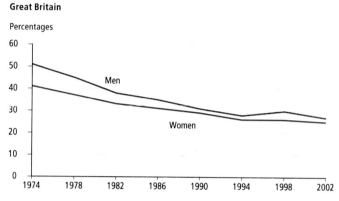

1 Adults aged 16 and over.
2 Data are presented in four-yearly intervals and are weighted in 2002.
Source: General Household Survey, Office for National Statistics

Among smokers the number of cigarettes smoked was also higher in men than in women. In 2003, male smokers smoked 15 cigarettes per day on average and female smokers smoked 13 cigarettes per day (Figure 4.2). The heaviest consumption was by those aged 35–59 among both male and female smokers. Ten per cent of male and 7 per cent of female smokers smoked more than 20 cigarettes per day.[7]

There are striking differences in the prevalence of cigarette smoking by social position as defined by the National Statistics Socio-Economic Classification. Prevalence was lowest among those in households where the household reference person was in a higher professional or higher managerial occupation (15 per cent in both cases) and greatest among those in a semi-routine (33 per cent) or routine (36 per cent) occupation.[7] Large and persistent differences in smoking prevalence between different socio-economic groups are considered to be an important contributory factor in health inequalities between different socio-economic groups.[2,3]

The regional pattern of smoking prevalence remained unchanged in 2003. As in previous years, smoking prevalence was higher in Scotland (31 per cent) than in Wales (27 per cent) and England (25 per cent). Between 1998 and 2003 the

Figure **4.2**

Average daily cigarette consumption: by age and sex of smokers, 1998 and 2003

Great Britain

Number smoked

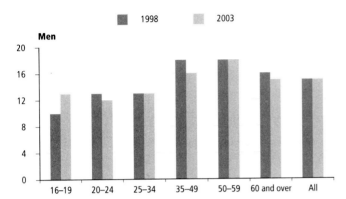

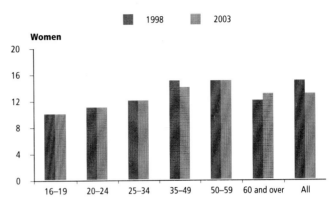

Source: General Household Survey, Office for National Statistics

proportion of cigarette smokers in England fell from 28 to 25 per cent. In Scotland and Wales it was fairly stable over this period.[7]

Smoking among schoolchildren

Most people who have ever smoked started smoking when teenagers.[7] The *Smoking Kills* White Paper set a target for England of reducing the proportion of young people aged 11–15 smoking at least one cigarette per week from 13 per cent in 1996 to 11 per cent by 2005 and 9 per cent or less by 2010.[2] The survey of Smoking, Drinking and Drug-use among Secondary School Pupils showed that in 2004 around 10 per cent of children in England aged 11–15 were smokers; a similar level to that observed since 1999.[9] Since 1986 the proportion of girls who were regular smokers (smoking at least one cigarette a week) exceeded the proportion of boys (Figure 4.3). In 2004, 26 per cent of girls and 16 per cent of boys aged 15 smoked regularly.

In Scotland, the percentage of girls aged 13 and 15 smoking regularly in 2004 also exceeded that of boys.[10] Among 15-year-olds the proportion of girls (24 per cent) and boys (14 per cent) who smoked regularly was slightly lower than in England (26 per cent of girls, 16 per cent of boys). There are no recent comparable statistics for Northern Ireland or Wales. An earlier 2000 survey, Young Persons' Behaviour and Attitudes in Northern Ireland showed that 33 per cent of 11- to 15- year-olds were regular smokers.[11]

Between 1982 and 2002, the average number of cigarettes smoked per week by regular smokers aged 11–15 in England fluctuated from year to year, but was higher for boys (between 50 and 52) than for girls (between 44 and 48) (Figure 4.4 – see

overleaf). During the same period the average weekly consumption by occasional smokers was between four and seven cigarettes for girls, and between seven and 14 for boys. The method of measuring 'cigarette consumption in the last week' changed in 2003, so the results are not comparable with estimates from previous surveys, and are not included here.[12]

All pupils, regardless of their smoking status, were asked about their family's attitude towards their smoking. Non-smokers were asked how they thought their family would feel if they started smoking. Smokers were asked how their family felt about the fact that they smoked. Two-thirds of pupils in England aged 11–15 in 2002 thought that their families would try to stop them smoking.[13] In Scotland nearly nine out of 10 of 13- and 15-year-olds in 2004 reported that their families would stop them smoking or persuade them not to smoke.[10]

Figure **4.3**

Regular smokers:[1] by sex for children aged 11–15, 1982–2004[2]

England

Percentages

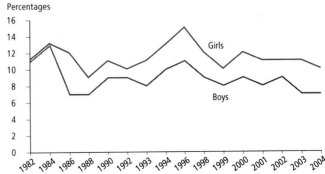

1   Regular smokers defined as those who usually smoke at least one cigarette a week.
2   Data presented for every year available.

Source: Survey of Smoking, Drinking and Drug Use among Young People in England, Department of Health

Figure **4.4**

Average cigarette consumption in the last week:[1] by smoking status and sex for children aged 11–15, 1982–2002[2]

England

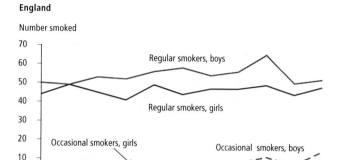

Number smoked
70
60
50
40
30
20
10
0
Regular smokers, boys
Regular smokers, girls
Occasional smokers, girls
Occasional smokers, boys
1982
1984
1986
1988
1990
1992
1994
1996
1998
2000
2002

1 *The method of measuring the number of cigarettes smoked in the last 7 days changed in 2003.*
2 *Data presented for every alternate year to 2002.*

Source: Survey of Smoking, Drinking and Drug Use among Young People in England, Department of Health

Smoking-related mortality

The estimated proportion of male deaths in the UK attributable to smoking between 1998 and 2002 was double that of female deaths, 23 and 12 per cent respectively (Figure 4.5). It was highest in Scotland (26 per cent of male deaths and 14 per cent of female deaths) and lowest in Northern Ireland (21 per cent of male deaths and 10 per cent of female deaths). The estimated number of deaths from smoking-attributable disease decreased in the UK from 120,000 in 1995, to an average of 106,000 between 1998 and 2002 – or from just over one in five deaths to just under one in six.[4]

Figure **4.5**

Deaths attributable to smoking: by sex and country, 1998–2002

United Kingdom

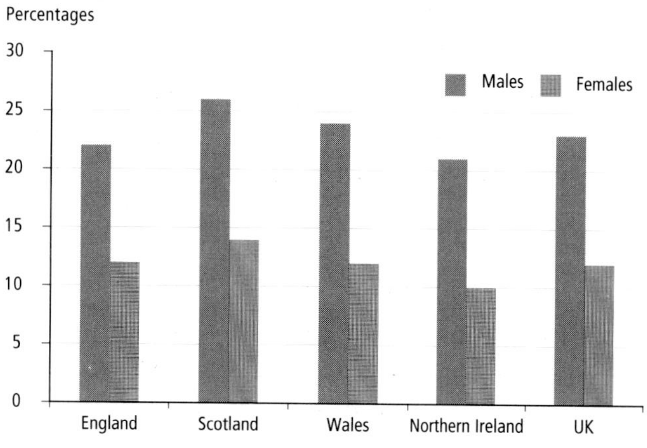

Percentages
30
25
20
15
10
5
0
Males
Females
England
Scotland
Wales
Northern Ireland
UK

Source: Health Development Agency

Smokers are more at risk than non-smokers or ex-smokers of dying from respiratory, circulatory, and digestive disorders and various cancers. The Health Development Agency (HDA) estimated that in England between 1998 and 2002, smoking caused nine out of ten deaths from lung cancer in men, and eight out of 10 in women.[4]

The HDA calculated the relative mortality risks by type of disease for current and ex-smokers in England, compared with those who had never smoked.[4] A male smoker was 27 times, and a female smoker 14 times, more likely to die from lung cancer than a person who had never smoked. Smokers also had a higher mortality risk of cancers in other parts of the body including upper respiratory tract, oesophagus, bladder, kidney, stomach, and pancreas. A smoker was also 14 times more likely to die from chronic obstructive lung disease. The risks for ex-smokers were reduced.

Drinking

Drinking among adults

In 1995, the government changed its guidelines on sensible drinking from weekly to daily benchmarks, because binge drinking was recognised as a growing problem. The advice for men is not to consistently drink more than three to four units per day, and for women two to three units per day. Regular moderate drinking of between one and two units per day can protect men over the age of forty and post-menopausal women against the risk of death from coronary heart disease and ischaemic stroke.[5, 14]

Alcohol consumption in the previous week is measured in the annual General Household Survey series. In 2003, three-quarters of men and three out of five women in Great Britain drank alcohol in the previous week. Men were more likely than women to exceed the daily benchmarks on at least one day during the previous week – 40 per cent of men compared with 23 per cent of women (Figure 4.6).

Younger people were more likely than older people to exceed the daily benchmarks (Figure 4.6). Just over half (51 per cent) of men aged 16–24 had drunk more than four units on at least one day during the previous week compared with 19 per cent of men aged 65 and over. Among women, 40 per cent of those aged 16–24 had exceeded three units on at least one day in the past week compared with only 4 per cent of those aged 65 and over.

Among both men and women, those in large employer/ higher managerial households were the most likely to have drunk alcohol in the previous week, and those in households where the household reference person was in a routine occupation

Figure 4.6

Drinking more than the recommended guidelines on at least one day last week: by age and sex, 2003

Great Britain

Percentages
60
50
40
30
20
10
0
Men
Women
16–24
25–44
45–64
65 and over

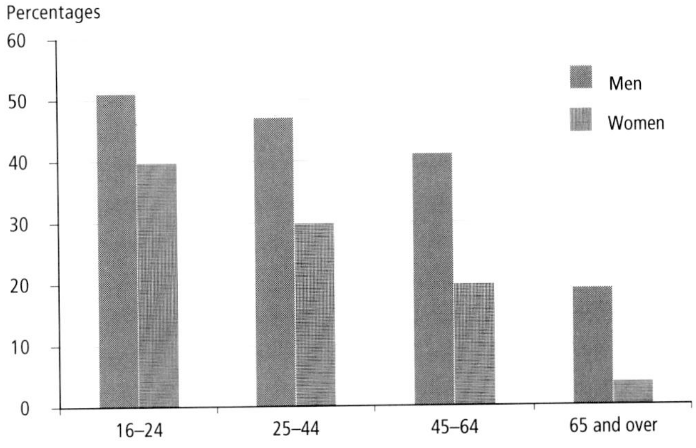

Source: Omnnbus Survey, Office for National Statistics

Figure 4.7

Average weekly alcohol consumption: by alcohol type, age and sex, 2004

Great Britain

Number of units
Men
65 and over
45–64
25–44
16–24
Women
65 and over
45–64
25–44
16–24
0
5
10
15
20
25
Strong beer, lager, cider
Normal strength beer, lager, cider
Spirits
Fortified wine
Wine
Alcopops

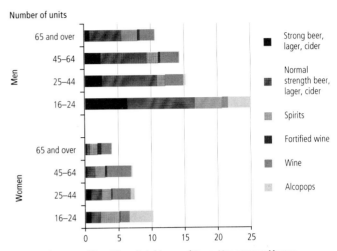

Source: Survey of Smoking, Drinking and Drug Use among Young People in England, Department of Health

the least likely.[15] Variations in the amount drunk were less marked. The proportion of men and women in the managerial and professional occupational group who had exceeded the daily benchmarks, on at least one day in the previous week, was higher than for men and women in the routine and manual groups, but these differences were not statistically significant.

Heavy drinking (defined as more than eight units a day for men and six units a day for women) on at least one day during the previous week was much more common among men (23 per cent) than women (9 per cent).[7] Heavy drinking decreased as age increased: from 37 per cent of men and 26 per cent of women aged 16–24, to 6 per cent of men and 1 per cent of women aged 65 and over.[7]

Beer, lager and cider were the most popular alcoholic drinks among men, accounting for two-thirds of all alcohol drunk by men (10 units each on average per week), and a quarter by women (less than two units each on average per week) (Figure 4.7). Wine was the next most popular drink, accounting for 16 per cent of all alcohol drunk by men and 37 per cent by women (two and a half units each on average per week).

The number of units of beer, lager, cider, spirits and alcopops consumed decreased as age increased, except for wine which increased with age up to 65 then fell (Figure 4.7). Alcopops were most popular with people aged 16 to 24 (drunk by 14 per cent of men and 35 per cent of women) with an average consumption of three and a half units per week. Spirits were most popular with the youngest and oldest age groups, but the younger age group drank more units – four per week by men and three by women aged 16–24, compared with two by men and one by women aged 65 and over.

Drinking more than the recommended levels and heavy drinking were more common among both men and women in Scotland than in England or Wales, and in the North of England rather than the South.[7] Scotland therefore set a target to reduce the proportion of adults exceeding weekly limits from 33 per cent in 1995 to 31 per cent by 2005 and to 29 per cent by 2010.[16]

Surveys of adults' knowledge of sensible drinking recommendations, conducted in 1997 and 2004, reported that the proportion of people who had heard of daily benchmarks increased from 54 per cent in 1997 to 61 per cent in 2004.[17] Having heard of daily recommended levels did not necessarily mean that people knew what they were. For example, 14 per cent thought that the recommended daily maximum levels for men was five units or more and 10 per cent thought that for women it was four units or more. There was no statistically significant change in the knowledge of benchmark levels between 1997 and 2004.

When questioned about 'drink-driving' in the 2002 Omnibus Survey, one in eight drivers admitted to driving after drinking what they believed was a sufficient amount to take them 'over the limit', increasing to one in four of 16- to 29-year-old men.[18] Men and frequent drinkers were more likely to drive when 'over the limit' than women or infrequent drinkers. Nearly one in five people who admitted to driving while 'over the limit' did so at least once a month. The average amount drunk by 'over the limit' drivers was five units.

Drinking among schoolchildren

Figure 4.8

Drinking in past week: by age and sex for children aged 11–15, 2004

England

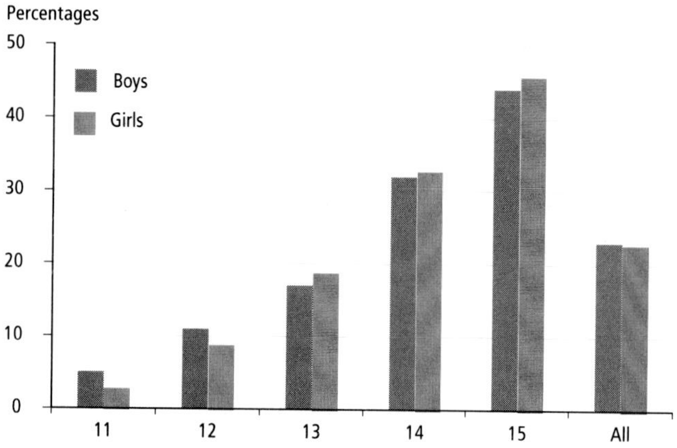

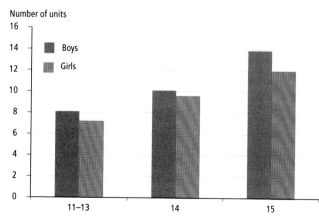

Percentages
50
40
30
20
10
0
Boys
Girls
11
12
13
14
15
All

Source: Survey of Smoking, Drinking and Drug Use among Young People in England, Department of Health

The 2004 survey of schoolchildren in England aged 11–15 showed that 23 per cent of both boys and girls aged 11–15 drank alcohol (Figure 4.8). The proportion of drinkers increased with age from 4 per cent of 11-year-olds to 45 per cent of 15-year-olds. Boys drank more units in the previous week than girls in each age group. On average, the number of units consumed by 11- to 13-year-olds was eight by boys and seven by girls, while the equivalent amounts for 15-year-olds were 14 and 12 units respectively (Figure 4.9).

More boys than girls drank alcohol until 2004, when the proportions were equal (Figure 4.10). The mean number of units consumed by young people who drank 'last week'

Figure 4.9

Average alcohol consumption: by age and sex for children aged 11–15 who drank last week, 2004

England

Number of units
16
14
12
10
8
6
4
2
0
Boys
Girls
11–13
14
15

Source: Survey of Smoking, Drinking and Drug Use among Young People in England, Department of Health

Figure 4.10

Drinking in past week: by sex for children aged 11–15, 1990–2004[1]

England

Percentages
30
25
20
15
10
5
0
Boys
Girls
1990
1992
1994
1996
1998
2000
2002
2004

1 Data are presented in two-yearly intervals.

Source: Survey of Smoking, Drinking and Drug Use among Young People in England, Department of Health

doubled from 5.3 to 10.7 between 1990 and 2004. The greatest increase was among girls (Figure 4.11).

Among those who drank last week, in 2004 boys drank more beer, lager and cider (6.3 units) than any other drink, followed by alcopops (1.9 units) and spirits (1.8 units) (Figure 4.12). Girls drank 3.6, 2.7 and 2.3 units respectively.

In Scotland, the percentage of children aged 13 who 'drank in the last week' doubled from 10 to 20 per cent between 1990 and 2004.[10] Among those aged 15, the proportion who drank increased from 30 to 40 per cent of boys and from 25 to 46 per cent of girls. In 2004, among those who drank in the previous week, 13-year-olds drank nine units and 15-year-olds drank 12 units per week. Beer, lager and cider were the most

Figure 4.11

Average alcohol consumption: by sex for children aged 11–15 who drank last week, 1990–2004[1]

England

Number of units
14
12
10
8
6
4
2
0
Boys
Girls
1990
1992
1994
1996
1998
2000
2002
2004

1 Data are presented in two-yearly intervals.

Source: Survey of Smoking, Drinking and Drug Use among Young People in England, Department of Health

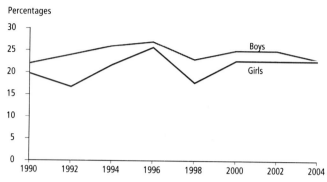

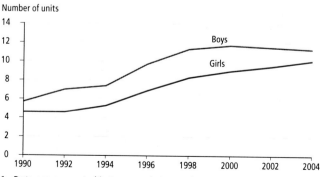

Figure **4.12**

Average alcohol consumption: by alcohol type and sex for children aged 11–15 who drank last week, 2004

England

Number of units

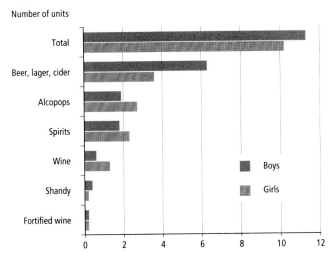

Source: Survey of Smoking, Drinking and Drug Use among Young People in England, Department of Health

popular drinks for both sexes, accounting for about a third of units drunk, followed by spirits, wine and alcopops.

Nearly one in five young people aged 11–16 in 2000 in Northern Ireland reported that they were currently drinking weekly or more frequently. More than two in five reported having been drunk on more than one occasion.[19]

Alcohol-related ill-health

People who drink large amounts of alcohol regularly are at increased risk of a variety of health harms such as cirrhosis of the liver (which has nearly doubled in the last 10 years), cancer, and haemorrhagic stroke.[5] In addition, health and social harms caused by alcohol misuse increase for a range of vulnerable groups. These include problem drinkers from vulnerable groups such as ex-prisoners, street drinkers, those who suffered abuse as children, children of those who misuse alcohol, and young drinkers. As well as alcohol problems they are more likely to experience a whole range of other problems, such as mental illness, drug use and homelessness.[5]

The ONS Survey of Psychiatric Morbidity among Adults in Great Britain in 2000 found that women with significant levels of neurotic symptoms were more likely than those without to be hazardous or harmful drinkers. Of the neurotic disorders examined, both men and women with obsessive compulsive disorder were most likely to have a drink problem. The likelihood of being a harmful drinker was greater for people presenting with multiple disorders rather than a single disorder. Showing evidence of anti-social personality disorder was

significantly associated with higher rates of hazardous drinking, compared with both the general population, and to those with a personality disorder other than an anti-social one.[20]

The ONS survey of the mental health of children and young people in 2004 showed that, among those aged 11–16, young people with emotional, conduct or hyperkinetic disorders were more likely to be regular drinkers than those with no such disorder.[21]

The number of NHS hospital admissions in England with a diagnosis (primary or secondary) of 'mental and behavioural disorders due to alcohol' rose from 71,900 in 1995/96 to 90,900 in 2002/03.[22] Over the same period, diagnoses of alcoholic liver disease almost doubled from 14,100 to 28,000.

In 1997, about one in six accident and emergency (A&E) patients in England were estimated by staff to have an alcohol-related attendance.[23] Up to 70 per cent of all admissions to A&E at peak times (between midnight and 5.00 am) are alcohol-related.[24] There are more than 30,000 hospital admissions a year for alcohol dependence syndrome.

The number of admissions due to alcohol-related accidents, with a primary diagnosis of 'injuries' and secondary mention of 'mental and behavioural disorders due to use of alcohol', increased from 16,700 in 1995/96 to 21,000 in 2002/03.[22] Males accounted for nearly three quarters of these admissions in 2002/03. The number of accidents involving 'accidental poisoning by exposure to alcohol' nearly doubled from 600 in 1995/96 to 1,100 in 2002/03.[22]

The legal limit for driving, set out in the Road Safety Act 1967, is 80 mg of alcohol per 100 ml blood. The absorption of alcohol in the blood is known to vary by factors such as age, sex and body weight and it is difficult for individuals to know precisely when they are over the legal limit. An estimated 7 per cent of road traffic accidents involved alcohol levels that were over the legal limit. In Great Britain in 2003, these accidents resulted in around 19,000 casualties.[25] In 2003, Department of Transport estimates showed there were 2,600 serious injuries where at least one of the drivers involved was over the legal limit.[25]

Alcohol-related mortality

Estimates of the annual total number of deaths in which alcohol has played a role can vary widely depending on the criteria used. The ONS definition of alcohol-related mortality only includes those causes regarded as being most directly due to alcohol consumption.[26] The definition includes deaths from chronic liver disease and cirrhosis, even when alcohol is not specifically mentioned on the death certificate. It also includes deaths due to accidental poisoning with alcohol. It does not include diseases where alcohol has been shown to have some causal relationship, such as pancreatitis or cancers of the mouth, pharynx, larynx, oesophagus and liver. The definition also excludes external causes of death, such as road traffic deaths and other accidents, and alcohol-related suicides and homicides. The definition used by ONS allows for consistent comparisons over time for those deaths most clearly associated with alcohol consumption.

Using the ONS definition, the rate of alcohol-related mortality in England and Wales more than doubled for men and nearly doubled for women over the last quarter century, from 5.9 per 100,000 men in 1979 to 15.8 in 2003 and from 3.9 to 7.6 per 100,000 women (Figure 4.13). Deaths from chronic liver disease and cirrhosis comprised the largest proportion of all alcohol-related deaths.

Between 1999 and 2002, deaths from alcoholic liver disease increased by 40 per cent for males and 26 per cent for females. Deaths from cirrhosis increased by 10 per cent among males and did not change among females. Deaths from accidental poisoning by and exposure to alcohol increased by 21 per cent for men and 4 per cent for women (Table 4.14).

Chronic drinkers are also at higher risk of premature death from causes not directly linked to alcohol consumption. In 1995

Figure **4.13**

Alcohol-related mortality (age-standardised): by sex, 1979–2003[1]

England & Wales

Rates per 100,000

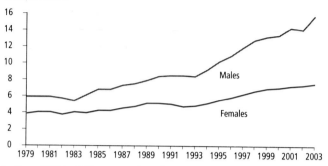

1 From 1979 to 1992 rates are based on year of registration and from 1993 onwards on year of occurrence.

Source: Office for National Statistics

up to 22,000 premature deaths, and up to 1,000 suicides in England were estimated to be linked with alcohol misuse.[5,27] In 2001 about 4,000 deaths due to acute incidents (eg, accidents) and between 11,300 and 17,900 deaths from chronic diseases were attributable to longer term alcohol abuse.[5] In 2002 17 per cent of road deaths in Great Britain involved at least one of the drivers being over the legal limit.[22] In 2003 there were 580 such fatalities in England and Wales.[25]

Table **4.14**

Alcohol-related deaths: by selected causes[1] and sex, 1999,[2] 2001–2003[3]

England & Wales

Number of deaths

	1999	2001	2002	2003
Males				
Mental and behavioural disorders due to alcohol (F10)	316	332	311	339
Alcoholic cardiomyopathy (I42.6)	111	103	90	97
Alcoholic liver disease (K70)	1,928	2,292	2,418	2,700
Chronic hepatitis, not elsewhere specified (K73)	16	23	17	14
Fibrosis and cirrhosis of liver (K74)	928	956	919	1,021
Accidental poisoning by and exposure to alcohol (X45)	91	94	60	110
Females				
Mental and behavioural disorders due to alcohol (F10)	149	145	124	130
Alcoholic cardiomyopathy (I42.6)	31	17	29	11
Alcoholic liver disease (K70)	1,026	1,172	1,199	1,291
Chronic hepatitis, not elsewhere specified (K73)	65	55	60	46
Fibrosis and cirrhosis of liver (K74)	772	736	763	772
Accidental poisoning by and exposure to alcohol (X45)	47	45	43	49

1 Coded to ICD-10.
2 Data for 1999 are death registrations.
3 Data for 2001 onwards are deaths occurring in each year.

Source: Office for National Statistics

Drug use

Under the Misuse of Drugs Act, drugs have been classified into three categories, A, B and C depending upon their harmfulness: drugs in Class A being most harmful followed by Class B and Class C. The classification of well known drugs is set out below.

Drug	Mode of use	Classification
Speed and other amphetamines	Inject	A
	Oral	A
Ecstasy	Sniff or inject	A
Cocaine	Inject or smoke	A
Crack	Smoke, sniff or inject	A
Heroin	Oral	A
LSD	Oral	A
Magic Mushrooms	Oral	A
Methadone		
Speed and other amphetamines	Sniff or oral	B
Tranquillisers	Oral or inject	B/C (depends on drug)
Anabolic steroids	Oral or inject	C
Cannabis	Smoke or oral	C
Poppers	Sniff	It is an offence to supply these substances if it is likely that the product is intended for abuse
Glue	Sniff	
Gas	Sniff	

The classification of certain drugs depends on the method of delivery used. For example, amphetamines are a Class B drug if taken orally and a Class A drug if injected. Cannabis was reclassified from Class B to C in January 2004.[28]

In 1998, the government launched a 10-year national strategy for tackling drug misuse. It states that 'the most effective way of reducing the harm drugs cause is to persuade all potential users, particularly the young, not to use drugs'. This commitment was reaffirmed in the revised drug strategy, published in 2002, with a new emphasis on vulnerable young people.[29]

Drug use among adults

Results from the 2003/04 British Crime Survey show that 12 per cent of people aged between 16 and 59 reported having taken illicit drugs in the last year.[30] Young people aged 16–24 were far more likely to have used drugs than older people, with 28 per cent of them reporting using drugs during the last year (Figure 4.15). Prevalence was far higher among young men (33 per cent) than among young women (23 per cent).

Among adults aged 16–59 in England and Wales, cannabis was the most commonly used drug with 11 per cent reporting its use in the last year. Cocaine use was reported by 2.4 per cent, closely followed by ecstasy (2.0 per cent), amphetamines (1.5 per cent) and amyl nitrite (1.3 per cent). Less than 1 per cent reported using other drugs.

Figure 4.15

Drug use in the last year: by age and drug type, 2003/04

England & Wales

Percentages

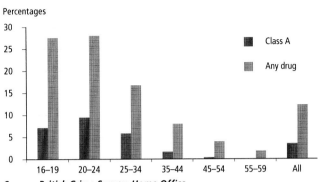

Source: British Crime Survey, Home Office

Drug use patterns among young people aged 16–24 were somewhat different.[30] Cannabis was the drug most likely to be used, with 24.8 per cent reporting its use in the last year. Ecstasy was the next most commonly used drug (5.3 per cent), followed by cocaine (4.9 per cent), amyl nitrite (4.4 per cent), amphetamines (4.0 per cent) and hallucinogens (2.9 per cent). Less than 1 per cent reported using other drugs.

During the period 1996 to 2003/04, drug-taking in the year prior to interview largely remained stable at around 12 per cent of the population aged 16–59 (Figure 4.16). However, the type of drug taken has changed over the period. There has been an increase in the use of Class A drugs. This was mainly due to an increase in the use of cocaine and ecstasy. Over the same period the use of amphetamines, LSD, glues and steroids has declined.[30]

Following an upward trend during the early 1990s, there are some indications to suggest that the overall drug use among young people may well have peaked and stabilised. During the

Figure 4.16

Drug use in the last year:[1] by drug type, 1996–2003/04

England & Wales

Percentages

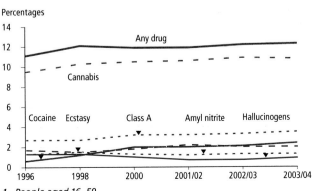

1 People aged 16–59.

Source: British Crime Survey, Home Office

period 1998 to 2003/04, the proportion of 16- to 24-year-olds taking 'any drug' decreased from 32 per cent to 28 per cent.[30] In particular, there have been decreases in the use of amphetamines, LSD, methadone and glue. Over the period, although the use of Class A drugs has remained stable, there have been increases in the use of cocaine.

Young people aged 16–24 were far more likely to be frequent drug users than other age groups.[30] More than one in ten took drugs at least once a month, compared with two per cent of all adults aged 16–59.

The self-reported prevalence of drug use among those aged 15–64 in Northern Ireland in 2002/03 was much lower than in England and Wales, with 6.2 per cent using any illegal drugs in the last year and 5.3 per cent using cannabis.[31]

Drug use among schoolchildren

Data from the 2004 survey of Smoking, Drinking and Drug Use among Children in England show that 10 per cent of pupils aged 11–15 had taken drugs during the last month and 18 per cent had taken drugs during the last year.[9] The prevalence of drug use in the last month was almost as high among girls (9 per cent) as among boys (11 per cent); and drug use in the last year was also similar between the sexes – 17 per cent and 18 per cent, respectively.

The likelihood of drug taking increased sharply with age.[9] In 2004 5 per cent of 11-year-olds had taken drugs in the last year compared with 32 per cent of 15-year-olds. Likewise, 3 per cent of 11-year-olds had taken drugs in the last month compared with 21 per cent of 15-year-olds.

Consistent with the pattern of many years, in 2004 the drug most commonly taken was cannabis with 11 per cent of children having taken it in the last year, followed by volatile substances (6 per cent) and poppers (3 per cent) (Figure 4.17). Cannabis use was slightly higher among boys (12 per cent) than girls (10 per cent). There was little difference between the proportions of boys and girls taking other drugs.

The most commonly used drug among older pupils (aged 13–15) was cannabis while among younger pupils (11–12) it was volatile substances.[9] In terms both of prevalence, (potentially fatal) hazard to health and the relative youth of users, volatile substance abuse (VSA) is a more serious problem than any other drug, 'soft' or 'hard',[32] among children.

The use of volatile substances was fairly similar across all ages (4 per cent among those aged 11 to 6 per cent aged 15).[9] On the other hand, the use of cannabis increased sharply with age: 1 per cent of 11-year-olds reported its use in the last year, increasing to 7 per cent of 13-year-olds, and 26 per cent of 15-year-olds.

Figure **4.17**

Drug use in the last year: by drug type for children aged 11–15, 1998–2004[1]

England

Percentages

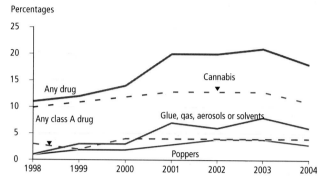

1 Estimates from 2001 onwards are not strictly comparable with previous estimates because of changes in the measurement of drug taking.

Source: Survey of Smoking, Drinking and Drug Use among Young People in England, Department of Health

All drug use carries risks, but the use of Class A drugs and the frequent use (i.e. at least 2–3 times a month every month in the last year) of any drug carries the greatest risk. Young people who do so are the most likely to go on to become problematic drug users.[29] Four per cent of pupils were frequent users with 2 per cent taking drugs two or three times a month, 1 per cent taking drugs at least once a week and 1 per cent taking drugs most days.[9]

Since 2001 (when the current definitions of drug use were introduced), there are some indications that the prevalence of drug taking may well have peaked (Figure 4.18). In 2004, 18 per cent of pupils had taken drugs in the last year, down from 20

Figure **4.18**

Drug use in the last year: by sex for children aged 11–15, 1998–2004[1]

England

Percentages

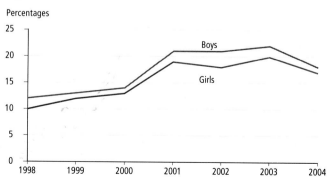

1 Estimates from 2001 onwards are not strictly comparable with previous estimates because of changes in the measurement of drug taking.

Source: Survey of Smoking, Drinking and Drug Use among Young People in England, Department of Health

per cent in 2001. Lately there has been some decrease in drug use both among boys (22 per cent in 2003, 18 per cent in 2004) and among girls (20 per cent in 2003, 17 per cent in 2004).

The pattern of drug use among pupils in Scotland is generally similar to that in England.[10] Northern Ireland has slightly lower prevalence rates than England.[11]

Correlation between smoking, drinking and drug use among children

Smoking, drinking and drug use are all highly related behaviours.[11, 12] Among children, regular or recent use of one substance was found to be strongly associated with regular or recent use of other substances. The strongest correlation coefficients in England in 2003 were found between cigarette smoking and cannabis use, cigarettes and alcohol consumption, and cannabis and Class A drug use. This however does not imply that any of these behaviours – smoking, drinking, cannabis or Class A drug use – leads to the other. Slightly weaker relationships existed between consumption of alcohol and cannabis, cigarettes and Class A drugs, and volatile substances and Class A drugs. The weakest associations were found between all other substances and volatile substances.

Pupils with a younger age of initiation into smoking or drinking were more likely to have used drugs before they were aged 15.[10] In Scotland three-fifths of 15-year-old pupils who started smoking aged 11 or younger had used drugs before they were aged 15, compared with just over a quarter of 15-year-olds who reported first smoking at age 14. Almost half of 15-year-old pupils who reported first drinking alcohol aged 11 or younger also reported using drugs before they were aged 15,

compared with 14 per cent of those who reported first drinking alcohol at age 14.

Drug use and ill health

Drug misuse carries risks, particularly when used frequently and over a long period. It is generally accepted that there is an association (not necessarily causal) between taking drugs and prevalence of mental disorders.

Analysis of combined data from the surveys of the mental health of children and young people in 1999 and 2004 showed that young people aged 11–16 having emotional, conduct or hyperkinetic disorders, were about three times as likely to have taken drugs at some time as those with no such disorder.[21] Cannabis was the most widely used drug: 16 per cent of those with an emotional disorder, 23 per cent of those with a conduct disorder and 18 per cent of those with a hyperkinetic disorder had used cannabis compared with 6 to 7 per cent of those with no such disorders. (Table 4.19)

Likewise, data from the ONS Survey of Psychiatric Morbidity Survey 2000 among adults (aged 16–74) showed that both men and women with significant levels of neurotic symptoms as measured by Revised Clinical Interview Schedule (CIS-R score of 12 or above) were more likely to have used drugs or to be dependent on them.[20] For example, people who had a CIS-R score of at least 12 were more than twice as likely to have used any drug in the last month, than those who scored less (12 per cent compared with 5 per cent).

People with neurotic disorders, such as depression, anxiety or phobia, showed greater rates of drug use and dependency than those without a neurotic disorder. Those with obsessive

Table **4.19**

Drug use: by mental disorder and drug type[1] for young people aged 11–16, 1999 and 2004 combined

Great Britain   Percentages

	Emotional disorders	No emotional disorder	Conduct disorders	No conduct disorder	Hyperkinetic disorders	No hyperkinetic disorder
Cannabis	16	7	24	6	18	7
Inhalants	1	1	4	1	3	1
Ecstasy	1	0	2	0	0	1
Amphetamines	3	1	5	1	4	1
LSD	1	0	2	0	0	0
Tranquilisers	1	0	1	0	0	0
Cocaine	0	0	1	0	0	0
Heroin	0	0	1	0	0	0
Any drugs	20	8	28	8	23	8

1 The total of individual drugs exceed the percentage of 'Any drugs' because young people may take more than one type of drug.

Source: Survey of Mental Health of Children and Adolescents in Great Britain, Office for National Statistics

compulsive disorder were the most likely to use drugs or have signs of dependence; in comparison to the general population they were three times more likely to have used drugs in the last month (15 per cent compared with 5 per cent) and were more likely to be dependent on drugs other than cannabis (7 per cent compared with 1 per cent).

Injecting drug users (IDUs) are vulnerable to a diverse range of infectious diseases including viral infections (such as hepatitis C and HIV) and bacterial infections (such as tetanus and Staphylococcus aureus).[33] Hepatitis C is currently the most significant infectious disease affecting IDUs. More than two in five IDUs have been infected with hepatitis C. Around 80 per cent of those acquiring hepatitis C develop chronic infection and are at risk of developing cirrhosis and liver cancer. There had been around 60,000 reported laboratory diagnoses of hepatitis C in the UK by the end of 2003. The majority of these reports are associated with injecting drug use.

Drug-related mortality

Drug-related poisoning

Deaths related to drug poisoning include accidents and suicides involving drug poisoning, as well as poisonings due to drug abuse and drug dependence, but not other adverse effects of drugs.[34] Deaths in England and Wales with mentions of selected substances on the death certificate – those controlled under the 1971 Act (eg, cocaine and heroin), prescription drugs (eg, antidepressants) or over-the-counter medications (eg, paracetamol and aspirin) – increased during the 1990s, reaching 2,967 in 2000. Since then total deaths of this type have fallen to 2,445 in 2003.

In 2003, heroin and morphine (591 deaths) were the most frequently mentioned drugs in drug-related poisoning deaths, followed by paracetamol and paracetamol compounds (466), anti-depressants (424) and benzodiazepines (211). But it should be noted that where more than one drug is mentioned on the death certificate, the death is included in the figures for each drug. In these cases it is not possible to determine which drug was primarily responsible for the death. Hence the figures mentioned above are not mutually exclusive.

As in previous years, in 2003 the age-standardised drug poisoning death rates were higher for males (6.0 per 100,000) than for females (3.0 per 100,000) (Table 4.20). Between 1993 and 2000, drug-related poisoning death rates increased from 5.3 to 7.9 per 100,000 for males, but remained fairly stable among females. Since 2000, rates for both males and females have been falling.

Table 4.20

Mortality rates (age-standardised) from drug-related poisoning and drug misuse:[1] by sex, 1993–2003[2]

England & Wales | | | | Rate per 100,000 population

	Drug-related poisoning			Drug misuse
	Males	Females	Persons	Persons
1993	5.3	3.2	4.3	1.6
1994	5.9	3.2	4.5	1.9
1995	6.4	3.3	4.8	2.1
1996	7.0	3.3	5.1	2.4
1997	7.5	3.4	5.4	2.5
1998	7.5	3.5	5.5	2.8
1999	7.9	3.2	5.5	3.0
2000	7.9	3.3	5.6	3.2
2001	7.7	3.1	5.4	3.1
2002	6.9	3.1	5.0	3.0
2003	6.0	3.0	4.5	2.4

1 Deaths where the underlying cause is poisoning, drug abuse or drug dependence and where any of the substances controlled under the Misuse of Drugs Act (1971) are mentioned on the death certificate.
2 Rates based on year of occurrence.

Just over half (57 per cent) of all drug-poisoning related deaths in 2003 related to drug misuse. Drug misuse related deaths are a subset of all drug poisoning deaths and include deaths where the underlying cause is poisoning, drug abuse or drug dependence and where any of the substances controlled under the Misuse of Drugs Act (1971) are involved.[34] Within this category of deaths, 'mental and behavioural disorders due to drug use' formed the largest proportion. Between 1993 and 2000 there was a steady increase in the age-standardised rates for drug misuse mortality for all persons, but rates have since begun to decline (Table 4.20).

Volatile substance abuse

VSA is the deliberate inhalation of a volatile substance (gas, aerosol propellants, solvents in glue and other solvents) to achieve a change in mental state[35] and deaths from these are not included in deaths related to drug poisoning described above.

The Intoxicating Substances Supply Act 1985, in England and Wales (Northern Ireland has similar legislation), makes it an offence for a person to supply or offer to supply to someone under the age of 18 a substance (other than a controlled drug) 'if he knows or has reasonable cause to believe that the substance or its fumes are likely to be inhaled for the purpose of causing intoxication'. An amendment to the Consumer Protection Act (The Cigarette Lighter Refill (Safety) Regulations 1999) made it an offence to 'supply any cigarette lighter refill canister containing butane or a substance with butane as a constituent part to any person under the age of eighteen years.'

There were 51 deaths associated with VSA in the UK in 2003. The cumulative number of VSA deaths in the UK every year from 1971 onwards now exceeds 2,100. VSA deaths peaked in 1990 (152 deaths) and then fell rapidly. This fall was associated in part with an advertising campaign in 1992. Half the deaths between 1971 and 2003 were among children aged 7–17. In 2003, however, more than half of VSA deaths were of people aged 20–34. VSA deaths continue to be more common among males than females, although the proportion of female deaths has been rising, and in 2002 reached one-quarter of all VSA deaths.

Conclusion

The recent trends in smoking, drinking and drug-taking suggest that the prevalence of these has remained relatively stable, but there are differences between sexes, age groups and occupational classes.

Among adults, the overall prevalence of smoking, drinking and drug taking is higher in men than in women. In contrast, among children (aged 11–15) the prevalence of smoking is higher in girls than in boys, the prevalence of drinking in girls is about the same as in boys and the prevalence of drug-taking is only marginally lower in girls than in boys.

Cigarette smoking is more common among adults aged 20–34 than other age groups, but those aged 35–59 are the heaviest smokers. Exceeding the benchmarks for drinking alcohol, and heavy drinking, was most common among adults aged 16–24 and decreased with age. Drug use was most common among young people aged 16–24.

Smoking, drinking to excess, and drug-taking place individuals at higher risk of developing a range of diseases. Smokers are at a far higher risk of developing a number of cancers (notably lung cancer), chronic obstructive pulmonary disease, heart disease, respiratory and circulatory diseases and a multitude of other diseases. Chronic drinkers are at increased risk of developing diseases such as cirrhosis (which has nearly doubled in the last ten years), cancer and haemorrhagic stroke. Drug-taking is highly correlated with mental disorders, particularly in school children.

Each year, smoking, drinking and drug-taking cause or contribute to a large number of deaths. It was estimated that in 2002 that there were around 106,000 deaths attributable to smoking in the UK (17 per cent of all deaths); these include deaths from causes directly related to smoking (such as lung cancer) as well as those where smoking is thought to contribute to excess mortality (such as deaths due to heart diseases). There were 6,580 deaths directly related to alcohol misuse and 1,388 deaths related to illicit drug use in England and Wales in 2003. In recent years while deaths related to smoking and drug misuse have been falling, those related to alcohol have been increasing.

References

1. Department of Health/NHS (November 2004) *Choosing Health: Making healthier choices easier,* Department of Health/NHS.

2. Department of Health (1998) *Smoking Kills: A White Paper on Tobacco,* Cm 4177, TSO: London.

3. Department of Health (2000) *The NHS Plan: a plan for investment, a plan for reform*, Department of Health, at: www.dh.gov.uk

4. Health Development Agency (2004) *The smoking epidemic in England,* Health Development Agency.

5. *Alcohol Harm Reduction Strategy for England* (March 2004) Prime Minister's Strategy Unit at: www.strategy.gov.uk

6. *Department of Health Technical Note for the Spending Review 2004: Public Service Agreement 2005–2008 at:* www.dh.gov.uk.

7. Results of the 2003/04 General Household Survey at: www.statistics.gov.uk/ghs

8. Evandrou M and Falkingham J (2002) Smoking behaviour and socio-economic status: a cohort analysis, 1974 to 1998. *Health Statistics Quarterly* **14**, 30–38.

9. National Centre of Social Research/ National Foundation for Education Research (2005) *Smoking, drinking and drug use among young people in England in 2004*, National Centre of Social Research/ National Foundation for Education Research.

10. Adolescent Health Research Unit (CAHRU) (2005) *Scottish Schools Adolescent Lifestyle and Substance Use Survey (SALSUS) National Report: Smoking, Drinking and Drug Use among 13 and 15 year olds in Scotland in 2004*, TSO: London.

11. Central Survey Unit, Northern Ireland Statistics and Research Agency (2004) *Young Person's Behaviour and Attitudes Survey 2000.*

12. Boreham R and Blenkinsop S (eds.) (2004, revised 17th December) *Drug use, smoking & drinking among young people in England in 2003*, TSO: London.

13. Boreham R and McManus S (eds.) (2003) *Smoking, drinking & drug use among young people in England in 2002*, TSO: London.

14. Department of Health (December 1995) *Sensible Drinking: the Report of an Inter-Departmental Working Group*

15. Richards L *et al* (2004) *Living in Britain No. 31 Results from the 2002 General Household Survey 2002,* TSO: London.

16. Scottish Department of Health (February 1999) *Towards a Healthier Scotland – a White Paper on Health* Cm 4269, TSO: Edinburgh.

17. Lader D and Goddard E (2004) *Drinking: Adults' Behaviour and Knowledge in 2004*, Office for National Statistics: London.

18. Brasnett L (2002) *Drink-driving: prevalence and attitudes in England and Wales*, Findings 258, Home Office: London

19. Information and Analysis Directorate (May 2004) *Health And Social Care: Comparative Data for Northern Ireland and Other Countries*, at: www.dhsspsni.gov.uk

20. Coulthard M *et al* (2002) *Tobacco, Alcohol and Drug Use and Mental Health,* TSO: London.

21. Green H *et al* (2005) *Mental health of children and young people in Great Britain,* 2004, Palgrave Macmillan: Basingstoke.

22. *Statistics on alcohol: England* (2004) Department of Health statistical bulletin 2004/15.

23. Waller S *et al* (1998) Perceptions of alcohol-related attendances in accident and emergency departments in England: a national survey. *Alcohol and Alcoholism* **33 (4)**: 354–61 cited in *Prevention and reduction of alcohol misuse*, Evidence briefing, June 2002, Health Development Agency.

24. Stategy Unit Alcohol Harm Reduction project (2003) *Interim Analytical Report* at: www.strategy.gov.uk/downloads/su/alcohol/index.htm

25. Campbell R (2005) Drinking and Driving Road Accidents in (Department for Transport) *Road Casualities Great Britain 2004*, Annual Report, TSO; London, pp 24–36

26 Baker A and Rooney C (2003) Recent trends in alcohol-related mortality, and the impact of ICD-10 on the monitoring of these deaths in England and Wales. *Health Statistics Quarterly* **17**, 5–14.

27. White and Nanchahal (1998) *The number of deaths and person-years of life lost attributable to alcohol consumption in England and Wales in 1995*, unpublished report: London School of Hygiene and Tropical Medicine, cited in Strategy Unit Alcohol Harm Reduction project *Interim Analytical Report.*

28. Home Office Circular 05/2004 at: www.homeoffice.gov.uk

29. Cabinet Office (1998) *Tackling drugs to build a better Britain*, Cm 3945, TSO: London. The strategy update published in December 2002, can be found at: www.drugs.gov.uk

30. Chivite-Matthews N and Richardson N *et al* (2005) *Drug misuse declared: findings from the 2003/04 British Crime Survey,* Home Office at: www.drugs.gov.uk

31. National Advisory Committee on Drugs (NACD) & Drug and Alcohol Information and Research Unit (DAIRU) (October 2003) *Drug Use in Ireland & Northern Ireland Bulletin 1: First Results from the 2002/2003 Drug Prevalence Survey,* NACD: Dublin.

32. Miller R and Dowds L (2002) *Drug and Alcohol Use among Young People in Northern Ireland: A Secondary Analysis of Drug and Alcohol Use Surveys*, Final Report, ARK Northern Ireland, Queen's University, Belfast and the University of Ulster.

33. Health Protection Agency, SCIEH, National Public Health Service for Wales, CDSC Northern Ireland, CRDHB, and the UASSG (October 2004) *Shooting Up; Infections among injecting drug users in the United Kingdom 2003*, Health Protection Agency: London.

34. Office for National Statistics (2005) Report: Deaths related to drug poisoning: England and Wales, 1999–2003. *Health Statistics Quarterly* **25**, 52–59.

35. Field-Smith M E, Butland B K, Ramsey J D, Anderson H R (June 2004) *Trends in Death Associated With Abuse of Volatile Substances 1971–2003*, Department of Community Health Sciences, St George's Hospital Medical School, Report 18 at: www.vsareport.org

Obesity, eating and physical activity

Emmanuel Stamatakis

Chapter 5

Introduction

Certain behaviours such as smoking, excessive alcohol drinking, poor eating habits and a physically inactive lifestyle multiply the risk for certain types of disease, as well as premature death. Physical activity and diet are the behaviours most closely linked to the development and maintenance of obesity, which is an important disease risk factor in its own right. Obesity develops as a result of an energy imbalance, when energy taken in through eating exceeds energy expended during physical activity. Although genes seem to play a role, the rapid increases in obesity worldwide in recent decades cannot be explained by genetic or metabolic abnormalities alone.[1]

Besides the human costs in terms of disease, premature death and quality of life; obesity, poor diet, and inactivity have severe economic consequences as they cost the economy approximately £20 billion a year (£6.6 billion–7.4 billion for obesity,[2] £8.2 billion for inactivity[3] and £4 billion for poor diet[4]).

The public health White Paper *Choosing Health: Making Healthier Choices Easier*[5] set out the Government commitments for action on obesity. *Choosing Health White Paper Delivery Plan*,[6] *Food and Health Action Plan*,[4] and *Physical Activity Plan2*[7] specified the action that needs to be taken at national, regional and local level to improve people's health through better diet and nutrition and increasing physical activity.

The main aim of this chapter is to provide an overview of the key national statistics on obesity and the two associated behaviours, eating and physical activity. Geographical coverage is the UK where data sources permit. The chapter covers both the most recent publicly available evidence and time trends over the last 10–15 years.

Key terms

Overweight and obesity are terms that refer to an excessive accumulation of body fat. The two terms, however, denote different degrees of excess fatness, and so being overweight can be thought of as a stage where an individual is at risk of becoming obese. Although principally concerned with obesity this chapter also presents key estimates for overweight. Overweight and obesity prevalence is estimated using the body mass index (BMI). BMI is calculated as weight in kilograms divided by height in metres squared (kg/m^2). Physical activity is defined as any bodily movement produced by skeletal muscles that results in energy expenditure above resting level.[8] Exercise and sport is a subset of physical activity that is distinguished by being done in a planned, structured and repetitive manner.[8]

Obesity and overweight in early life

Obesity in early life is linked to persistence of the condition into adulthood,[9] a compromised life quality[10] and an increased risk for asthma,[11] type 2 diabetes,[12] and raised blood pressure.[13] Obese children and adolescents have an increased risk of disease in mid-life, regardless of their weight as adults.[14, 15] The Government has set a target to halt the year-on-year rise of obesity in children under 11 by year 2010 in the context of a broader strategy to tackle obesity in the population as a whole.[16]

A child is classified as obese when their BMI is in the highest 5 per cent of values for boys or girls of their age based on the 1990 UK BMI reference data (above the 95th percentile). Children are classified as overweight if their BMI is in the 10 per cent below the top 5 per cent (that is, between the 85th and 95th percentiles).

Prevalence

The Health Survey for England has been collecting height and weight information for children since 1995. Although there are no marked differences in obesity between boys and girls, prevalence rates increase with age as shown in Figure 5.1. In total, 16 per cent of both boys and girls were obese and another 14 per cent of both sexes were overweight. Obesity is more common in older than in younger children. Obesity increased from 13 per cent in young boys (aged 2–5) to 20 per cent in older boys (aged 11–15). In girls, obesity prevalence increased from 10 to 19 per cent between these age groups.

Figure **5.1**

Obesity and overweight[1] prevalence estimates: by age and sex, 2001–02[2]

England

Percentages

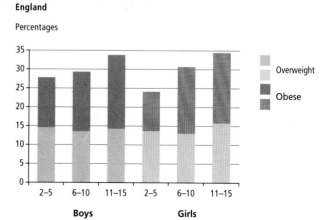

1 Obesity is defined as those who were in the top 5 per cent of boys or girls based on 1990 UK BMI measurement, overweight as those who were in the 10 per cent below the top 5 per cent.
2 Two years of data combined.

Source: Health Survey for England, Department of Health

Parental influences play an important role in early obesity development since parental BMI is the best predictor of children's obesity. Boys and girls with two obese parents are over ten times more likely to be obese than boys and girls with no obese parents. Even children with one obese parent are considerably more likely to be obese than children with no obese parents.[17] This is due to both genetic influences (a predisposition for fat accumulation), and the shared eating and physical activity habits within a family.[18]

Overall, the relationship between socio-economic status and obesity is complex and varies with age, sex, and cultural environment.[18] Socio-economic circumstances of the parents affect many other aspects of health in early life[19] and obesity is no exception. For both boys and girls obesity prevalence is lower in households where the household reference person is in a managerial or professional occupation (14 per cent for boys and 13 per cent for girls) than all other socio-economic groups, where obesity ranged from 17 to 19 per cent for boys and from 14 to 19 per cent for girls (Figure 5.2). Income also relates to obesity in children as financial constraints are a key obstacle with regard to access to a healthy diet.[20] The Health Survey for England found that boys and girls from households in the bottom 40 per cent of the household income distribution are more likely to be obese than boys and girls from higher income households.[17]

Time trends

Childhood obesity and overweight has increased rapidly in recent decades. Data from the National Study of Health and Growth indicate that the upward trend started no later than the mid-1980s. This study is now discontinued but more recent data are available from the Health Survey for England.[21] As Figure 5.3 shows, the prevalence of being overweight or obese among children in England continued to rise between 1995 and 2002. The percentage of obese boys increased from 10 per cent in 1995 to 17 per cent in 2002 and the percentage of obese girls increased from 12 per cent to 17 per cent over the same period. Similar increases occurred in the prevalence of being overweight (including obesity). A closer look at the figures shows that the prevalence of being overweight alone (that is, excluding obesity) remained stable at 14 per cent for both boys and girls, while obesity increased for both sexes.

It has been estimated that if the upward trend in childhood obesity continues unabated, obesity rates will increase dramatically in some age groups in the next few years. For example, 27 per cent of boys and 23 per cent of girls aged 11–15 will be obese by year 2010.[22]

Although the prevalence of obesity has increased over time among all age, sex, and social class groups, increases have been more pronounced among older children (aged 6–10 and 11–15) and children living in manual households (as classified using the Registrar General's occupational classification). For example, among girls aged 6–10 and 11–15 obesity increased by 7.0 and 4.3 percentage points between 1995 and 2002. The increase in the youngest age group, 2–5 years, over the same period was less severe at 3.5 percentage points.[17] Among children aged 2–10 obesity increased by five percentage points for those in manual households and by three percentage points for those in non-manual households between 1995 and 2003.

Figure **5.2**

Obesity[1] prevalence estimates[2] (age-standardised): by NS-SEC[3] and sex, 2001–02[4]

England

Percentages

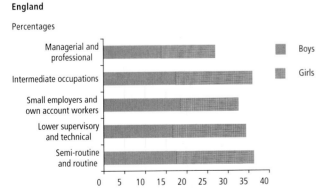

1 *Obesity is defined as those who were in the top 5 per cent of boys or girls based on 1990 UK BMI measurement.*
2 *For children aged 2–15.*
3 *NS-SEC of household reference person.*
4 *Two years of data combined.*

Source: Health Survey for England, Department of Health

Figure **5.3**

Trends in obesity and overweight[1] prevalence:[2] by sex, 1995–2002[3]

England

Percentages

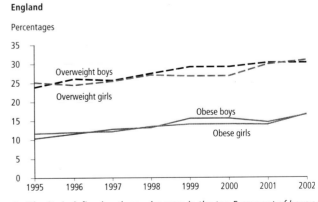

1 *Obesity is defined as those who were in the top 5 per cent of boys or girls based on 1990 UK BMI measurement, overweight as those who were in the 10 per cent below the top 5 per cent.*
2 *For children aged 2–15.*
3 *Estimates for 1999 and 2000 are based on the pooled average for the two years of data.*

Source: Health Survey for England, Department of Health

Increases in overweight (including obesity) followed the same pattern, increasing by seven percentage points for those in manual households and five percentage points for those in non-manual households between 1995 and 2003.[23]

Obesity and overweight in adulthood

In adult life obesity diminishes the overall quality of life and can lead to premature death[24] due to its association with serious chronic conditions such as type 2 diabetes, hypertension, and raised blood lipid levels, which are major risk factors for cardiovascular disease.[25, 26] It has been estimated that obesity is responsible for at least 9,000 premature deaths a year in England alone and decreases life expectancy by nine years on average.[27] An adult is classified as overweight when BMI is over 25 kg/m^2 and obese when BMI is over 30 kg/m^2.

Prevalence

The most recently available survey estimates for obesity and overweight prevalence in England, Scotland and Northern are shown in Figure 5.4. The rates are not directly comparable because the surveys were conducted in different years and obesity prevalence is changing rapidly. In all three constituent countries obesity rates are lower for men than for women. Sex differences range from one percentage point in England (21 versus 22 per cent), to two in Scotland (18 versus 20 per cent), and four in Northern Ireland (16 versus 20 per cent). English data show that obesity prevalence in men and women increases steeply with age to middle life (45–54 age group) where it remains relatively stable until the ages 65–74 and then drops for the eldest age group, 75 and over (Figure 5.5). Most notable sex differences occur in young adulthood (16–24) and late life (75 and over), where obesity rates are higher in women than in men by four and five percentage points respectively. In Scotland the general pattern is similar to that in England, except that the fall in obesity prevalence in men occurs earlier (from age 55 onwards) and for women obesity continues to rise until age 55–64.[28] The all ages overweight (including those who are obese) prevalence was greater than 60 per cent among English men and Scottish women, and ranged from over 50 but under 60 per cent for all other groups.

It has long been known that obesity prevalence in adulthood is inversely related to socio-economic status in women but not in men.[18] Women in higher socio-economic classes are more often engaged in weight-management behaviours such as dieting,[18] participate more often in walking and sports[29] and have better access to resources that facilitate dieting and healthy foods.[18] Figure 5.6 shows the age-standardised prevalence of obesity in England by socio-economic

Figure **5.4**

Obesity and overweight[1] prevalence estimates[2] (age-standardised): by country and sex

England, Scotland and Northern Ireland

Percentages

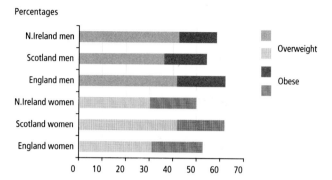

1   Obesity is defined as those who were in the top 5 per cent of boys or girls based on 1990 UK BMI measurement, overweight as those who were in the 10 per cent below the top 5 per cent.
2   For people aged 16 and over.

Source: Health Survey for England 2003, Department of Health; Scottish Health Survey 1998, Scottish Executive Department of Health; Northern Ireland Health and Social Wellbeing Survey 1997, Northern Ireland Statistics and Research Agency

Figure **5.5**

Obesity[1] prevalence estimates: by age and sex, 2003

England

Percentages

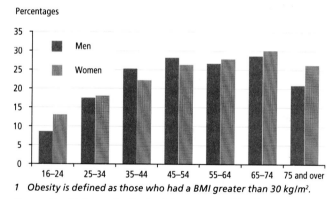

1   Obesity is defined as those who had a BMI greater than 30 kg/m^2.
Source: Health Survey for England, Department of Health

classification of the household reference person. No clear pattern emerged in men: prevalence is relatively similar in managerial and professional, intermediate, and semi-routine and routine occupations (19–20 per cent), while small employers and own account workers have the highest prevalence (24 per cent). Among women, 27 per cent in lower supervisory and technical occupation households were obese, 28 per cent in semi-routine and routine households, and between 17 and 19 per cent in other households.

Figure **5.6**

Obesity[1] prevalence estimates[2] (age-standardised): by NS-SEC[3] and sex, 2003

England

Percentages

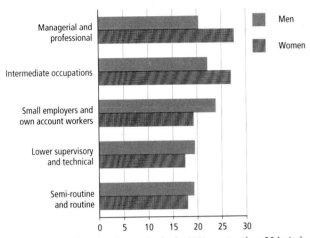

1 Obesity is defined as those who had a BMI greater than 30 kg/m[2].
2 For people aged 16 and over.
3 NS-SEC of household reference person.

Source: Health Survey for England, Department of Health

Time trends

As with children, adult obesity has increased sharply in recent years. Figure 5.7 shows obesity and overweight prevalence trends from 1994 to 2003 in England. Obesity prevalence among men increased from 14 per cent in 1994 to 23 per cent in 2003. The corresponding figures for women were 17 and 23 per cent, respectively. In men, increases greater than 10 percentage points over this period occurred in the age groups 35–54 and in the post-retirement years (65 and over). In women, obesity prevalence increased by more than 10 percentage points only for those aged 75 and over.[30]

There was no marked increase in the prevalence of overweight alone (a BMI of more than 25 but less than or equal to 30 kg/m[2]) over the period 1994–2003. Overweight alone (excluding obesity) increased by one percentage point in men (from 44 to 45 per cent) and by two percentage points in women (from 31 to 33 per cent). The upward trend in being overweight (including obesity) shown in Figure 5.7 reflects increases in obesity (a BMI of over 30 kg/m[2]), rather than in the prevalence of overweight alone.

Eating

Diet is closely related to many chronic conditions, such as cancer, cardiovascular disease and diabetes.[31] For example, it has been estimated that about a third of cancers can be

Figure **5.7**

Trends in obesity and overweight[1] prevalence:[2] by sex, 1994–2003

England

Percentages

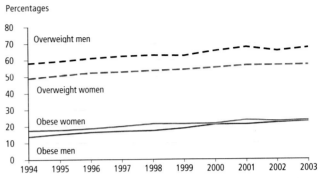

1 Obesity is defined as those who had a BMI greater than 30 kg/m[2], overweight as those who had a BMI greater than 25 and less than or equal to 30 kg/m[2].
2 For people aged 16 and over.

Source: Health Survey for England, Department of Health

directly attributed to poor eating habits.[4] Current guidelines for healthy eating prioritise reductions in total fat, saturated fat and added sugars and increases in fruit and vegetable consumption. A diet rich in fat contributes to obesity because fat is dense in terms of calories: a gram of fat contains over twice as many calories as a gram of protein or carbohydrate. Increased intake of saturated fat may increase the risk of type 2 diabetes.[32, 33] Added sugars (termed 'non-milk extrinsic sugars') are carbohydrates with usually little nutritional value in terms of vitamins and minerals. Foods high in added sugar can be high in fat as well. Low fruit and vegetable consumption is an important risk factor in chronic diseases, most notably cancer and cardiovascular diseases.[30]

Total energy intake

The National Diet and Nutrition Survey collected detailed information on the eating behaviours of British young people aged 4–18 in 1997,[34] and adults aged 19–64 in 2001.[35] Figure 5.8 (see overleaf) shows the total energy intake from all food and drink by sex and age group. Males consume consistently more energy than females. These sex differences range from 8 per cent at ages 4–6 to 33 per cent between the ages of 25 and 34. The average energy intake of young people reflects the different growth patterns of males and females. In males, energy intake increases through childhood and adolescence to age 15–18 and then remains relatively stable until age 50–64. In females increases cease earlier, during the ages of 11–14 years and energy intake remains relatively stable thereafter.

Figure **5.8**

Average daily energy intake: by age and sex, 1997[1] and 2001[2]

Great Britain

Kcal per day

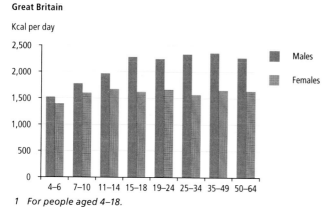

1 For people aged 4–18.
2 For people aged 19–64.

Source: National Diet and Nutrition Survey, Food Standards Agency

Fat, saturated fat and added sugars

Dietary reference values for added sugars, fat and saturated fatty acids have been formulated and are expressed as population averages. Current recommendations state that total fat should not contribute to more than 35 per cent of total food intake, and saturated fat and added sugars should not contribute to more than 11 per cent each of total food intake.[36] Table 5.9 shows the percentage of food energy taken from total fat, saturated fat, and added sugars by age and sex. While, for all age and sex groups total fat accounts for 35 to 36 per cent of total food intake, the contributions of saturated fat and added sugars clearly exceed the recommended limit of 11 per cent each. For both males and females, saturated fat

contribution to total food intake gradually decreased from 15 per cent at ages 4–6 to 13 per cent for adults aged 50–64. In both males and females, the contribution of added sugars to total food intake tended to decline with age, from 18 per cent among boys aged 7–10 and girls aged 4–6, to 12 per cent among men and 11 per cent among women aged 50–64.

Total fat and saturated fat consumption do not vary consistently with socio-economic classification.[35, 37] The average daily intake of added sugar is higher in households where the reference person is in semi-routine (96 grams per person per day), routine (94 grams), and lower supervisory and technical occupations (93 grams) than in other occupational groups where the average daily intake of added sugars varied between 84 and 88 grams per person per day.[37]

Time trends

UK food intake trends are available from the Expenditure and Food Survey (from 2001/02 onwards) and its predecessor, the National Food Survey (up to 2000) which collected information on food and drink purchased (and presumably consumed) in the household and food eaten out. Despite the marked increases in obesity in all age groups outlined in the previous section, there have been no marked increases in average daily energy intake (expressed as kcal per person) over the last decade in the UK. Table 5.10 shows that, in fact, there has actually been a small decrease, from 2,387 kcal in 1994 to 2,300 kcal in 2002/03. The contribution of total fat to total energy intake over the same period has fallen from 39 to 36 per cent, while the contribution of saturated fat has decreased slightly from 15 to 14 per cent and the contribution of added sugars has remained the same at 15 per cent.

Table **5.9**

Percentage of food energy from added sugars, saturated fat and total fat: by age and sex, 1997 and 2000/01

Great Britain

Percentages

	Males			Females		
	Added sugars	Saturated fat	Total fat	Added sugars	Saturated fat	Total fat
Aged 4–18[1]						
4–6	16	15	36	18	15	36
7–10	18	14	35	17	15	36
11–14	17	14	35	16	14	36
15–18	16	14	36	15	14	36
Aged 19-64[2]						
19–24	17	14	36	14	13	36
25–34	14	13	36	12	13	35
35–49	13	14	36	12	13	35
50–64	12	13	36	11	13	35

1 1997.
2 2000/01.

Source: National Diet and Nutrition Surveys, Food Standards Agency

Table **5.10**

Trends in energy intake[1], 1994–2002/03

United Kingdom[2] Kcal per day

	Percentages			
	Total fat	Saturated fat	Added sugars	Daily energy intake
1994	39	15	15	2,387
1995	38	15	15	2,383
1996	38	15	15	2,496
1997	37	15	15	2,433
1998	37	15	15	2,362
1999	37	15	15	2,311
2000	36	15	15	2,382
2001/02	37	14	15	2,301
2002/03	36	14	15	2,301

1 Including food eaten outside the home.
2 Northern Ireland is included from 1996 onwards.

Source: National Food Survey 1994-2000, Ministry of Agriculture, Fisheries and Food; Expenditure and Food Survey 2001/02-2002/03, Department for Environment, Food and Rural Affairs

Decreases in the total energy intake of adults have been found by the National Diet and Nutrition Surveys in 1986/87 and 2000/01.[35] Men aged 16–64 in 1986/87 reported a daily energy intake of 10.3 MJ (approximately 2,462 kcal), falling to 9.72 MJ (approximately 2,323 kcal) for men aged 19–64 in 2000/01. Women's decreases were less marked, from 7.0 MJ (1,685 kcal) per day in 1986/87 to 6.9 MJ (1,642 kcal) in 2000/01. Reductions over the same period were also observed in the contribution of total fat (from 38 to 34 per cent in men and from 39 to 34 per cent in women) and saturated fat (from 15 to 13 per cent in men and from 17 to 13 per cent in women) to total energy intake.

Fruit and vegetable consumption

In 2000, the Government initiated the 'Five-a-day' programme with a view to increasing fruit and vegetable consumption in the general population. The central message is that everyone should aim to consume five 80 gram portions of fruit, vegetables or pulses per day. The programme was designed to raise public awareness of the importance of fruit and vegetables to good health; to provide information and education; and to improve access to fruit and vegetables through programmes such as the National School Fruit and Vegetable Scheme and local community initiatives.[38] The School Fruit and Vegetable Scheme specifically aims to increase fruit and vegetable consumption among young children. Under the scheme, all four- to six-year-old children in publicly-funded

infant, primary and special schools are entitled to a free piece of fruit or vegetable on each school day. The scheme reaches almost two million children in over 16,000 schools.

Figure 5.11 shows the age-standardised proportions of children and adults in England who have less than two, at least two but less than five, and at least five portions of fruit and vegetables a day. Only one in seven boys and girls aged 2–15 (14 per cent) have a minimum of five portions of fruit and vegetables a day, while the majority (six in 10) consume two or more portions a day. Among adults aged 16 and over, one in five men (21 per cent), and one in four women (25 per cent) consumed at least five portions a day and seven in 10 consumed two or more portions a day. The Welsh Health Survey 2003/04 also included questions on fruit and vegetable consumption.[39] Substantially higher proportions of Welsh adults aged 16 and over reported eating at least five portions of fruit and vegetables a day compared to England (37 per cent of men and 41 per cent of women).

More individuals in managerial and professional households consume at least five portions a day than any other socio-economic group (Figure 5.12 – see overleaf). One in six children (17 per cent) living in managerial and professional households consumed the recommended amounts of fruit and vegetable compared with about one in 10 children in semi-routine and routine households. One in four men (26 per cent) and one in three women (32 per cent) in managerial and professional households consumed the recommended amounts, compared with one in six men (16 per cent) and women (17 per cent) in semi-routine and routine households.

Figure **5.11**

Fruit and vegetable consumption (age-standardised): by sex, 2001–02[1] and 2003[2]

England

Percentages

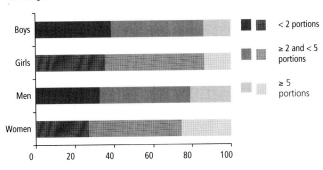

1 For children aged 2–15 and based on two years of data combined.
2 For people aged 16 and over.

Source: Health Survey for England, Department of Health

Figure **5.12**

Consumption of at least five portions of fruit and vegetables a day: by NS-SEC[1] and sex, 2001–02[2] and 2003[3]

England

Percentages

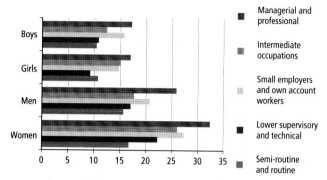

1 *National Statistics Socio-Economic Classification of household reference person.*
2 *For children aged 2–15 and based on two years of data combined.*
3 *For people aged 16 and over.*

Source: Health Survey for England, Department of Health

Time trends

Data from the National Food Survey and Expenditure and Food Survey show that more fruits and vegetables are being consumed in the UK today than in the 1970s. The long-term trend is a 23 per cent increase between 1975 and 2002/03 (from 1,868 to 2,305 grams per person per week).[37] During a comparable period to that for which obesity trends are presented in this chapter, the overall average household purchase (and presumably consumption) of fruits and vegetables in UK households has slightly increased by approximately 100 grams a week between 1995 and 2002/03 (from 2,219 to 2,305 grams per person).

Physical activity in early life

Physical activity is an important part of the physical and mental growth of children. The relationship between disease and physical activity in early life is difficult to study since children rarely suffer from lifestyle chronic disease (such as coronary heart disease) and generally do not have risk factors such as high blood lipids and hypertension. Less active children are more likely to have more body fat[40] and obese children are more likely to be inactive than their non-obese peers.[41]

Participation

The Chief Medical Officer recommends that children and young people should achieve a total of at least 60 minutes of at least moderate-intensity physical activity each day.[3] The

Health Survey for England in 2002 and the Scottish Health Survey in 1998 used comparable physical activity methodologies to examine children's activity levels. Assuming that the activity levels of Scottish children have not changed much since 1998, there seem to be no between-country differences in the age-standardised percentage of boys and girls who meet the recommendations. Overall, seven in 10 boys and six in 10 girls in England and Scotland met the recommendation. Sex differences in the proportion meeting the recommendation begin to appear after the age of seven and progressively widen to approximately 20 per cent by the age of 13 (69 per cent of boys and 50 per cent of girls).[17] This is in line with the decline in total time spent in physical activity by girls as they approach puberty.

The Health Survey for England collected information on children's participation in walking, sports and exercise (for example football, rugby, swimming, gymnastics) and active play (for example cycling, kicking a ball around, running about, playing active games) in the last seven days. Parents responded on behalf of children aged 2–12 whereas adolescents aged 13–15 answered the questions themselves.

Active play and sports and exercise are fundamental aspects of children's overall activity. Boys spend more time in sports and exercise, active play, and total activity than girls (Figure 5.13). Time spent in sports and exercise in the last seven days was 2.4 hours for boys and 1.7 hours for girls. Larger periods of time are spent in active playing by both boys (7.9 hours) and girls (6.4 hours). Boys engage in physical activity for 3.2 hours a week longer than do girls (14.2 versus 11.0 hours). Average walking times are the same for boys and girls (3.5 hours a week).

Figure **5.13**

Time spent in physical activity[1] (age-standardised): by sex, 2002

England

Hours per week

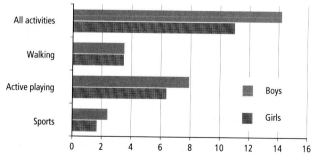

1 *For children aged 2–15.*

Source: Health Survey for England, Department of Health

Time spent in physical activity decreases in girls from the age of nine: girls aged two were active for 13.0 hours, girls aged nine for 12.7 hours, falling to 9.6 hours for girls aged 15. The same was not true for boys, whose total duration of activity was similar throughout childhood (from 13.5 hours a week at the age of two, to 13.8 hours at the age of nine and 14.3 hours at the age of 15).[17] The 1998 Health Survey for England indicated that although time spent in physical activity decreases with age for girls only, sedentary time (doing things like watching television, reading, or being read to) increases with age for both sexes. Sedentary time increased from approximately nine hours a week among boys and eight hours among girls at age two, to 17 hours among boys and 18 hours among girls at age 15.[42]

Time spent in physical activity varies with socio-economic classification of the household reference person. As Table 5.14 shows, boys and girls from semi-routine and routine households spend more time in physical activity (15.0 and 12.5 hours a week respectively) than those from any other social class. The lowest times of activity are observed in boys from managerial and professional (13.3 hours) and in girls from small employers and own-account workers' households (9.4 hours). This pattern in total activity is the result of a socio-economic variation in time spent in active play, as there is no consistent pattern in walking or time spent in sports.

Contrary to the pattern observed for all forms of activity, girls' participation in sports and exercise was the highest amongst those in managerial and professional households and lowest in semi-routine and routine households. It may be that participation in sports for girls, unlike free playing, involves costs (clothing, equipment, club fees, and so on) that parents

from semi-routine and routine occupations find difficult to bear. In support of this hypothesis, there are strong associations between children's participation in sports in the past week and household income.[17] For example, seven out of 10 girls aged 2–10 living in households in the top 20 per cent of the household income distribution participate in sports, but less than four out of 10 in the bottom 20 per cent do so. Sports participation rates for girls aged 11–15 in the highest and lowest 20 per cent of income distribution are seven out of 10 and just under five out of 10 respectively.[17] Parental socio-economic status and income is less of an issue for boys' participation in sports, where there is a less consistent pattern.

Journey to school

The journey to school is an important opportunity to increase everyday physical activity in children.[43] There have been many local and national initiatives to promote more walking, cycling, and bus use on the way to and from school, as outlined in the Travelling to School action plan.[44] The current policy target is that all schools in England should have travel plans by 2010.[7] In recent years walking to school has become less common and car use more common, among both younger children and adolescents. Figures 5.15 and 5.16 (see overleaf) illustrate the time trends in young children (aged 5–10) and adolescents' (aged 11–16) transportation to school between 1992/94 and 2002/03.

For young children, walking and car represent over 90 per cent of school journeys, but as children become adolescents the use of bus and bicycle becomes more common. Among young children, walking to school fell from six in 10 journeys (61 per cent) in 1992/94 to just over half (52 per cent) in 2002/03,

Table **5.14**

Time spent in physical activity[1] (age-standardised): by NS-SEC[2] and sex, 2002

Great Britain

Hours per week

	Boys				Girls			
	Sports	Active playing	Walking	All activities	Sports	Active playing	Walking	All activities
Managerial & professional	2.5	7.5	3.3	13.3	1.9	5.9	3.4	10.1
Intermediate occupations	2.0	7.6	3.5	13.6	1.6	6.3	3.7	10.7
Small employers & own account workers	2.3	8.3	3.0	14.6	1.7	6.2	2.8	9.4
Lower supervisory & technical	2.4	8.1	3.8	14.5	1.8	6.8	3.5	11.6
Semi-routine & routine	2.3	8.4	3.7	15.0	1.4	7.1	3.9	12.5

1 For children aged 2–15.
2 NS-SEC of household reference person.

Source: General Household Survey, Office for National Statistics

mirroring the equivalent 10 percentage point rise in the proportion of school journeys by car, from 30 per cent to 40 per cent, over the same period. Travelling to school by bicycle at this age represented a negligible proportion throughout the time span.

Among adolescents aged 11–16, bus travel accounted for about a third of school journeys (32 per cent) in all years during the period in question, while the proportion of such journeys on foot fell from 44 per cent in 1992/94 to 40 per cent in 2002/03. Increases in journeys by car over the same period (from 16 to 23 per cent) roughly equalled the decreases on foot and by bicycle combined (bicycle journeys fell from 4 to 2 per cent). Walking to school was more common in the mid-

Figure 5.15

Main mode of travel to school[1] for those aged 5–10, 1992–94 to 2002–03[2]

Great Britain

Percentage of jouneys

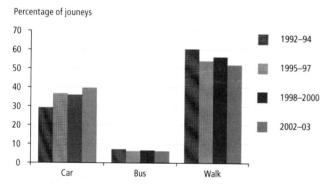

1 Excludes journeys of 50 miles or more.
2 Datapoints based on two or three combined years of data.

Source: National Travel Survey, Department of Transport

Figure 5.16

Main mode of travel to school[1] for those aged 11–16, 1992–94 to 2002–03[2]

Great Britain

Percentage of journeys

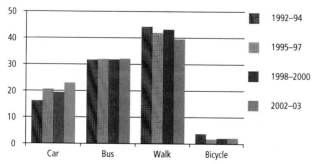

1 Excludes journeys of 50 miles or more.
2 Datapoints based on two or three combined years of data.

Source: National Travel Survey, Department of Transport

1980s (1985/86) when it accounted for 67 and 52 per cent of the journeys made by children aged 5–10 and 11–16 respectively.[45]

Physical activity in adulthood

Physical inactivity is associated with increased risk of many chronic conditions. Adults who are physically active have 20–30 per cent reduced risk of premature death, and up to 50 per cent reduced risk of developing the major chronic diseases, most notably cardiovascular disease (such as coronary heart disease and stroke), diabetes and cancers.[3] Beyond its role in the development of obesity, physical inactivity and associated poor cardiorespiratory fitness pose direct health risks. For example, lean unfit men may have higher risk for cardiovascular disease and death than obese fit men.[46, 47]

Participation

The Chief Medical Officer recommends that all adults (including the elderly) should achieve a total of at least 30 minutes a day of at least moderate-intensity physical activity on five or more days of the week.[3] This amount of activity is recommended for general health benefits but is not adequate for the prevention of weight gain, where 45–60 minutes of at least moderate-intensity activity a day are required. The recommended levels of activity can be achieved either by doing all the daily activity in one session, or through several shorter bouts of activity of 10 minutes or more. The activity can be part of everyday life (such as walking, cycling to work) or structured exercise or sport (such as aerobics, football, swimming), or a combination of these.

Currently less than four in 10 English men (39 per cent) and one in four women (26 per cent) meet these recommendations (age-standardised estimates). About one in three men (29 per cent) and over one in three women (36 per cent) fall into the sedentary category, that is they engage in activities of moderate intensity for less than 30 minutes a week. The proportions of adults meeting the physical activity recommendations in Wales were 36 per cent for men and 22 per cent for women[39] (unstandardised estimates).The decreases in physical activity occurring in childhood and adolescence continue into adulthood for both sexes. Table 5.17 shows that the proportion of English and Welsh men who meet the physical activity recommendations decreases steadily with age. The proportion of women doing at least five moderate-intensity activity sessions a week remains level to the age group of 45–54 (55–64 for Welsh women) and then gradually drops for those aged 75 and over. Sex differences narrow with age, for example, from 23 percentage points difference between English men and women aged 16–24, to four points at ages 65–74.

Table 5.17

Meeting physical activity recommendations:[1] by country, age and sex, 2003 and 2003/04

England & Wales   Percentages

	England		Wales	
	Men	Women	Men	Women
16–24	53	30	45	25
25–34	44	29	45	24
35–44	41	30	41	25
45–54	38	31	37	25
55–64	32	23	32	23
65–74	17	13	24	15
75 and over	8	3	15	8

1 A total of at least 30 minutes a day of at least moderate-intensity activity on five or more days a week.

Source: Health Survey for England 2003, Department of Health; Welsh Health Survey 2003/04, Welsh Assembly

Results from the 2003 Health Survey for England enable overall activity levels to be broken down into participation in specific activity types (walking, heavy housework, heavy manual/DIY, sports/exercise) for at least 30 continuous minutes over the last four weeks. Men's participation in sports/exercise and walking decreases from young adulthood (ages 16–24) onwards. While women's participation in sports and exercise also declines from an early age, participation in walking remains constant until ages 45–54 before it starts declining.[29]

In 2002 the General Household Survey collected information on participation in recreational (leisure-time) physical activity and sports.[48] Participation in recreational physical activity varies with socio-economic status. In contrast to children, where semi-routine and routine households were associated with greater participation in active play, more men and women from managerial and professional households participate in swimming, recreational cycling, and recreational walking than all other socio-economic categories (Table 5.18). Age-standardised participation in any recreational physical activity and sport (excluding walking) varied from six in 10 men (62 per cent) and five in 10 women (48 per cent) in managerial and professional households to four in 10 men (42 per cent) and three in 10 women (29 per cent) in semi-routine and routine households. Similarly, recreational walking for more than two miles varied from over four in 10 men (44 per cent) and women (43 per cent) in managerial and professional households to under three in 10 men (27 per cent) and women (29 per cent) in semi-routine and routine households. Similar socio-economic variations occur in cycling and swimming participation, as shown in Table 5.18.

When overall physical activity levels are considered (including sports and exercise, walking, housework and occupational activity) variations by socio-economic classification become less clear. For example, the age-standardised percentage of men who meet the physical activity recommendations is higher among small employers and own account workers (50 per cent), lower supervisory and technical (46 per cent), and semi-routine and routine workers (44 per cent) than among managerial and professional (33 per cent) and intermediate occupations (36 per cent). This may occur due to the nature of non-managerial/professional occupations that are more likely to involve manual work and therefore more physical activity on an everyday basis. No significant socio-economic classification variation is found in women's overall activity levels.[29]

Table 5.18

Participation in recreational physical activity[1,2] (age-standardised): by NS-SEC and sex, 2002

Great Britain   Percentages

	Men				Women			
	Swimming	Cycling	Walking[3]	Any activity[4]	Swimming	Cycling	Walking[3]	Any activity[4]
Managerial & professional	17.2	16.2	44.4	62.3	20.7	7.9	43.5	48.0
Intermediate occupations	12.2	11.5	39.1	57.6	16.1	5.3	33.0	41.4
Small employers & own account workers	9.3	10.2	28.6	52.7	16.2	6.2	32.5	40.0
Lower supervisory & technical	11.8	11.8	29.9	51.4	14.3	4.4	29.5	34.1
Semi-routine & routine	7.8	10.5	26.8	42.4	11.0	4.9	29.1	28.4

1 At least once in the last four weeks.
2 Adults aged 16 and over.
3 Recreational walking for two miles or more.
4 Excluding all walking but including swimming and cycling.

Source: General Household Survey, Office for National Statistics

Time trends

Figure 5.19 shows the time trends in participation in primarily recreational physical activity between 1990 and 2002 for men and women. Trends refer to participation in recreational walking or hiking for over two miles, cycling, swimming and all recreational physical activity and sport (excluding all walking)) in the last four weeks. Men's participation in any sport or recreational physical activity decreased from 58 per cent in 1990 to 50 per cent in 2002. Among women, a smaller decrease occurred, from 39 per cent to 37 per cent. Participation in recreational walking increased between 1990 and 1996 (from 44 to 49 per cent for men and from 38 to 41 per cent for women) but decreased sharply by 13 percentage points for men and by six percentage points for women between 1996 and 2002. Similarly, participation in cycling slightly increased up to 1996 and then decreased between 1996 and 2002 back to 1990 levels. A similar tendency for increased participation in swimming from 1990 to mid 1990s but decreases thereafter are seen for both men and women.[48]

Long-term trends in modes of travelling and transportation are provided by the National Travel Survey. Transportation to work provides an important opportunity to increase everyday physical activity. The trends in adults' transportation to work are clearer than their participation in recreational activities, where initial increases were followed by decreases over the 1990s. Figure 5.20 shows trends in mode of transport for journeys to work made by British adults between 1989/91 and 2002/03. The percentage of car trips over this period increased from 66 to 71 per cent while the percentage of trips on foot

Figure **5.20**

Trends in main mode of travel to work,[1] 1989–91 to 2002–03[2]

Great Britain

Percentage of journeys

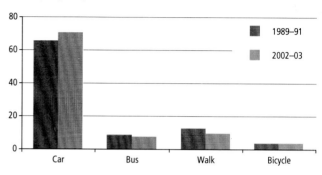

1 For people aged 17 and over.
2 Datapoints based on two or three combined years of data.
Source: National Travel Survey, Department of Transport

gradually decreased from 13 to 10 per cent. The use of bus has fallen slightly (from 9 to 8 per cent), while bicycle use has remained the same at 4 per cent.

Walking is the most common physical activity for British men and women. Cycling is the third most common activity for men and fourth most common activity for women.[48] Trends in walking and cycling provide a proxy measure of overall physical activity trends. The National Travel Survey provides information on the overall average distance walked and cycled between 1975 and 2003 in Britain. The survey records journeys on public highways but excludes recreational walking and cycling. The

Figure **5.19**

Trends in participation[1] in recreational physical activity:[2] by sex, 1990–2002[3]

Great Britain

Percentages

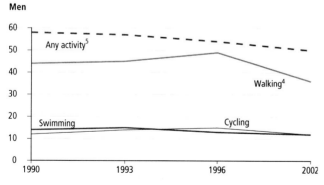

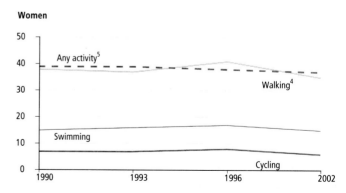

1 For people aged 16 and over.
2 At least once in the last four weeks.
3 Percentages prior to 2002 are based on unweighted data and for 2002 on weighted data. The weighting procedure adjusts for differential non-response in different population groups.
4 Recreational walking for two miles or more.
5 Excluding all walking but including swimming and cycling.

Source: General Household Survey, Office for National Statistics

total number of miles travelled per year per person on foot in Great Britain has decreased from 255 miles in 1975/76 to 199 miles in 1992/94 and 191 miles in 2002/03. Total miles cycled for the same years decreased from 51 miles in 1975/76 to 38 miles, and finally 34 miles in 2002/03.

Conclusion

Obesity is closely linked to numerous diseases, most notably cancer and cardiovascular and metabolic disease. Physical activity and eating behaviours are closely linked to the development and maintenance of overweight and obesity. Overall, one in six English children aged under 15 were obese in 2001/2002 and one in five English men and women were obese in 2003. One in six men and one in five women were obese in Scotland in 1998 and Northern Ireland in 1997.

The prevalence of obesity increased markedly among all age and sex groups during the 1990s and the early 2000s and there is no sign that this upward trend is easing. This increase could be the result of a decline in the population's physical activity, increases in calorific intake, or a combination of the two. Over the last three decades there has been a consistent increase in the use of car, and decreases in walking and cycling, for transportation to school and to work. Participation in recreational physical activities (such as recreational walking, swimming, and cycling) has also been declining. On the other hand, there seems to be no evidence that the total calorific intake, or the consumption of foods rich in fat and added sugar has increased over the same period. In contrast, there is evidence that more fruit and vegetables and less fat are now consumed in the UK than approximately 10–15 years ago.

Although the above findings suggest that reductions in physical activity may make a greater contribution to the recent rapid rise in obesity prevalence than changes in diet, the way in which diet is measured and changes in eating patterns also need to be considered. Experts argue that the contribution of nutrition to obesity may be masked by reliance on self-reported measures of consumption, since people may under-report what they eat. This under-reporting may be more common for foods that are regarded as 'bad' for the health, such as high-sugar and high-fat foods. Regardless of changes in the amount of calories taken, there have been changes in patterns of eating, such as increases in consumption of energy-dense snacks (foods that contain too many calories in relation to their weight)[2] and alcohol[35] and increased reliance on ready-meals.[2] For these reasons, the current evidence does not give clear answers as to whether it is changes in diet or physical activity that are primarily responsible for the marked increases in obesity.

Both obesity and physical activity are affected by socio-economic inequalities. Generally, living in managerial and professional households is linked to lower obesity rates for boys, girls, and women, but not for men. Adults in managerial and professional occupations participate more in recreational physical activities than adults in all other occupational groups. The opposite is true for children, where higher participation is seen in semi-routine and routine households. No socio-economic differences are found in total calories eaten or fat consumption, but children and adults from managerial and professional households tend to consume more fruit and vegetables and less added sugars than other socio-economic groups.

As far as obesity is concerned, both treatment and prevention are important. The Health Development Agency has reviewed the evidence on the best approaches to prevent and treat obesity.[49] The evidence base supports the use of school-based interventions (including nutrition education, physical activity promotion, reduction in sedentary behaviour, modification of school meals) to prevent obesity in children and adolescents. For the treatment of obesity in the young, family-based behaviour interventions involving increases in everyday physical activity, decreases in sedentary time, and improvements in diet represent the most promising approach. There is limited evidence to support the role of community based programmes for the prevention of obesity in adults. A wide range of evidence-based approaches to treating adult obesity exist, including several low-calorie diets, increased physical activity, combinations of physical activity and dieting, and a combination of behavioural therapy with other practices.

References

1. Weinsier R L, Hunter G R, Heini A F, Goran M I and Sell S M (1998) The etiology of obesity: relative contribution of metabolic factors, diet, and physical activity. *The American Journal of Medicine* **105**, 145–150.

2. Health Select Committee (2004) *Third Report of Session 2003-04, Obesity HC23-1*, TSO:London www.parliament.the-stationeryoffice.co.uk

3. The Chief Medical Officer (2004) *At least five a week: evidence on the impact of physical activity and its relationship to health*, Department of Health: London. www.dh.gov.uk

4. *Choosing a Better Diet: a Food and Health Action Plan* at: www.dh.gov.uk

5. Department of Health (2004) *Choosing Health: Making Healthy Choices Easier*, TSO: London. www.dh.gov.uk/PublicationsAndStatistics

6. *Delivering Choosing Health* at: www.dh.gov.uk/assetRoot/04/10/ 57/13/04105713.pdf

7. *Choosing Activity: a physical activity action plan* at: www.dh.gov.uk

8. Caspersen C J, Powell K E and Christensen G (1985). Physical activity, exercise and physical fitness: definitions and distinctions of health-related research. *Public Health Reports* **10**, 126–131.

9. Steinbeck K (2001) The importance of physical activity in the prevention of overweight and obesity in childhood: a review and an opinion. *Obesity Reviews* **2**, 117–130.

10. Schwimmer J B, Burwinkle T M and Varni J W (2003) Health-related quality of life of severely obese children and adolescents. *JAMA* **289**, 1813–1819.

11. Von Mutius E, Schwartz J, Neas L M, Dockery D and Weiss S T (2001) Relation of body mass index to asthma and atopy in children: the National Health and Nutrition Examination Study III. *Thorax* **56**, 835–838.

12. Fagot-Campagna A, Pettitt D J, Engelgau M M, Burrows N R, Geiss L S, Valdez R, Beckles G L A, Saaddine J, Gregg E W, Williamson D F and Narayan K M V (2000). Type 2 diabetes among North American children and adolescents: An epidemiologic review and a public health perspective. *Journal of Pediatrics* **136**, 664–672.

13. Ribeiro J, Guerra S, Pinto A, Oliveira J, Duarte J and Mota J (2003) Overweight and obesity in children and adolescents: relationship with blood pressure, and physical activity. *Annals of Human Biology* **30**, 203–213.

14. Gunnell D, Frankel S, Nanchahal K, Peters T J and Smith G D (1998) Childhood obesity and adult cardiovascular mortality: a **57**-y follow-up study based on the Boyd Orr cohort. *American Journal of Clinical Nutrition* **67**, 1111–1118.

15. Hoffmans M, Kromhout D and Coulander C D (1998) The impact of body-mass index of 78,612 18-year-old Dutch men on 32-year mortality from all causes. *Journal of Clinical Epidemiology* **41**, 749–756.

16. Department of Health. Public Service Agreement targets at: www.hm-treasury.gov.uk/media

17. Department of Health (2003) *Health Survey for England 2002: The health of children and young people*, TSO: London. www.official-documents.co.uk

18. Sobal J and Stunkard A J (1989) Socioeconomic status and obesity: a review of the literature. *Psychological Bulletin* **105**, 260–275.

19. Roberts H (1997) Socioeconomic determinants of health: Children, inequalities, and health. *British Medical Journal* **314**, 1122.

20. Drewnowski A and Specter S E (2004) Poverty and obesity: the role of energy density and energy costs. *American Journal of Clinical Nutrition* **79**, 6–16.

21. Stamatakis E, Primatesta P, Falascheti E, Chinn S, Ronna R. Overweight and obesity trends from 1974 to 2003 in English children: what is the role of socio-economic factors? *Archives of Disease in Childhood* **90**, 999–1004.

22. Joint Health Surveys Unit (2005) *Forecasting Obesity to 2010*. Department of Health: London.

23. Joint Health Surveys Unit (2005) *Obesity among children under 11*, Department of Health: London www.dh.gov.uk

24. Jonsson S, Hedblad B, Engstrom G *et al* (2002) Influence of obesity on cardiovascular risk. Twenty-three-year follow-up of 22,025 men from an urban Swedish population. *International Journal of Obesity* **8**, 1046–1053.

25. Kopelman PG (2000) Obesity as a medical problem. *Nature* **404**, 635–643.

26. Gensini G F, Comeglio M and Colella A (1998) Classical risk factors and emerging elements in the risk profile for coronary artery disease. *European Heart Journal* **19**, A53–A61.

27. The National Audit Office (2001) *Tackling Obesity in England*, TSO; London. www.nao.org.uk/publications/nao_reports

28. Scottish Executive Department of Health (2000) T*he Scottish Health Survey* 1998, TSO: Edinburgh. www.show.scot.nhs.uk/scottishhealthsurvey

29. Department of Health (2004) *Health Survey for England 2003: Cardiovascular Disease,* TSO: London. www.dh.gov.uk

30. Department of Health (2004) *Health Survey for England* 2003: Trends, at: www.dh.gov.uk/PublicationsAndStatistics

31. World Heath Organisation (2003) *Technical Report Series 916. Diet, nutrition and the prevention of chronic diseases. Report of a Joint WHO/FAO Expert Consultation*, World Heath Organisation: Geneva. www.who.int/nut/documents

32. Hu F B, van Dam R M and Liu S (2001) Diet and risk of Type II diabetes: the role of types of fat and carbohydrate. *Diabetologia* **44**, 805–817.

33. van Dam R M, Willett W C, Rimm E B, Stampfer M J and Hu F B (2002) Dietary fat and meat intake in relation to risk of type 2 diabetes in men. *Diabetes Care* **25**, 417–424.

34. Food Standards Agency (2000) *National Diet and Nutrition Survey: young people aged 4 to 18 years*, TSO: London.

35. Food Standards Agency (2003) *National Diet and Nutrition Survey: adults aged 19 to 64 years*, TSO: London.
www.food.gov.uk/science

36. Department of Health (1991) *Dietary reference values for food energy and nutrients for the UK*. Report on Health and Social Subjects 41, Department of Health: London.

37. Department of Environment Food and Rural Affairs (2004) *Family Food. A report on the 2002-03 Expenditure and Food Survey*, TSO: London.
www.statistics.defra.gov.uk/esg/publications

38. For information about the Five-a-day programme see the Department of Health website: www.dh.gov.uk/PolicyAndGuidance/HealthAndSocialCareTopics/FiveADay/fs/en

39. Welsh Assembly (2005) *Welsh Health Survey 2003/04, Welsh Assembly:* Cardiff.
www.wales.gov.ukkeypubstatisticsforwales/content/publication/health

40. Twisk J (2001) Physical activity guidelines for children and adolescents. A critical review. *Sports Medicine* **31**, 617–627.

41. Page A, Cooper A R, Stamatakis E, Griffiths L J, Crawne E and Shield J (2005) Physical activity patterns in non-obese and obese children and adolescents using minute-by-minute accelerometry. *International Journal of Obesity* **29**, 1070–1076.

42. Department of Health (1998) *Health Survey for England 1995–97: The health of children and young people*, TSO: London.

43. Cooper A, Page A and Foster L (2003) Commuting to school. Are children who walk more physically active? *American Journal of Preventive Medicine* **25**, 273–276.

44. Department for Education and Skills and Department of Transport (2003) *Travelling to School Action Plan*, Department for Education and Skills: London.
www.dft.gov.uk/stellent/groups

45. Department of Transport (2004) *Transport Trends: 2004 Edition*, Department of Transport: London.
www.dft.gov.uk/stellent/groups

46. Lee C D, Blair S N and Jackson A S (1999) Cardiorespiratory fitness, body composition, and all-cause and cardiovascular disease mortality in men. *American Journal of Clinical Nutrition* **69**, 373–380.

47. Stevens J, Evenson K R, Thomas O, Cai J and Thomas R (2004) Associations of fitness and fatness with mortality in Russian and American men in the lipids research clinics study. *International Journal of Obesity* **28**, 1463–1470.

48. Office for National Statistics (2004) *General Household Survey 2002. Sport and Leisure*, TSO: London.
www.statistics.gov.uk

49. Health Development Agency (2003). *The management of obesity and overweight. An analysis of reviews of diet, physical activity and behavioural approaches*. NHS Health Development Agency: London.
www.hda.nhs.uk/documents

Sexual behaviour and health

Susan Westlake

Chapter 6

Introduction

There has been a change in sexual behaviour, and attitudes towards sex and sexuality, over the last thirty years. The third report of the Government's *Select Committee Report on Sexual Health* 2003 refers to the rapid decline in sexual health as a major public health issue.[1]

Information about risks from Human Immunodeficiency Virus (HIV), open access to Genitourinary Medicine (GUM) clinics, and measures such as needle-exchange schemes, have resulted in the UK having one of the lowest rates of HIV in Western Europe.[2]

There is a clear relationship between sexual ill health, poverty and social exclusion. Information about contraception and the avoidance of Sexually Transmitted Infections (STIs) is widely available, but the quality of service provision remains uneven across the country. The first national strategy for sexual health and HIV services[2] was published by the Department of Health in 2001 with the aim of improving services, information and support, reducing inequalities and improving sexual health.

Sexual behaviour

Age at first intercourse

Early first intercourse is thought to be linked to unplanned, unprotected sex and therefore to a greater risk of unintended pregnancy and STIs. Alcohol and drug use have a clear association with early first intercourse, which is likely to be unintended and unprotected.[3–5]

The National Survey of Sexual Attitudes and Lifestyles II (Natsal II) was carried out in Great Britain between 1999 and 2001, among men and women aged 16–44 living in private households.[6] In both Natsal II and the Northern Ireland Health and Social Wellbeing Survey 2001,[7] respondents were asked how old they were when they first had sexual intercourse. In Great Britain 27 per cent of men and 20 per cent women were younger than 16 years of age (up from 22 per cent and 10 per cent respectively in Natsal I carried out between 1989 and 1990). In Northern Ireland 18 per cent of men and 7 per cent of women were younger than 16 at first intercourse (Figure 6.1).

People in non-manual occupations were much less likely to have first sex at an early age than those in manual occupations.[6, 7] In Great Britain, 8 per cent of men and 9 per cent of women in professional occupations were younger than 16, compared to 38 per cent of men and 24 per cent of women in unskilled occupations (Figure 6.2).

Figure **6.1**

Under 16 at first heterosexual intercourse: by sex for people aged 16–44, 1989/1990 and 1999/2001

Great Britain

Percentages

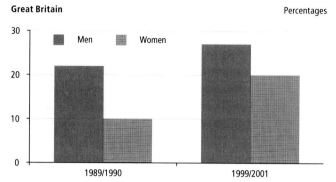

Source: National Survey of Sexual Attitudes and Lifestyles II, National Centre for Social Research

The Health Behaviour of School-aged Children Survey (HBSC), carried out in 2001/02 in Great Britain, asked 15-year-olds about age at first intercourse, the first HBSC survey to collect such information.[8] In all three countries, a larger proportion of girls than boys had experienced intercourse by the age of 15: 40 per cent versus 36 per cent in England, 40 per cent versus 29 per cent in Wales and 35 versus 33 per cent in Scotland.

Figure **6.2**

Under 16 at first heterosexual intercourse: by social class[1] and sex for people aged 16–44, 1999/2001

Great Britain

Percentages

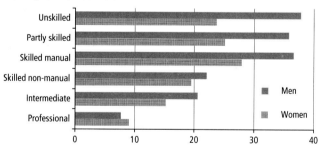

1   *Using the Registrar General's Social Class based on occupation of informant and excluding those not working in past ten years.*

Source: National Survey of Sexual Attitudes and Lifestyles II, Department of Health

Number of sexual partners

ONS Omnibus surveys in Great Britain regularly ask women aged less than 50, and men aged less than 70, how many sexual partners they have had in the previous year. Between 1997/98 and 2003/04 the proportions of men and women having none, one, two/three or four or more partners were fairly stable. Results from the most recent survey show that younger age groups tend to have larger numbers of sexual partners than older age groups. For example, 11 per cent of men and 5 per cent of women aged 16–19 reported having four or more partners in the previous year, compared with only 3 per cent of men and 1 per cent of women aged 35–39.[9] Overall 4 per cent of men reported having this number of partners, compared with 1 per cent of women. At the opposite end of the scale, around three-quarters of both men and women had one partner in the previous year and 13 per cent had been celibate.

The Natsal surveys I and II asked respondents how many partners of the opposite sex they have ever had. In 1999/2001 nearly half of those aged 16–17 had not yet had any partners (Table 6.3). Unsurprisingly the number of partners increased with age and after age 19 men had more partners than women. However in every age group a higher percentage of men than women reported never having a partner of the opposite sex. In 1989/90 half of all men interviewed reported a total of at least four partners and this had increased to six by the time of the second survey in 1999/2001. The corresponding figures for women were two and four partners. The proportion

of those having had ten or more partners increased significantly for both sexes in the decade between the surveys: up from 26 per cent to 35 per cent for men and from 8 to 19 per cent for women.

Concurrent partnerships increase the probability that any STIs will be passed on to more than one person. In 1999/2001 more men (15 per cent) had concurrent partners than did women (9 per cent). Proportions ranged from 21 per cent of men and 15 per cent of women aged 16 to 24, to 10 per cent of men and 7 per cent of women aged 35–44 (Figure 6.4 – see overleaf).

Alcohol and sexual practices

People who abuse alcohol, that is drink heavily, are more likely to engage in risky behaviours such as unprotected sex. In addition, a recent study showed that alcohol abuse may increase susceptibility to HIV infection during receptive oral sex.[10] There is also evidence that alcohol abuse is common among people who are HIV positive.[11]

Natsal II asked about usual weekly alcohol consumption and sexual practices. Proportions of men practising vaginal intercourse, oral sex or anal sex with women were lowest for

Table **6.3**

Number of opposite sex partners ever had: by age and sex for people aged 16–44, 1989/1990, 1999/2001

Great Britain

Percentages

	1989/1990[1]	1999/2001					
	All	All	16–17	18–19	20–24	25–34	35–44
Men							
0	8	7	50	17	7	4	2
1	17	11	13	21	14	8	11
2	10	8	8	10	8	7	7
3–4	18	15	11	18	19	14	13
5–9	21	25	15	20	24	25	28
10 or more	26	35	4	15	29	41	39
Median number of partners[2]	4	6	1	3	5	7	7
Women							
0	7	5	48	14	6	1	1
1	33	18	21	22	16	16	21
2	17	11	7	14	12	11	11
3–4	20	20	12	16	20	20	22
5–9	15	27	9	21	27	30	27
10 or more	8	19	3	14	20	23	19
Median number of partners[2]	2	4	1	3	4	5	4

1 Weighted to be comparable with 1999/01 results.
2 Half of respondents had this number or fewer partners and half had this number or more.

Source: National Survey of Sexual Attitudes and Lifestyles II, National Centre for Social Research

Figure **6.4**

Concurrent sexual partnerships in the last year: by age and sex, 1999/2001

Great Britain

Percentages

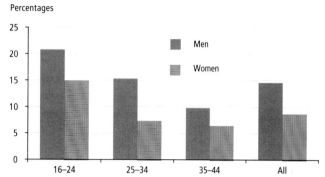

Source: National Survey of Sexual Attitudes and Lifestyles II, National Centre for Social Research

those who did not drink alcohol at all, and increased with the amount of alcohol consumed up to 49 units per week, and then slightly decreased. For women the proportions increased with the amount of alcohol for vaginal intercourse, but among those consuming 35 or more units per week they decreased slightly for oral sex and more than halved for anal sex.

The Young Persons' Behaviour and Attitudes Survey was carried out in Northern Ireland in 2000. Pupils aged 11–16 were asked 'Have you ever had so much alcohol that you were drunk?' Results show that the proportion of pupils who had had sexual intercourse increased with the number of times they had felt drunk (Figure 6.5). Five per cent of pupils who had never been drunk had had sexual intercourse, compared with 52 per cent of those who had felt drunk more than 10 times.

Figure **6.5**

Number of times ever felt drunk: by sexual experience for people aged 11–16, 2000

Northern Ireland

Percentages

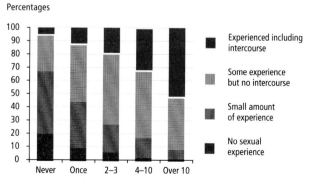

Source: The Young Persons' Behaviour and Attitudes Survey, Northern Ireland Statistics and Research Agency

Conceptions

The estimated number of conceptions (pregnancies leading to maternities or legal abortions) in England and Wales began to decrease over the 1990s from 2.50 million in the three-year period 1991 to 1993, to 2.36 million in 2001 to 2003.[12] The conception rate decreased from 77.7 per 1,000 females aged 15–44 in 1991 to 73.7 in 2003. Conception rates varied across England and Wales, from 66.0 per thousand women living in the North East to 90.0 in London.[13]

In England and Wales, nearly four-fifths of the conceptions result in a maternity and this proportion has remained fairly stable over the past 13 years.

Conception rates for women aged 30 and over have increased significantly since 1990, particularly among the oldest age groups (35–39 and 40 and over). In contrast, conception rates for women aged under 20 fell in the early 1990s but rose between 1995 and 1998 and have been falling again since then (Figure 6.6).

Figure **6.6**

Relative changes in age-specific conception rates, 1990–2003

England and Wales

Percentages

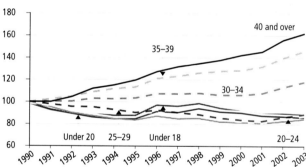

Source: Office for National Statistics

Teenage pregnancy

Teenage pregnancy is associated with increased risk of adverse health and social outcomes for both mothers and their babies, and there is also an association between teenage pregnancies and deprivation.[14] The Department of Health's *Public Service Agreement 2005–08* set a target in England of reducing the conception rate of girls aged less than 18 by 50 per cent by 2010, using 1998 as the base year.[15] So far, rates have fallen from 46.6 per thousand girls aged 15–17 in 1998, to 42.1 in

Figure **6.7**

Teenage conception rates: by age at conception and country, 1996–2002

England, Wales, Scotland

Rates per 1,000

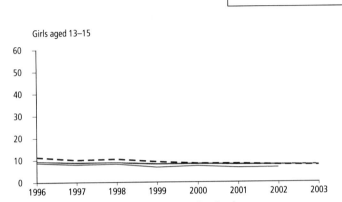

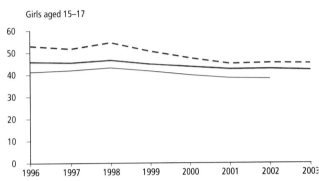

Source: Office for National Statistics; ISD Scotland

2003. For girls aged 13–15, conception rates were 8.8 per thousand in 1998, decreasing to 7.9 in 2003 (Figure 6.7).

Towards a Healthier Scotland[16] set a target to reduce pregnancies among girls aged 13–15 by 20 per cent between 1995 and 2010. So far rates in this group have fallen from 8 per thousand in 1995/96 to 7 in 2002/03.

Contraception

In Great Britain, data from the General Household Survey (GHS) show that the proportion of women aged 16–49 who do not use contraception has remained fairly stable in recent years (28 per cent in 2002). The most common method of contraception used by women in 2002 was the contraceptive pill (26 per cent), followed by condoms (19 per cent) and reliance on partners' sterilisation (12 per cent). The proportion using at least one method of non-surgical contraception increased from 46 per cent in 1991 to 51 per cent in 2002.[17]

There are differences in the method of contraception between age groups. Use of the pill, condom and injection was more common in younger age groups in 2002 (Table 6.8 – see overleaf). Among women aged 20–24, 52 per cent used the pill and 30 per cent the male condom. Rates of sterilisation increased with age: from two per cent of women and one per cent of men aged 25–29, to 21 per cent and 23 per cent respectively of those aged 45–49.

The Continuous Household Survey (CHS) carried out in 2003/04, shows a similar pattern of contraceptive use in Northern Ireland (Table 6.9 – see overleaf). As in Great Britain, the pill was the most popular form of contraception (chosen by 29 per cent of women aged 16–49), followed by condoms (20 per

cent). However in contrast to Great Britain, it was more common for the woman in a relationship to be sterilised than the man. The proportion of women aged 16–49 in Northern Ireland who were sterilised was twice the corresponding rate in Great Britain, whereas the proportion relying on male sterilisation was half that in Great Britain. Again use of the pill, condom and injection was more common in the younger age groups. In Great Britain only 3 per cent of women liable but not seeking to become pregnant were not using contraception; the corresponding figure in Northern Ireland was 5 per cent.

The Health Behaviour of School Children survey carried out across Europe in 2000/01 asked 15-year-olds who had had sex about the use of contraception during their last intercourse.[18] In both England and Wales a higher proportion of girls than boys had used at least one form of contraception: in England 88 per cent compared with 80 per cent and in Wales 85 per cent compared with 82 per cent. In Scotland the situation was reversed and boys were more likely to have used contraception than girls (81 and 74 per cent respectively).

Emergency contraception

Two forms of emergency contraception are available for women to use after intercourse: hormonal emergency contraception (the 'morning after pill') and the emergency intrauterine device (IUD). In Great Britain, data from the 2002 GHS show that six per cent of women aged 16–49 used the morning after pill once during the previous 12 months, and 1 per cent used it twice. The highest proportion of users was among those aged 18–19. One per cent of women aged 16–24 used it more than twice. Less than half a per cent used an emergency IUD.[9]

Table **6.8**

Current use of contraception in Great Britain: women aged 16–49, 2002

Great Britain

Percentages

Using method(s)[1]	16–17	18–19	20–24	25–29	30–34	35–39	40–44	45–49	Total
Non-surgical:									
Pill	24	46	53	45	28	20	10	9	26
IUD	0	1	2	6	6	5	5	4	4
Condom	23	21	30	24	22	17	13	12	19
Cap	0	1	0	0	1	1	1	1	1
Withdrawal	3	1	2	4	5	4	4	3	4
Safe period	0	1	1	1	2	1	2	1	1
Spermicides	0	0	0	0	0	0	0	0	0
Injection	3	8	6	5	4	3	2	1	3
Surgical sterilisation:									
Female	0	0	0	2	6	12	17	21	9
Male	1	0	1	1	7	17	22	23	12
Total using at least one method	40	61	75	78	72	75	74	71	72
Total not using a method	60	39	25	22	28	25	26	29	28

1 Percentages add to more than 100 because of rounding and because some women used more than one non-surgical method.

Source: General Household Survey, Office for National Statistics

Table **6.9**

Current use of contraception in Northern Ireland: women aged 16–49, 2003/04

Northern Ireland

Percentages

Using method(s)[1]	16–17	18–19	20–24	25–29	30–34	35–39	40–44	45–49	Total
Non-surgical:									
Pill	29	33	53	49	33	24	14	6	29
IUD	0	0	2	3	8	6	7	2	5
Condom	18	17	25	31	19	19	14	15	20
Cap	4	0	2	1	2	1	1	0	1
Withdrawal	0	3	7	6	6	6	4	5	5
Safe period	0	0	2	3	3	7	4	5	4
Spermicides	0	0	1	0	0	0	0	0	0
Injection	2	10	11	6	5	2	3	1	4
Surgical sterilisation:									
Female	0	0	0	5	13	23	32	32	17
Male	0	0	0	1	7	10	13	8	6
Total using at least one method	29	53	74	80	73	71	71	56	69
Total not using a method	71	47	26	21	27	31	30	46	32

1 Percentages add to more than 100 because of rounding and because some women used more than one non-surgical method.

Source: Continuous Household Survey, Northern Ireland Statistics and Research Agency

In 2001 the morning after pill became available over the counter at pharmacies and chemists to women aged 16 and over. In 2002 nearly half of women aged 16–49 in Great Britain obtained it from their own GPs (47 per cent), followed by chemists or pharmacies (23 per cent) and family planning clinics (17 per cent). The proportions varied according to age, marital status and socio-economic classification.[9]

In Northern Ireland, data from the 2003/04 CHS show that 11 per cent of women aged 16–49 used emergency contraception within the previous two years, 7 per cent using it only once. Less than one per cent used an IUD as emergency contraception. Most women obtained emergency contraception from their own GPs (61 per cent), or family planning clinics (28 per cent).[19]

Homosexual partners

In the 2001 Census, 85,210 people in the UK identified themselves as cohabiting in a same-sex couple, 0.2 per cent of all people aged 16 and over living in households (Figure 6.10). The proportion varied within the UK: 0.20 per cent in England, 0.15 in Scotland, 0.12 in Wales and 0.05 in Northern Ireland.

Figure **6.10**

Individuals living in a same-sex couple as a proportion of all individuals[1] aged 16 and over: by country, 2001

United Kingdom

Percentages

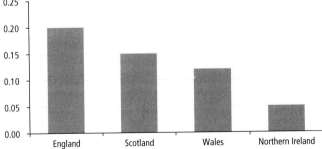

1 Individuals living in households.

Source: Census 2001, Office for National Statistics; Census 2001, General Register Office for Scotland; Census 2001, Northern Ireland Statistics and Research Agency

The areas with the largest proportions of people cohabiting in a same-sex couple in each country were London (0.38 per cent, comprising 0.60 in Inner London and 0.24 in Outer London), Edinburgh (0.40 per cent), Cardiff (0.27 per cent) and Belfast (0.11 per cent). The places with the largest proportions were Brighton and Hove in the South-East of England (1.29 per cent), followed by the City of London (1.16 per cent).

Figure **6.11**

People aged 16–44 having had at least one same-sex partner: by sex, 1989/1990 and 1999/2001

Great Britain

Percentages

Source: National Survey of Sexual Attitudes and Lifestyles II, National Centre for Social Research

The Natsal surveys asked people aged 16–44 how many partners of the same sex they had ever had (Figure 6.11). The proportion of women who had at least one same-sex partner trebled in the decade between the two surveys (from 1.9 to 5.6 per cent) while the male rate nearly doubled (from 3.5 to 6.1 per cent).

Natsal II found that, up to the age of 24 women were more likely than men to have had a homosexual partner. For example at ages 18–19 the female rate was 4.5 per cent, compared with 2.1 percent for males. However by ages 35–44 the situation was reversed with 7.9 per cent of men having had a homosexual partner compared with 5.9 per cent of women.

Anal sex

Anal sex is associated with an increased risk of HIV and STIs.[20, 21] The proportions of both men and women aged 16–44 who reported having anal sex with partners of the opposite sex within the previous five years nearly doubled between 1989/90 and 1999/2001 (Table 6.12 – see overleaf). In 1999/2001 age variations for prevalence of heterosexual anal sex were similar for men and women, with the highest rate being in the 25–34 age group (24.5 per cent for men and 22.9 for women). This age group also reported the highest prevalence of men having homosexual anal sex (2.5 per cent). The overall rate for men aged 16–44 was 1.8 per cent.

Sexual health

Sexually transmitted infections

Chlamydia is the most common bacterial STI in the UK. It is often undiagnosed, since it is asymptomatic in 70 per cent of infected women and 50 per cent of infected men. Levels of awareness of chlamydia have greatly increased in recent years.[9]

Table **6.12**

Prevalence of anal and oral sex in the last five years: by age and sex, 1989/1990, 1999/2001

Great Britain

Percentages

		1989/1990	1999/2001			
		All	All	16–24	25–34	35–44
Men same sex	Anal		1.8	1.3	2.5	1.5
	Oral		2.4	1.8	3.1	2.2
Men opposite sex	Anal	10.9	21.1	17.4	24.5	20.1
	Oral	70.0	84.4	77.0	89.6	87.3
Women opposite sex	Anal	10.2	18.4	17.1	22.9	14.6
	Oral	65.0	83.7	75.2	90.0	82.8

Source: National Survey of Sexual Attitudes and Lifestyles II, National Centre for Social Research

Most genital herpes is caused by herpes simplex virus type 2. It typically affects the genital area and is most frequently a result of penetrative intercourse.

Syphilis is transmitted through direct contact with a syphilis sore during vaginal, anal, or oral sex.

Genital warts are the commonest of all viral STIs and are almost always transmitted by sexual contact.

Gonorrhoea is mainly transmitted through sexual contact but infected mothers can pass the disease to their children during delivery.

Among a wide variety of other conditions presenting to clinics and requiring specialist investigation and treatment are urinary tract infection, dermatological and psycho-sexual problems and infections caused by fungi such as vaginal candida (thrush). In addition, the hepatitis B virus can be sexually transmitted, though not normally by vaginal intercourse; hepatitis A and C are rarely sexually transmitted.[1]

Treatment and trends

In 1999/2001 Natsal II found that 11 per cent of men and 13 per cent of women aged between 16 and 44 reported having had an STI at least once. Among this group, three-quarters of men and more than half of women had attended a GUM clinic, demonstrating the extensive use of these clinics for the diagnosis and treatment of such infections.[22] Attendance at a GUM clinic varied by specific STI and was highest for those with a history of gonorrhoea, among whom 90 per cent of both sexes reported attending. Of those diagnosed with chlamydia in the past five years, 78 per cent of men and 54 per cent of women reported having their most recent episode treated in a GUM clinic.

Between 2000 and 2004 there were large increases in the rates of new episodes of chlamydia and syphilis diagnosed in GUM

clinics in the UK (Figure 6.13). The rate of chlamydia increased from 116 to 175 per thousand population, and the rate of syphilis increased more than five-fold but from a very low base: the number of new diagnoses in 2004 for example was four per thousand population. Rates for other STIs changed less dramatically over the period: in 2004 the rates per thousand population were 134 for genital warts, 38 for gonorrhoea and 32 for herpes. For all STIs except syphilis by far the highest increase in rates was among those aged under 16. There were large increases in the rate of new episodes of syphilis for all age groups 16 and over, although in all age groups this disease is much less common than the other STIs.

Looking at the 2004 rates in more detail shows that the female rates for chlamydia, gonorrhoea and genital warts all peaked for the 16–19 age group, whereas for men the highest rate was among those aged 20–24.[23] For both men and women the

Figure **6.13**

New episodes of selected sexually transmitted infections: 2000–2004

United Kingdom

Rate per 100,000 population[1–3]

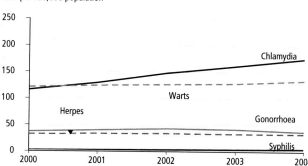

1 Diagnoses are calculated based on GUM clinics in the region, rates are calculated for the region's resident population.
2 2003 mid-year population estimates were used for 2004.
3 KC60 (England, Wales and Northern Ireland) and ISD(D)5 (Scotland) codes are used.

Source: Health Protection Agency

Figure **6.14**

STIs¹ among MSM² as percentage of all diagnoses³ in men, 2000–2004

United Kingdom

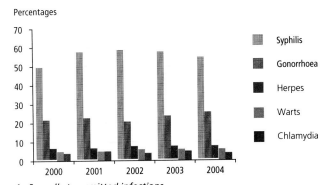

Percentages

Legend:
Syphilis
Gonorrhoea
Herpes
Warts
Chlamydia

1   Sexually transmitted infections.
2   Men who have sex with men.
3   Numbers of diagnoses were adjusted for missing clinic data.

Source: Health Protection Agency

highest rate for new diagnoses of herpes was among those aged 20–24. The highest female rate for syphilis was also at ages 20– 24 but the highest male rate was for ages 25–44.

Of all STI diagnoses in men, the proportion accounted for by men who have sex with men (MSM) fluctuated by type of STI and over the period 2000 to 2004 (Figure 6.14). Proportions for syphilis were the highest and also showed the greatest variation within this time interval (ranging between 49 and 58 per cent). Proportions for gonorrhoea ranged between 20 and 25 per cent. Proportions for herpes, genital warts and chlamydia were all much lower and showed little variation.

In the 2003 analysis of the Gonorrhoea Resistance to Antimicrobials Surveillance Programme (GRASP), Black-Caribbean heterosexual men accounted for 44 per cent and

women for 32 per cent of diagnoses in England and Wales in 2003. The majority of diagnoses in MSM are in the White ethnic group.[24]

HIV/AIDS

Human Immunodeficiency Virus (HIV) prevents the immune system from working properly. Around a quarter of new HIV cases are resistant to one or more of the antiviral drugs now available. If untreated, almost all HIV infected people will develop Acquired Immune Deficiency Syndrome (AIDS) and die.[1]

HIV is usually transmitted through sexual intercourse, in the womb (mother to foetus), or through blood and blood products, including the use of contaminated needles by intravenous drug users. There is substantial biological evidence demonstrating that the presence of STIs increases the likelihood of both transmitting and acquiring HIV.[25]

Apparent trends over time must be interpreted with care, as each data source is subject to reporting delay which varies over time. Also, diagnosis depends upon risk recognition, willingness to have an HIV test and test accessibility.

Number of HIV diagnoses

The number of diagnosed HIV-infected patients seen for care in the UK in 2003 was 37,079: 34,103 in England, 1,651 in Scotland, 575 in Wales and 189 in Northern Ireland, with over half of those infected living in Greater London (Table 6.15).

The distribution of diagnosed cases by exposure category varied with place of residence, with 45 per cent of all diagnoses in the UK being among heterosexuals (ranging from 35 per cent in Scotland to 45 in England) and 43 per cent among

Table **6.15**

Diagnosed HIV-infected patients seen for care: by exposure category and country, 2002

United Kingdom   Percentages

	Overall UK total	England	Scotland	Wales	N Ireland	Greater London
Heterosexual men and women	45	45	35	38	41	43
Men who have sex with men	43	44	37	48	51	46
Injecting drug users	4	3	22	3	3	3
Mother to infant	3	3	0	4	3	4
Blood / blood products	1	1	2	5	1	1
Other / not reported	4	4	3	2	2	4
Total Numbers	37,039	34,103	1,651	575	189	19,071

1 Includes 49 diagnosed individuals resident in England for whom SHA of residence was not known.
2 Scotland includes Grampian, Greater, Glasgow, Lothian, Tayside, Argyll and Clyde, Ayrshire and Arran, Borders, Dumfries and Galloway, Fife, Forth
   Valley, Highland, Lanarkshire, Orkney, Shetland and Western Isles NHS boards.
3 Total includes those resident abroad, 'other', or not known

Source: Health Protection Agency

MSM (ranging from 37 in Scotland to 51 in Northern Ireland). In England and Scotland the heterosexual and MSM proportions were similar but in both Wales and Northern Ireland the MSM proportion was 10 percentage points higher than the heterosexual rate.

The largest difference between countries within the UK was among injecting drug-users. This category accounted for 4 per cent of all diagnoses in the UK, but accounted for 22 per cent of diagnoses in Scotland compared to 3 per cent in each of the other countries. Other known exposure routes included blood and blood products and mother to infant.[24]

Many people are infected with HIV but are unaware of the fact. The Health Protection Agency has calculated undiagnosed HIV infection; the method of calculation is set out in *Focus on Prevention*.[24] Among those infected through heterosexual activity in 2003, 58 per cent were women. However a far higher percentage of men were estimated to be undiagnosed: 39 per cent compared with 22 per cent of women. In terms of ethnicity, twice as many African women were infected as were non-Africans. The difference for men was less dramatic, with 59 per cent being African. Africans of both sexes were more likely to be diagnosed than were non-Africans. Some 86 per cent of African women were diagnosed compared with 62 per cent of non-Africans, the corresponding rates for men being 67 and 48 per cent respectively (Figure 6.16).[24]

Trends in HIV and AIDS cases

HIV is mainly transmitted through sex. Sex between men was the main route of HIV infection until 1999 in the UK, after which heterosexual transmission predominated.[26] Diagnoses of

Figure **6.16**

Estimates of HIV cases among heterosexuals:[1] by ethnicity and sex, 2003

United Kingdom

Numbers

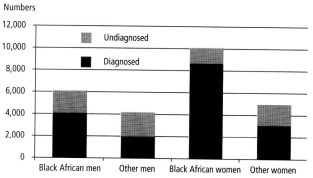

1   Adults aged 16–44.

Source: Health Protection Agency

HIV among MSM exceeded 1,700 in 1991, after which the number fell gradually during the 1990's to less than 1,400 in 1999. Subsequently the annual figure has again been on the increase, exceeding 1,700 once more by 2001. By contrast, diagnoses among heterosexuals rose gradually from around 500 in 1990, to exceed 1,000 by 1997. After this date the number more than doubled over the next three years, and nearly doubled again during the following three, to reach approximately 3,800 by 2003. Round figures only are quoted for HIV diagnoses because these counts are subject to change as further reports are received (Figure 6.17).

Figure **6.17**

HIV diagnoses,[1] in MSM[2] and heterosexuals, 1989–2003

United Kingdom

Numbers

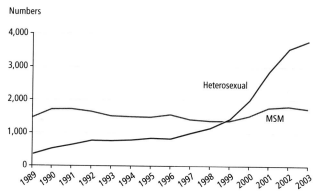

1   Numbers, particularly for recent years, will rise as further notifications are received.
2   Men who have sex with men.

Source: Health Protection Agency

Samples from pregnant women are tested anonymously for HIV infection, around 85 per cent of pregnant women being covered in 1993. The rate of infections in those tested in England greatly increased between 1993 and 2003, but hardly varied in Scotland. During this time the rate for London was mostly at least twice that for the rest of England. However from the year 2000 onwards there have been sharp increases in the rate for the rest of England, to the extent that by 2003 it had reached 55 per 10,000 population, compared to 45 for London (Figure 6.18).

Diagnoses of AIDS increased from 1,083 in 1989 to 1,852 in 1994 then decreased to 766 in 2003, fluctuating in the last four years. The number of deaths from AIDS rose from 744 in 1989 to 1,719 in 1995. However the number halved between 1996 and 1997 and continued to fall, with some fluctuations, reaching 475 in 2003.

Figure **6.18**

HIV prevalence[1] in females giving birth: by region[2] of mother's residence, 1993–2003

England and Scotland

Rate per 10,000

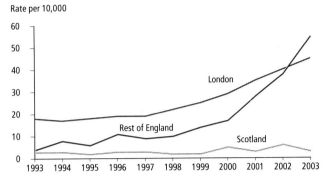

1 Data provided from the Unlinked anonymous dried blood spot survey.
2 Rates for 'Rest of England', may be slightly overestimated because data from Yorkshire and Humberside include some from the antenatal survey.

Source: Health Protection Agency

Conclusion

Over the last ten years there have been clear changes in sexual behaviour, (or in the proportion of people who report them), especially among younger people. Many of these behaviours, such as anal sex and promiscuity, are high-risk in terms of sexual health particularly when people do not use condoms. Use of alcohol increases the likelihood of high-risk behaviour. More people had heterosexual sex before they were aged 16, the legal age of consent, and increasing numbers of people have had ten or more sexual partners. There are differences in sexual behaviour between men and women, and within the UK.

The results of high-risk behaviour can be seen in the use of the 'morning-after pill' and increases in STIs. Teenage pregnancies are falling, but high rates are associated with deprivation and urban areas.

The rates of STIs increased significantly in recent years, particularly for syphilis and chlamydia. Rates varied with age, sex, ethnicity, sexual orientation and area of residence.

There are an increasing number of people living with HIV, with the number of diagnosed cases tripling over 15 years. From 1995 heterosexual sex replaced MSM as the most common route of exposure. AIDS diagnoses and deaths have fallen over the last eight years.

References

1. House of Commons Health Select Committee (2003) *House of Commons Health Select Committee Report on Sexual Health*, TSO: London.

2. Department of Health (2001) *Better Prevention, Better Services, Better Sexual Health: the national Strategy for Sexual Health and HIV.*

3. Flanigan B J and Hitch M A (1986) Alcohol use, sexual intercourse and contraception: an exploratory study. *Journal of Alcohol and Drug Education* **31(3)**, 6–40.

4. Robertson J A and Plant M A (1988) Alcohol, sex and risks of HIV infection. *Drug and Alcohol Dependence* **22(1)**, 75–78.

5. Traeen B and Lundin Kvalem I (1996) Sex under the influence of alcohol among Norwegian adolescents. *Addiction* **9(7)**, 995–1006.

6. Erens B *et al* (2003) *National Survey of Sexual Attitudes and Lifestyles II: Reference tables and summary report*, National Centre for Social Research: London.

7. *Northern Ireland Health and Social Wellbeing Survey 2001*, Northern Ireland Statistics and Research Agency

8. Currie C *et al* (eds.) (2004) *Young people's health in context Health Behaviour in School-aged Children (HBSC) study: international report from the 2001/2002 survey*, World Health Organisation: Denmark.

9. Dawe F and Rainford L (2004) *Contraception and Sexual Health, 2003:* A report on research using the ONS Omnibus Survey produced by the Office for National Statistics on behalf of the Department of Health, Office for National Statistics: London.

10. Zheng J *et al* (2004) Ethanol Stimulation of HIV Infection of Oral Epithelial Cells. *Journal of Acquired Immune Deficiency Syndromes* **37(4)**, 1445–1453.

11. Petry N M (1999) Alcohol use in HIV patients: what we don't know may hurt us. *International Journal of STD & AIDS* **10: 9**, 561–570.

12. Chamberlain J and Corbin T (2004) Trends in reproductive epidemiology and women's health, in Lewis G (ed.) *Why mothers die 2000-2002 - Report on confidential enquiries into maternal deaths in the United Kingdom*, RCOG Press: London.

13. Office for National Statistics (2005) Report: Conceptions in England and Wales, 2003 *Health Statistics Quarterly* **26**, 58–61.

14. Botting B *et al* (1998) Teenage mothers and the health of their children. *Population Trends 93*, 19–28.

15. *Technical Note for the Spending Review 2004: Public Service Agreement 2005-2008*, Department of Health at: www.dh.gov.uk.

16. Scottish Office Department of Health (1999) *Towards a Healthier Scotland - A White Paper on Health*, TSO: Edinburgh.

17. Office for National Statistics (2004) *Living in Britain* No. 31, Results from the 2002 General Household Survey, TSO: London

18. Ross J, Godeau E and Dias S (2004) Sexual Health, in Currie C *et al* (eds.) *Young people's health in context Health Behaviour in School-aged Children (HBSC) study: international report from the 2001/2002 survey*, World Health Organisation: Denmark.

19. Northern Ireland Statistics and Research Agency (2004) *Continuous Household Survey: Bulletin 3*.

20. Terence Higgins Trust at: www.tht.org.uk/press_desk and www.tht.org.uk/gaymen

21. Johnson A M *et al* (2001) Sexual behaviour in Britain: partnerships, practices, and HIV risk behaviours. *The Lancet* **358**, 1835–1842.

22. Fenton K A *et al* (2001) Sexual behaviour in Britain: reported sexually transmitted infections and prevalent genital Chlamydia trachomatis infection. *The Lancet* **358**, 1851–1854.

23. Health Protection Agency, Diagnoses and rates of selected STIs seen at GUM clinics, United Kingdom: 2002–2004, National, Regional and Strategic Health Authority Tables.

24. The UK Collaborative Group for HIV and STI Surveillance (2004) *Focus on Prevention. HIV and other Sexually Transmitted Infections in the United Kingdom in 2003*, Health Protection Agency Centre for Infections: London.

25. Fleming D T and Wasserheit J N (1999) From epidemiological synergy to public health policy and practice: the contribution of other sexually transmitted diseases to sexual transmission of HIV infection. *Sexually Transmitted Infections* **75**, 3–17.

26. Health Protection Agency, AIDS/HIV Quarterly Surveillance Tables No. 63: 04/2, London.

Morbidity

Velda Osborne

Chapter 7

Introduction

This chapter looks at the prevalence of 11 selected chronic diseases. Seven of the conditions (coronary heart disease (CHD), stroke, hypertension, diabetes, chronic obstructive pulmonary disease (COPD), asthma and epilepsy) are included because they feature in the quality and outcomes framework of the new General Medical Services Contract, introduced in April 2004.[1] The framework also includes cancer and mental health and these are dealt with in separate chapters of *Focus on Health*. The remaining four (arthritis, back problems, hay fever and migraine) are included because they are common and significantly impair the quality of life of people who suffer from them.

The Department of Health has developed national service frameworks (NSFs) for the management of CHD and diabetes. NSFs are long term strategies for improving specific areas of care. They set measurable goals within set time frames. The NSF for CHD was launched in March 2000 and sets standards for improved prevention, diagnosis and treatment, and goals aimed at securing fair access to high quality services.[2] The standards are to be implemented over a 10-year period. The first part of the NSF for diabetes was published in December 2001 and sets out a framework of care for the next 10 years.[3]

Most of the prevalence rates have been calculated on the basis of self-reported illness, as recorded by the General Household Survey (GHS). The GHS was chosen in preference to the Health Survey for England because of it's wider geographical coverage – Great Britain. During the GHS interview those who answer yes to the question 'Do you have any long-standing illness, disability or infirmity? By long-standing I mean anything that has troubled you over a period of time or that is likely to affect you over a period of time' are then asked 'What is the matter with you?' Details of up to six different disorders are then recorded for each informant. The rates reported are thus not directly comparable with, for example, those based on General Practitioner (GP) records. Further limitations of the data are that the sample size is small for the purpose of estimating disease prevalence and conditions may not be reported if for example they are well-controlled by medication, or are sporadic in occurrence or have symptoms which are mild or of short duration.

In fact the GHS was found to severely under-estimate the prevalence of hay fever and migraine when compared with other data sources, possibly for reasons connected with medication, duration and frequency. Accordingly rates for these conditions have been estimated using the Fourth National Morbidity Study from General Practice (MSGP4), which uses consultation data directly recorded by GPs.[4] MSGP4

also collected information about the socio-economic characteristics of patients, including occupation and ethnic group. Reasons for consulting were coded according to the Ninth Revision of the International Classification of Diseases (ICD-9). Variations in consulting patterns by social class (based on occupation) and ethnic group are described. Due to the nature of the data source these variations will also be related to health-seeking behaviours.

Demographic variations

Coronary heart disease

Several of the diseases included in this chapter are characterised by rapidly increasing prevalence above the age of 45 and by the disease being more common in men than in women in these age groups. Coronary heart disease typifies this pattern (Figure 7.1). The term CHD covers a number of more specific conditions including myocardial infarction (heart attack) and angina; the rates reported here are based on respondents coded into the GHS category 'heart attack/ angina'. In the 2003 sample the rate more than doubled for men in Great Britain aged 65–74 (184 per thousand population), compared to those aged 55–64 (84 per thousand population). The corresponding rates for women were 124 and 56.

Figure 7.1

CHD prevalence: by age and sex, 2003

Great Britain

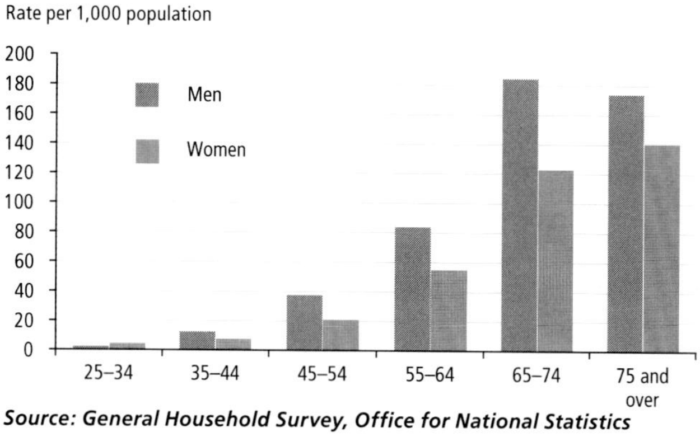

Source: General Household Survey, Office for National Statistics

CHD is preventable and the most important lifestyle risk factors are smoking, poor diet and lack of exercise. In England approximately 20 per cent of CHD related deaths in men and 17 per cent in women are attributable to smoking.[2] CHD has major economic consequences for the UK and cost the health care system just under £1,750 million in 1999.[5] However the total cost is much greater because production losses and informal care associated with CHD cost a further £5,300 million. This represents a cost higher than for any other single disease for which a comparable analysis has been undertaken.

Stroke

A stroke occurs when the blood supply to the brain is disturbed in some way. As a result, brain cells are starved of oxygen causing some cells to die and leaving others damaged. The condition shows a similar pattern of prevalence to CHD, although the rates are much lower. The 2003 GHS found prevalence rates for stroke of 11 or less per thousand population for all age groups under 65 in men and women in Great Britain. Beyond age 64 rates rose rapidly for both sexes, reaching 37 per thousand for men aged 75 and over and 27 for women in this age group. The after-effects of a stroke vary widely, depending on how much and which part of the brain is damaged. However it is the largest single cause of severe disability in England and Wales, with over 250,000 people being affected at any one time.[6] Hypertension is a major risk factor for stroke. Smoking and excessive drinking are the major lifestyle risk factors, with smokers having double the risk of stroke as non-smokers.[7] Stroke patients occupy around 20 per cent of all acute hospital beds and 25 per cent of long term beds.[6]

Hypertension

Hypertension, also known as high blood pressure, occurs when blood is forced through the arteries at an increased pressure. Blood pressure itself depends on how forcefully the heart pumps blood around the body and the width of the arteries through which the blood passes. There is a natural tendency for blood pressure to rise with age due to the reduced elasticity of the arterial system. Hypertension has a similar prevalence pattern to CHD as far as age is concerned but generally it is more common in women than in men. In the 2003 GHS sample the condition was found to be more prevalent in women for every age group except 45–54 (Figure 7.2). The major problem with high blood pressure is that it rarely causes

Figure **7.2**

Hypertension prevalence: by age and sex, 2003

Great Britain

Rate per 1,000 population

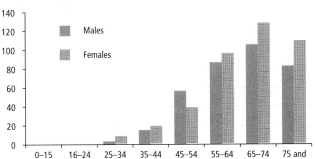

Source: General Household Survey, Office for National Statistics

symptoms but the consequences, if the condition is left untreated, can be severe and include stroke, heart attack, kidney failure and eye damage. Lifestyle factors which can aggravate hypertension and increase the risk of complications are smoking, heavy drinking, excessive salt intake, poor diet and lack of exercise.

Diabetes

Diabetes is a condition where the blood sugar level is higher than normal. There are two main types: type 1, which usually onsets in youth, and type 2, usually seen in adults over 40 and the overweight. Type 2 diabetes often has few symptoms in the early stages and it is estimated that half of those with the disease are as yet undiagnosed.[8] The GHS does not distinguish between type 1 and type 2 diabetes. Figure 7.3 shows that, over the age of 55, the disease is generally more common among males than females, although for this sample the situation was reversed for those who were 75 and over.

Both types of diabetes carry the risk of major complications and all diabetics require careful monitoring to both determine efficacy of treatment and test for longer term complications, such as eye or kidney disease. Eating a well-balanced diet, taking regular exercise and giving up smoking are all important factors in disease control.

Figure **7.3**

Diabetes prevalence: by age and sex, 2003

Great Britain

Rate per 1,000 population

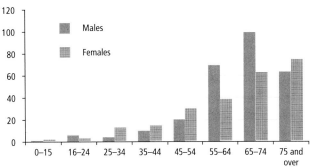

Source: General Household Survey, Office for National Statistics

Chronic obstructive pulmonary disease

Chronic obstructive pulmonary disease is the medical term for chronic bronchitis once the damage to the lungs results in airflow restriction. Chronic bronchitis is an inflammation in the lungs that causes the respiratory passages to be swollen and irritated, increases mucus production and may damage the lungs. The rates reported in this chapter are based on respondents coded into the GHS category 'bronchitis/

emphysema' and hence are a proxy for COPD. However the wording of the initial question ensures that sufferers from an isolated episode of bronchitis are unlikely to be included.

The prevalence pattern is similar to that for CHD and stroke but the rates are much lower than those for CHD: COPD rates were 14 or less for all age groups under 65 in Great Britain. The male rate for both the age groups over 64 was 28 per thousand population. For females the highest prevalence, 19 per thousand, was found among women aged 65–74, followed by a fall to 13 per thousand for the oldest age group. Smoking is the most important cause of COPD but air pollution and allergy can also exacerbate the condition. COPD accounts for about 7 per cent of all working days lost due to sickness and also accounts for more annual NHS staff resources than asthma.[9] Whereas the airway obstruction in asthma is reversible with treatment, in COPD it is largely irreversible.

Asthma

Asthma is a condition that affects the airways, the small tubes that carry air in and out of the lungs. People with asthma have airways that are almost always sensitive and inflamed. When someone with the condition comes into contact with an asthma trigger, the muscles around the walls of the airways tighten and the lining of the airway becomes inflamed and starts to swell. These reactions mean the sufferer has difficulty in breathing and may also experience attacks of coughing. Triggers include exertion, cold weather, tobacco smoke, traffic fumes and allergies (for example to pollen, house dust mites, domestic animals and certain drugs).

Asthma is quite unlike the other diseases discussed in this chapter in that it is most common among children. Figure 7.4 shows that boys tend to recover spontaneously from the condition more frequently than girls. Whereas asthma was found to be some 50 per cent more common among boys than

girls aged 0–15, the rates for 16- to 24-year-olds in Great Britain in 2003 were 29 and 54 per thousand population respectively. Treatment takes the form of relieving immediate symptoms and longer term prevention to reduce inflammation but even so around 1,400 people die from asthma each year in the UK.[10] Approximately 30–50 per cent of the risk of developing asthma is due to hereditary factors. If one parent has asthma, the chance of their child developing asthma is approximately double that of children whose parents do not have asthma. Children whose parents smoke are 1.5 times more likely to develop asthma than children of non-smokers. Over 12.7 million working days are lost to asthma each year in the UK.

Epilepsy

Epilepsy is a neurological condition in which patients have recurrent seizures. An epileptic attack happens when an abnormal electrical discharge occurs in the brain, disturbing its normal function. These attacks are usually brief, lasting from seconds to a few minutes, but can sometimes last much longer. Once the attack is over the normal electrical activity of the brain resumes. Because epilepsy is a relatively uncommon condition, demographic variation to the level of detail included in this chapter is susceptible to sampling error if the GHS is used. For this reason the rates shown in Figure 7.5 use data from the General Practice Research Database (GPRD) and are for England and Wales. There is a gradual increase in prevalence with age and little difference between male and female rates until age 75 and over, where the condition is around 40 per cent more common in men than in women. The condition is treatable with medication and around 50 per cent of people with epilepsy are seizure free.[11] The vast majority of people with epilepsy can take part in the same activities as everyone else, with the help of simple safety measures.

Figure **7.4**

Asthma prevalence: by age and sex, 2003

Great Britain

Rate per 1,000 population

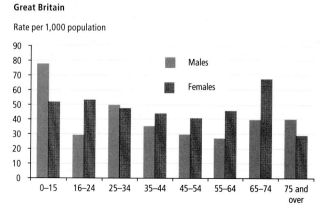

Source: General Household Survey, Office for National Statistics

Figure **7.5**

Epilepsy prevalence: by age and sex, 1998

England & Wales

Rate per 1,000 population

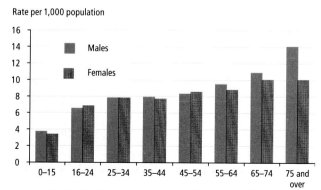

Source: Key Health Statistics from General Practice, Office for National Statistics

Arthritis

There are numerous different forms of arthritis and the symptoms can affect many parts of the body. The two most common forms are osteoarthritis and rheumatoid arthritis. In osteoarthritis, the smooth cartilage that takes the strain in a healthy joint becomes rough, brittle and weak and the bone beneath becomes deformed. The synovial membrane surrounding the joint thickens and the fluid-filled cavity within it becomes smaller. There is often inflammation and a great deal of pain. The condition is most common in the hands, knees, hips and feet. It is uncommon before the age of 40 and being overweight is a risk factor. An injury, operation or repeated strain on a joint may lead to osteoarthritis in later life. In rheumatoid arthritis, the immune system starts attacking the joints and sometimes other parts of the body. It is not yet known why this happens. The affected joints become inflamed and the sufferer may experience flare-ups where the inflammation increases in severity and the joint becomes swollen and painful. It is vital to treat inflammation quickly because any resulting joint damage cannot be reversed. People of all ages can have the condition, but it most commonly starts between the ages of 30 and 50. There are a variety of treatments available for arthritis including medication (for example non-steroidal anti-inflammatory drugs and disease-modifying drugs), physiotherapy and surgery.

The prevalence rates for arthritis reported here (Figure 7.6) are based on respondents coded into the GHS category 'arthritis/rheumatism' and thus are a proxy for arthritis. All forms of arthritis will be included if the symptoms are sufficiently severe to have troubled the informant over a period of time. The condition is more common in women than in men. This is increasingly the case with age and the 2003 GHS found the rate for women aged 65–74 to be twice the corresponding rate for men (227 per thousand population compared with 113).

Figure **7.6**

Arthritis/rheumatism prevalence: by age and sex, 2003

Great Britain

Rate per 1,000 population

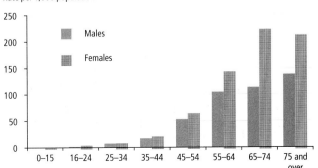

Source: General Household Survey, Office for National Statistics

Back problems

Back pain affects the majority of people at some time in their lives but many episodes will be either too infrequent or too transitory for the respondent to mention them in the context of a question on long-standing illness. Back problems have a different relationship to age than the diseases so far described, since for both sexes the GHS found the highest prevalence to be among those aged 45–64. In most age groups men are more likely to suffer back problems than women (Figure 7.7).

Figure **7.7**

Back problems prevalence: by age and sex, 2003

Great Britain

Rate per 1,000 population

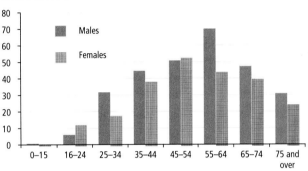

Source: General Household Survey, Office for National Statistics

Occupation is the major risk factor for back pain and it is most common in those with skilled manual, partly skilled and unskilled jobs. Particular occupations which lead to high levels of back pain include: those involving driving high mileages, driving a train, work involving intensive use of the telephone without headsets and being a supermarket cashier.[12] A study of occupational morbidity using data from MSGP4 compared the prevalence of back pain between workers aged 16–64 years in different occupations in England and Wales.[13] For both men and women, the job groups with raised prevalence largely reflected the work-related physical risk factors commonly associated with back pain (whole body vibrations, physically demanding work, frequent twisting or bending, heavy lifting, repetitive movements and work requiring long periods of concentration). For men there was a five-fold difference in prevalence between the least and most healthy jobs and for women the difference was four-fold. The female study population prevalence was significantly higher than the equivalent male prevalence (86 per thousand population compared with 64). This was due to the large numbers of women working in high risk jobs such as other medical & health care related occupations, cleaners & related occupations and catering.

The economic consequences of back pain are extremely high: in 1999 the total cost was in excess of £6,800 million, second only to CHD.[5] One in eight unemployed people say that back pain is the reason they are not working.[12] The longer someone is off work with back pain, the lower their chances of returning to work (50 per cent will return at six months but only five per cent after an absence of a year).[14]

Hay fever

Hay fever is caused by an allergy to pollen or sometimes mould spores. In hay fever the body's immune system over reacts to the presence of external substances, as if they were toxic. This results in irritation and inflammation of the upper respiratory passages and the eyes. The name is misleading because symptoms do not just occur in the autumn when hay is gathered and never include fever. A tendency to suffer allergies is often hereditary and the condition is related to asthma and eczema. Data from MSGP4 show that in 1991/92 in England and Wales, hay fever prevalence reached a peak for those aged 16–24, being 56 per thousand for women and 42 per thousand for men, after which there was a steady decline to rates of 6 and 8 respectively at age 75 and over. In childhood the condition was more common among boys than girls, whereas in adults it was more common among women for all age groups, except those aged 75 and over (Figure 7.8). The symptoms of hay fever can be controlled through treatment, but the allergy will remain. However the condition is usually more of a nuisance than a health hazard in that it is neither infectious nor does it lead to further complications.

Figure **7.8**

Hay fever prevalence: by age and sex, 1991/92

England & Wales

Rate per 1,000 population

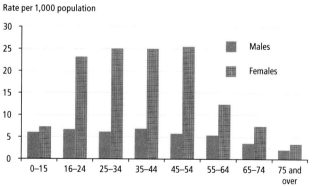

Source: Fourth National Morbidity Study from General Practice, Office for National Statistics

Migraine

A migraine is a form of headache which is severe and usually one sided, frequently associated with nausea and vomiting. This is sometimes preceded by warning symptoms such as visual disturbance (for example zigzag lines or flashing lights),

feeling depressed or even unusually happy or hungry. Every person is different but some common triggers are tiredness, stress, climatic change, hormones and certain foods (for example caffeine, cheese, chocolate, citrus fruits, red wine). The condition can have a very disruptive effect on the lives of sufferers because severe episodes can last as long as three days, during which the person is unable to carry out any of the activities of daily life. Measures of health-related quality of life have been found to be worse for migraine sufferers than for people with asthma.[15] One in three sufferers believe that the condition controls their life.[16]

Migraine prevalence varies more dramatically between the sexes than any of the other conditions described in this chapter. Between the ages of 16 and 54 the illness is some three or four times more common in women than in men. This female preponderance is commonly assumed to be associated with fluctuating hormonal levels during the female menstrual cycle. A recent study has found evidence for an association between high oestrogen states and attacks of migraine with aura and also between oestrogen withdrawal and migraines without aura.[17] This underlying cause is supported by the age variation in female rates shown in Figure 7.9, obtained from MSGP4. Beyond the age of 54 the rate falls gradually from 13 per thousand population for those aged 55–64 to four for the oldest age group. This contrasts with rates around the 25 level for the adult reproductive years. The male rate is relatively stable and less than seven per thousand population throughout the life span.

Figure **7.9**

Migraine prevalence: by age and sex, 1991/92

England & Wales

Rate per 1,000 population

Source: Fourth National Morbidity Study from General Practice, Office for National Statistics

Socio-economic and ethnic variations

Due to the small sample size it is not possible to analyse specific diseases by socio-economic factors using data from the GHS. However it is feasible to describe co-morbidities, in the form of a count of the number of long-standing illnesses suffered by each informant (informants were able to give the interviewer details of up to six disorders).

An analysis of age-standardised rates from the 2003 GHS shows the usual relationship between general measures of health and socio-economic status: those in higher status jobs tend to enjoy better health than those in lower status occupations (Table 7.10). In excess of 70 per cent of men and women in managerial and professional jobs said they had no long-standing illness, compared with around 64 per cent of those working in lower supervisory and technical and semi-routine and routine jobs. A similar pattern of variation is exhibited among those who claim to have one or more long-standing illnesses. The unemployed and those who have never worked stand out as being in particularly poor health: only 49 per cent of men and 58 per cent of women in this category had no long-standing illness. These high rates are in spite of this category being relatively young compared to those who were working or retired. This is illustrated by the fact that 63 per cent of unemployed men and 43 per cent of unemployed women were under 35 years of age, compared with 35 per cent of men and 28 per cent of women in intermediate occupations (the NS-SEC category with the highest proportion of young people).

Socio-economic variation in disease prevalence within England and Wales can be examined using MSGP4 by comparing the proportion of people in different groups who consulted at least once during the study year (1991–92) for a particular group of diseases. Results from this study again exhibit the usual social gradient found in health statistics. Those in professional, managerial and technical occupations enjoy reduced prevalence of a range of diseases and suffer very little raised prevalence, whereas the reverse is true of those working in semi-skilled

and unskilled manual occupations. The patterns of raised and lowered age-standardised patient consulting ratios (SPCRs) are shown in Table 7.11 (see overleaf). It should be noted that in this analysis, the social class of married and cohabiting women is based on the occupation of their partner. The ratios for married/cohabiting women aged 16–64, based on their own social class, show the same significance pattern as those discussed here with one minor exception; the SPCR for diseases of the nervous system is still lowered, but not significantly so.

Professional men have an SPCR of 115 for neoplasms (malignant and benign cancers). This means that they were 15 per cent more likely to consult for these conditions during the course of the study year than were all men aged 16–64 in the MSGP4 sample (the 'reference' population). In fact this is the only disease group which runs counter to expectations regarding health and social class. Both male and female professionals have a raised SPCR, whereas both male and female workers in semi-skilled and unskilled manual occupations have a lowered SPCR (84 and 91 respectively). This means that men in these types of job were 16 per cent less likely to consult for cancers than were men generally.

Professional men and women had reduced SPCRs for six different disease groups (ICD-9 chapters): mental (the most commonly occurring mental disorders in the reference populations were neuroses and depression); circulatory system (mainly hypertension, haemorrhoids, varicose veins and ischaemic heart disease); digestive system; musculoskeletal (principally back problems, rheumatism and joint disorders); symptoms (the most common of which involved the abdomen and pelvis, the respiratory system and the head and neck); and finally injury and poisoning.[13]

Table 7.10

Number of co-morbidities (age-standardised): by NS-SEC and sex,[1] 2003

Great Britain   Percentages

	Men				Women			
	0	1	2	3 and over	0	1	2	3 and over
Managerial & professional	72.5	20.9	4.6	2.0	70.5	20.0	6.7	2.7
Intermediate occupations	69.4	22.0	5.5	3.1	69.8	20.8	5.9	3.5
Small employers & own account workers	66.1	23.7	7.7	2.4	67.3	21.2	7.8	3.7
Lower supervisory & technical	65.0	23.1	7.6	4.3	63.6	23.7	7.0	5.7
Semi-routine & routine	63.8	24.0	8.0	4.3	64.0	22.7	7.9	5.5
Long-term unemployed & never worked	48.9	41.9	7.5	0.4	57.8	25.5	11.2	5.5

1 For people aged 16 and over, and based on last job if retired.

Source: General Household Survey, Office for National Statistics

Table **7.11**

Patient consulting ratios[1] (age-standardised): by ICD-9 chapter, social class[2] and sex, 1991/92

England & Wales

Ratios

		Men					Women				
		I & II	IIIN	IIIM	IV & V	Other	I & II	IIIN	IIIM	IV & V	Other
I	Infectious and parasitic diseases	103	104	99	99	93	101	98	104	105	93
II	Neoplasms	115	102	92	84	112	109	104	96	91	89
III	Endocrine, nutritional and metabolic diseases and immunity disorders	97	104	98	108	92	83	94	117	118	107
IV	Diseases of blood and blood-forming organs	89	104	102	111	111	84	99	113	116	96
V	Mental disorders	78	101	99	128	144	83	92	109	122	110
VI	Diseases of the nervous system and sense organs	98	99	99	103	109	95	99	102	104	103
VII	Diseases of the circulatory system	90	101	103	111	110	87	95	110	115	103
VIII	Diseases of the respiratory system	99	102	99	102	98	96	97	105	109	97
IX	Diseases of the digestive system	87	93	107	115	90	86	98	108	115	100
X	Diseases of the genitourinary system	96	102	99	108	100	95	99	106	108	93
XI	Complications of pregnancy, childbirth and the puerperium	-	-	-	-	-	107	97	112	103	83
XII	Diseases of the skin and subcutaneous tissue	100	101	99	98	106	91	100	103	106	104
XIII	Diseases of the musculoskeletal system and connective tissue	80	93	113	118	87	89	94	114	118	93
XIV	Congenital anomalies	99	97	81	112	162	95	93	73	112	121
XV	Certain conditions originating in the perinatal period	146	-	149	-	-	127	82	196	96	48
XVI	Symptoms, signs and ill-defined conditions	89	100	104	114	93	88	99	105	117	93
XVII	Injury and poisoning	80	92	114	119	82	92	95	113	116	92

░ Indicates significantly raised ratios.

▓ Indicates significantly lowered ratios.

1 Baseline ratio equals 100 for each sex.
2 For people aged 16–64.

Source: Fourth National Morbidity Study from General Practice, Office for National Statistics

Female professionals additionally had reduced ratios for a further six chapters: endocrine (the most common endocrine disorders in the female reference population were obesity and thyroid disorders); blood (mainly various forms of anaemia); nervous system (principally diseases of the ear and eye); respiratory system (the most common disorders being upper respiratory tract infections, bronchitis, pharyngitis and sinusitis); genitourinary system and lastly diseases of the skin.[13] However women in professional occupations did suffer a raised SPCR for complications of pregnancy. The full title of this ICD-9 chapter is complications of pregnancy, childbirth and the

puerperium, hence it includes a period of six weeks after the birth.

At the other end of the social scale both men and women in semi-skilled and unskilled occupations had significantly raised SPCRs for a range of disease groups, women more so than men. Women in this social class had raised ratios for 13 ICD-9 chapters; all the chapters for which women in the highest social class had lowered ratios and additionally infectious and parasitic diseases. The most common infectious and parasitic diseases in the female reference population were candidiasis, intestinal diseases and herpes.[13] Men in this social class had raised SPCRs for seven ICD-9 chapters; again all the chapters for which male professionals had lowered SPCRs and additionally endocrine disorders. The prevalence pattern for individual diseases in this chapter is rather different for men than for that already noted for women. Among men the most common diseases in this group are lipoid metabolism disorders (conditions characterised by high blood cholesterol), diabetes and gout.

Those categorised as 'other' with respect to social class were full time carers, students, those of independent means, the permanently sick and so on. The unemployed were classified according to their last main occupation. The heterogeneity of those classed as 'other' means that it is difficult to draw general conclusions about their health: a mixture of raised and lowered ratios are exhibited.

Table **7.12**

Patient consulting ratios[1] (age-standardised): by ICD-9 chapter, ethnicity[2] and sex, 1991/92

England & Wales   Ratios

		Men					Women				
		White	Black Afro-caribbean	Indian	Pakistani/ Bangladeshi	Other	White	Black Afro-caribbean	Indian	Pakistani/ Bangladeshi	Other
I	Infectious and parasitic diseases	100	110	101	126	93	100	106	91	96	89
II	Neoplasms	101	48	72	108	75	101	67	57	40	102
III	Endocrine, nutritional and metabolic diseases and immunity disorders	99	111	158	208	91	100	141	120	166	77
IV	Diseases of blood and blood-forming organs	99	124	152	81	144	97	209	332	262	127
V	Mental disorders	100	89	68	95	101	100	96	68	74	88
VI	Diseases of the nervous system and sense organs	100	87	108	114	103	100	100	110	129	88
VII	Diseases of the circulatory system	100	117	125	119	104	100	141	113	72	99
VIII	Diseases of the respiratory system	99	114	124	142	107	100	97	104	115	101
IX	Diseases of the digestive system	99	125	116	184	93	100	100	114	239	93
X	Diseases of the genitourinary system	100	108	90	154	93	100	106	82	107	88
XI	Complications of pregnancy, childbirth and the puerperium	-	-	-	-	-	100	95	80	137	95
XII	Diseases of the skin and sub-cutaneous tissue	100	93	120	161	103	100	109	115	136	107
XIII	Diseases of the musculoskeletal system and connective tissue	100	95	104	129	94	99	118	150	166	94
XIV	Congenital anomalies	101	122	135	-	20	100	102	133	52	60
XV	Certain conditions originating in the perinatal period	103	-	-	-	-	100	-	-	741	-
XVI	Symptoms, signs and ill-defined conditions	99	143	140	168	109	99	144	131	188	122
XVII	Injury and poisoning	100	103	93	83	78	100	112	86	108	80

    Indicates significantly raised ratios.

    Indicates significantly lowered ratios.

1 *Baseline ratio equals 100 for each sex.*
2 *For people aged 16–64.*
Source: Fourth National Morbidity Study from General Practice, Office for National Statistics

MSGP4 also enables comparison of SPCRs between ethnic groups in England and Wales. The reference group was again taken as all those aged 16–64 included in the study, the vast majority of whom were White. This is why the White ethnic group has no significantly raised or lowered ratios in this analysis. Both male and female Indians and Pakistani/Bangladeshis have a raised SPCR for a number of ICD-9 chapters, as do Black females (Table 7.12). Endocrine, musculoskeletal and blood disorders are the most commonly occurring of these disease groups. The magnitude of some of the raised ratios is notable, the highest being an SPCR of 332 for blood disorders in Indian women. These raised ratios are much greater than those found when making comparisons between the social classes, demonstrating that there is a greater disparity between ethnic minorities and the general population than is the case for the various social classes. The two disease groups which stand out as being less common among the ethnic minorities than the reference population are cancers and mental illnesses. As always, when drawing conclusions from GP datasets, the fact that the derived rates are influenced by health-seeking behaviours needs to be borne in mind.

Trends

The GHS permits the examination of trends in specific disease prevalence in Great Britain. Trends from 1995 to 2003 are described, with the omission of 1997 and 1999 when the survey was not carried out. Due to the sampling error inherent in sample surveys such as the GHS, these trends may not be as smooth as those which might be obtained from a larger data source. Of the diseases that seem to be on the increase, diabetes shows the most marked upward trend (Figure 7.13). The increase is particularly striking for females, nearly doubling, from 11 to 20 per thousand population (age-standardised rates). The corresponding rates for males were 16 and 23 per thousand population and both rises were significant.

The prevalence of hypertension also increased significantly for both men and women between 1995 and 2003. The male rate increased from 19 to 31 per thousand population and the female rate from 23 to 33 per thousand (Figure 7.14).

CHD is more common in men than in women but there is some evidence from the GHS that the prevalence among women has increased from the mid-1990s onwards. The rate in 1995 was 23 per thousand population whereas by 2003 it was 28, though the difference is not statistically significant due to the small sample size. The corresponding male prevalence rates were 35 and 38 per thousand population (Figure 7.15).

Figure **7.13**

Trends in diabetes prevalence (age-standardised): by sex, 1995–2003[1]

Great Britain

Rate per 1,000 population

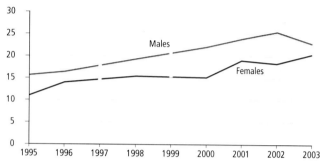

1 Data not available for 1997 and 1999. Rates prior to 2000 are based on unweighted data and from 2000 onwards on weighted data. The weighting procedure adjusts for differential non-response in different population groups.

Source: General Household Survey, Office for National Statistics

Figure **7.14**

Trends in hypertension prevalence (age-standardised): by sex, 1995–2003[1]

Great Britain

Rate per 1,000 population

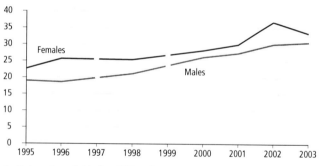

1 Data not available for 1997 and 1999. Rates prior to 2000 are based on unweighted data and from 2000 onwards on weighted data. The weighting procedure adjusts for differential non-response in different population groups.

Source: General Household Survey, Office for National Statistics

COPD shows a similar pattern of demographic variation to CHD but is much less prevalent and so a larger sample size is required to reliably detect changes over time. However there is no evidence from the GHS that the condition was on the increase between 1995 and 2003, either in men or women (Figure 7.16).

There is some indication from the GHS that the prevalence of asthma, at least in terms of it being considered a long-standing illness, disability or infirmity by the person concerned, is decreasing. The male rates during the period in question fell from 52 to 45 per thousand and the female rates from 55 to

Figure **7.15**

Trends in CHD prevalence (age-standardised): by sex, 1995–2003[1]

Great Britain

Rate per 1,000 population

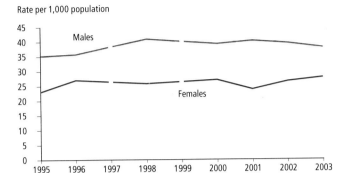

1   Data not available for 1997 and 1999. Rates prior to 2000 are based
    on unweighted data and from 2000 onwards on weighted data. The
    weighting procedure adjusts for differential non-response in
    different population groups.

Source: General Household Survey, Office for National Statistics

48 per thousand, but neither decrease was statistically significant (Figure 7.17). Results from the GPRD showed a steady and significant increase in the prevalence of treated asthma between 1994 and 1998 for both sexes in England and Wales.[18] These two sets of results are not necessarily contradictory; they may just reflect the fact that the disease is becoming increasingly better controlled through medication and that sufferers are less likely to find it troubling.

No trends in prevalence of stroke were evident from the GHS; the condition has a relatively low overall prevalence and, like COPD, requires a larger sample size to reliably identify a trend. The GPRD did in fact record a significant decrease in female stroke prevalence rates between 1994 and 1998 in England

Figure **7.16**

Trends in COPD prevalence (age-standardised): by sex, 1995–2003[1]

Great Britain

Rate per 1,000 population

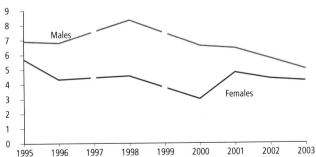

1   Data not available for 1997 and 1999. Rates prior to 2000 are based
    on unweighted data and from 2000 onwards on weighted data. The
    weighting procedure adjusts for differential non-response in
    different population groups.

Source: General Household Survey, Office for National Statistics

Figure **7.17**

Trends in asthma prevalence (age-standardised): by sex, 1995–2003[1]

Great Britain

Rate per 1,000 population

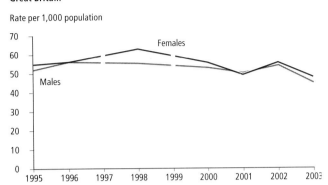

1   Data not available for 1997 and 1999. Rates prior to 2000 are based
    on unweighted data and from 2000 onwards on weighted data. The
    weighting procedure adjusts for differential non-response in
    different population groups.

Source: General Household Survey, Office for National Statistics

and Wales and a non-significant decrease for males.[18]   There was no apparent change in the prevalence of arthritis or back problems between 1995 and 2003, according to the GHS.

Conclusion

A number of the diseases covered by the quality and outcomes framework of the General Medical Services Contract are characterised by rapidly rising prevalence in the older age groups and being more common among men than women: CHD, stroke, COPD and diabetes. Smoking is a risk factor for the first three of these and those with diabetes are advised to cease smoking if possible because this disorder carries the risk of further complications. Poor diet and lack of exercise are risk factors for CHD and again diabetics need to pay attention to these aspects of life style. Excessive drinking is implicated in the occurrence of strokes. Hypertension, migraine and hay fever are generally more common among women. Hypertension prevalence increases rapidly with age whereas migraine is most common during the child-bearing years. All the previously mentioned risk factors can aggravate hypertension.

Prevalence rates based on GP consultations display the usual social gradient, with professionals consulting less than those in manual occupations, with the exception of cancer where the gradient is reversed. A similar analysis on the basis of ethnic group shows that there is a greater disparity between ethnic minorities and the general population than is the case for the various social classes. Diabetes and hypertension prevalence both increased significantly between 1995 and 2003 for men and women. The only encouraging message from the data examined is the possibility that asthma may be regarded less often as a troubling disorder.

References

1. Department of Health (2004) General Medical Services contract at: www.dh.gov.uk/policyandguidance/humanresourcesandtraining

2. Department of Health (2000) National Service Framework (NSF) for coronary heart disease at: www.dh.gov.uk/policyandguidance/healthandsocialcaretopics

3. Department of Health (1999) National Service Framework (NSF) for diabetes at: www.dh.gov.uk/policyandguidance/healthandsocialcaretopics

4. Royal College of General Practitioners, Office of Population Censuses and Surveys and Department of Health (1995) *Morbidity Statistics from General Practice Fourth National Study 1991-92*, HMSO: London.

5. British Heart Foundation (2004) *Coronary heart disease statistics 2004*.

6. The Stroke Association at: www.stroke.org.uk/media_centre/facts_and_figures

7. www.netdoctor.co.uk/diseases/facts/stroke

8. www.netdoctor.co.uk/diseases/facts/diabetes

9. www.netdoctor.co.uk/diseases/facts/smokerslung

10. Asthma UK at: www.asthma.org.uk/journalists/facts

11. Epilepsy Action at: www.epilepsy.org.uk/press/facts

12. Back Care at: www.backcare.org.uk

13. Fleming D M, Charlton J H, Osborne V A and Fear N T (2005) *A Study of Occupational Related Morbidity Presenting in General Practice*, Health and Safety Executive, at: www.hse.gov.uk

14. Clinical Standards Advisory Group (1994) *The Epidemiology and Cost of Back Pain*, HMSO: London.

15. Terwindt G, Ferrari M, Tijhus M *et al* (2000) The impact of migraine on quality of life in the general population. The GEM study, *Neurology* **55**, 624–629.

16. Dowson A and Jagger S (1999) The UK migraine patient survey: quality of life and treatment. *Current Medical Research and Opinion* **15(4)**, 241–253.

17. MacGregor E A (2004) Oestrogen and attacks of migraine with and without aura. *The Lancet Neurology* **3**, 354–361.

18. Office for National Statistics (2000) Key *Health Statistics from General Practice 1998*, Office for National Statistics: London.

Cancer

Steve Rowan, Helen Wood, Nicola Cooper and Mike Quinn

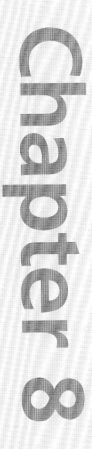

Chapter 8

Introduction

This chapter summarises information on cancer incidence (as measured by recorded cases, or registrations, of cancer) and mortality in England and Wales, and survival in England. It describes trends in the incidence of all malignant cancers (combined) over the period 1971–2001, and mortality from all cancers over the period 1950–2003. Trends in the incidence of some of the most common cancers are discussed in detail along with associated possible causes and risk factors. Trends in both survival and mortality from these cancers are also described.

Background

Cancer is a major cause of morbidity and mortality in England and Wales. One in three people are diagnosed with cancer during their lifetime, and one in four people die from cancer.[1]

Although mortality from infectious disease declined rapidly to very low rates during the 1950s, and mortality from heart disease and stroke fell more gradually in both males and females during the second half of the 20th century, mortality from cancer in both males and females changed relatively little. When grouped to Chapters of the International Classification of Diseases (ICD), all cancers are now the second most common cause of death among males and females, after circulatory diseases. If ischaemic heart disease and stroke are regarded as separate diseases, all cancers became the most common cause of death in females in 1969 in England and Wales, and in males in 1995.[1] However, no single cancer is more common as a cause of death than ischaemic heart disease.

More is known about the incidence of, and survival from, cancer than for most other diseases. This is because in England and Wales, there is a population-based cancer registration system with 100 per cent geographical coverage and mechanisms in place to follow up cases.

Cancer registration in England is conducted by nine regional cancer registries, which submit notifications to the National Cancer Intelligence Centre (NCIC) at the Office for National Statistics. In Wales, cancer registration is carried out by the Welsh Cancer Intelligence and Surveillance Unit. The quality of cancer registration data including levels of ascertainment, completeness, accuracy and timeliness have been discussed in detail elsewhere.[1, 2]

Details of the deaths registration system for England and Wales have been published.[3] Cancer mortality trends from 1950 are described here. The trends in mortality have, however, been affected by coding and classification changes over the years.

Discussions of the effects of some of the more recent changes have been published,[4–7] giving an indication of the likely effect on cancer registrations.

Both for investigations of the aetiology (causes and risk factors) of cancer, and for health care planning, incidence is the measure of primary interest, while mortality data are of value in planning resources for palliative care and hospices. Cancer incidence and mortality data each have their own advantages and disadvantages. For example, diagnostic accuracy is generally better for incidence than for mortality, but incidence data may not be as complete or timely as mortality data. The trends in mortality data, however, reflect a combination of the incidence and survival rates – and for cancers with moderate or good survival, deaths in any one year result from cases diagnosed and treated many years earlier. So mortality data on their own do not provide reliable indicators of trends and patterns related to the causes of cancer.[8]

The latest available cancer survival rates, summarised in this chapter, refer to patients diagnosed in England. Survival rates for patients diagnosed in England are representative of patients diagnosed in England and Wales because:

- The population of England accounts for almost 95 per cent of the total population of England and Wales.

- Survival rates in Wales have generally been closely similar to those in England.[9,10]

Figures in this chapter for 'all cancers' exclude non-melanoma skin cancer because the registration practices for it have varied both among the regional cancer registries, and within registries over time, and in general this cancer is believed to be under-recorded.[11]

Cancer incidence and mortality – all malignant cancers (excluding non-melanoma skin cancer)

In England and Wales in 2001, there were around 240,000 newly diagnosed cases of malignant cancer: 120,400 in males and 119,500 in females. The directly age-standardised incidence rate of all cancers was about 400 per 100,000 population in males and 340 per 100,000 in females (Appendix Tables 8A and 8B).

Cancer is, however, predominantly a disease of elderly people, and these overall rates conceal large differences between the sexes and across age groups. In 2001, after a small decrease following early childhood, age-specific incidence rates rose continuously across the age range, to peak in the most elderly group (Figure 8.1). Of the total number of cases diagnosed in 2001, only around 1,240, or 0.5 per cent, occurred in children aged 0–14; of these around a third were leukaemias. Cancers in people aged under 45 accounted for just over 5 per cent of cases in males and just under 9 per cent in females. The greater proportions of cases in females between the ages of 30 and 59 were largely due to the influence of cancers of the breast and cervix. The peak in the age distribution occurred in the 70–79 age range in both sexes.

In 2003, cancer accounted for about 28 per cent of all deaths in males and 23 per cent in females.[3] There were around 135,500 deaths from malignant cancer: 70,600 in males and 65,000 in females. The age-standardised mortality rate was about 220 per 100,000 in males and 160 per 100,000 in females (Appendix Tables 8C and 8D). The pattern of age-

specific mortality was broadly similar to that for incidence, that is, increasing steeply with age (Figure 8.2). About 95 per cent of cancer deaths occurred in people aged 50 and over, and only around 0.4 per cent in those aged under 25.

The incidence of cancer increased steadily between 1971 and the mid-1990s in both sexes. The age-standardised rate in males rose from about 330 to 400 per 100,000 over this period – an increase of around 20 per cent, while in females there was an increase of around 40 per cent, from about 240 to 340 per 100,000 (Figure 8.3). However, some of the apparent increases, particularly in the 1970s, will have arisen from improved ascertainment of cases by the cancer registries.[1]

Mortality from cancer in both males and females has changed relatively little since 1950. The age-standardised rate in males rose from about 240 per 100,000 in the early 1950s to around 290 in the mid-1970s, fell gradually until the 1990s, and then fell more steeply thereafter reaching its lowest rate ever in 2003 – around 220 per 100,000. In females, the age-standardised rate fell slightly from about 180 per 100,000 in 1950 to around 170 throughout the 1950s and 1960s before rising to a peak in the 1980s of just over 180 per 100,000. As for males, mortality decreased more steeply in the 1990s and reached its lowest rate ever in 2003 – just under 160 per 100,000 (Figure 8.3).

Figure **8.1**

Incidence of all cancers:[1] by age at diagnosis and sex, 2001

England & Wales

Rate per 100,000

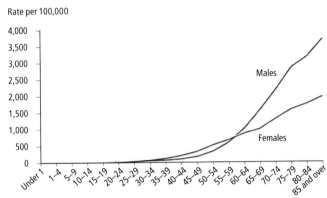

1 *All malignant neoplasms excluding non-melanoma skin cancer.*

Source: Office for National Statistics

Figure **8.3**

Incidence and mortality from all cancers[1] (age-standardised): by sex, 1950–2003

England & Wales

Rate per 100,000

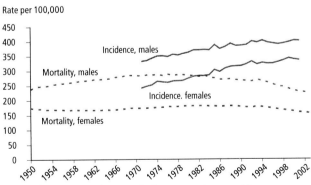

1 *All malignant neoplasms excluding non-melanoma skin cancer.*

Source: Office for National Statistics

Figure **8.2**

Mortality from all cancers:[1] by age at death and sex, 2003

England & Wales

Rate per 100,000

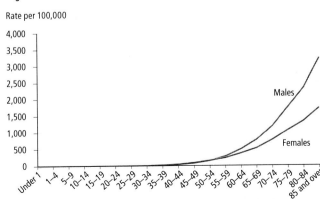

1 *All malignant neoplasms excluding non-melanoma skin cancer.*

Source: Office for National Statistics

Cancer incidence and mortality – the major cancers

In 2001, the most common cancers were prostate, lung and colorectal in males, and breast, colorectal and lung cancer in females (Figures 8.4a and 8.4b). Together these cancers accounted for more than 50 per cent of all cases in each sex.

Thirty years earlier, in 1971, the three most common cancers in males were lung, colorectal and stomach, accounting for just over 55 per cent of all cases.[12] Subsequently, both lung and

stomach cancer rates declined, and those for prostate and colorectal cancer increased (see cancer site-specific sections below). In females, the three most common cancers were breast, colorectal and lung (as in 2001) but these formed just under 50 per cent of all cases. Subsequently, the trends in breast and lung cancer increased, but colorectal cancer showed little change.[12]

The most common causes of cancer death in 2003 were lung, prostate and colorectal cancer in males, and breast, lung and colorectal in females (Figures 8.5a and 8.5b). Together these

Figure **8.4a**

Incidence of selected major cancers (age-standardised): males, 2001

England & Wales

Rate per 100,000

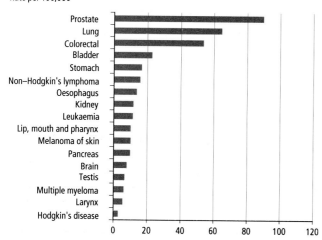

Source: Office for National Statistics

Figure **8.4b**

Incidence of selected major cancers (age-standardised): females, 2001

England & Wales

Rate per 100,000

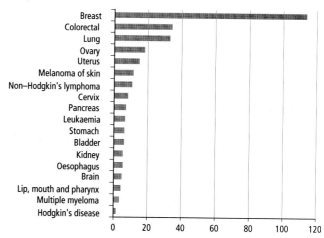

Source: Office for National Statistics

Figure **8.5a**

Mortality from selected major cancers (age-standardised): males, 2003

England & Wales

Rate per 100,000

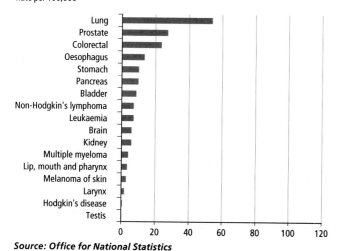

Source: Office for National Statistics

Figure **8.5b**

Mortality from selected major cancers (age-standardised): females, 2003

England & Wales

Rate per 100,000

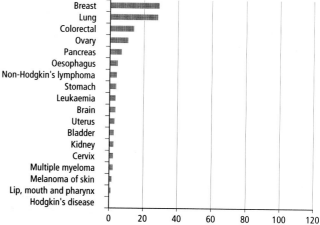

Source: Office for National Statistics

cancers accounted for 48 and 45 per cent of all cancer deaths in males and females, respectively. Just over 30 years earlier, in 1971, the three most common causes of cancer death in males were lung, colorectal and stomach and these accounted for over three in five of all cancer deaths.[12] The most common causes of cancer death in females in 1971 were breast, colorectal and lung and these formed just under half of all cancer deaths. Subsequently, mortality from breast cancer declined from the late 1980s onwards, and lung cancer mortality rates increased almost to the level of breast cancer. Colorectal cancer mortality among females also declined over the three decades resulting in a shift from being the second to the third most common cause of cancer death by the early 1980s.[12]

Five-year cancer survival rates for adults in England diagnosed during the periods 1971–75, 1986–90 and 1998–2001 are given in Table 8.6, separately for men and women. Survival from some cancers, such as melanoma of the skin and testicular cancer, has improved dramatically since the early 1970s, while survival from some of the highly fatal cancers, such as those of the pancreas and lung, has shown little change.

Breast (females)

There were over 36,000 newly diagnosed cases of breast cancer in females in 2001 and the age-standardised rate was 114 per 100,000 (Figure 8.7 – see overleaf). Breast cancer has always been the most common cancer in females – in 1971, at a rate of 67 per 100,000, incidence was double that of colorectal cancer. There was a gradual rise in incidence throughout the 1970s and early 1980s, but a more rapid increase from the late 1980s onwards, following the introduction of the NHS breast screening programme in 1988[13] (full population coverage was reached around 1994).

The effect of screening has been three-fold:

- raised incidence levels in females aged 50–54, who were being screened for the first time;

- a steep increase in females aged 55–64, as prevalent cases were diagnosed, although the rates in this age range subsequently returned to around the expected levels based on earlier trends; and finally,

Table 8.6

Five-year relative survival from selected major cancers: by sex, for patients diagnosed during 1971–2001

England   Percentages

	Patients diagnosed 1971–1975[1]		Patients diagnosed 1986–1990[1]		Patients diagnosed 1998–2001[1]	
	Men	Women	Men	Women	Men	Women
Bladder	44	42	62	57	60.3	53.2
Brain	7	9	13	15	13.3	15.4
Breast	-	52	-	66	-	79.9
Cervix	-	52	-	61	-	63.1
Colon	22	23	38	39	49.4	50.2
Kidney	28	28	38	36	44.9	44.9
Larynx	60	-	64	-	62.4	-
Leukaemia	15	14	27	27	38.2	39.1
Lung	4	4	5	5	6.3	7.5
Melanoma of skin	47	65	68	82	79.0	88.2
Multiple myeloma	13	13	19	19	25.6	25.6
Non-Hodgkin's lymphoma	27	31	41	45	50.9	54.7
Oesophagus	3	5	5	8	8.1	10.7
Ovary	-	20	-	28	-	38.3
Pancreas	1	2	2	2	2.5	2.2
Prostate	31	-	41	-	70.8	-
Rectum	25	28	37	39	50.0	53.5
Stomach	4	5	9	11	12.6	15.4
Testis	69	-	90	-	96.6	-
Uterus	-	61	-	70	-	76.2

1 Data for 1998–2001 available to 1 decimal place; data for 1971–1975 and 1986–1990 only available as integers.

Source: Office for National Statistics

- in females aged 70 and over there was a gradual upward trend throughout the 1970s and 1980s, which has continued since the introduction of screening.

Most of the risk factors for breast cancer relate to a woman's reproductive history – early onset of menstrual periods, late first pregnancy, low number of children and late menopause. Part of the increase in incidence could be related to the decline in birth rates and increase in maternal age at first birth since the 1960s. Oral contraceptives and hormone replacement therapy (HRT) have both been linked to increased risk, and the use of these increased in the 1980s and 1990s.[14] The increasing prevalence of obesity[15] may have contributed to the increase in incidence in older women, as overweight and obesity have been linked to post-menopausal breast cancer.

Figure **8.7**

Breast cancer incidence and mortality (age-standardised): females, 1950–2003

England & Wales

Rate per 100,000

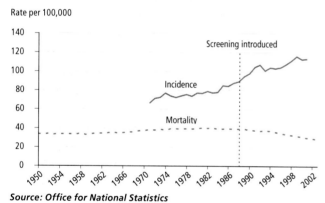

Source: Office for National Statistics

There were 11,200 deaths from breast cancer in females in 2003 accounting for about one-sixth of all female cancer deaths.[3] Since the early 1950s, it has been the most common cause of cancer death in females, but in 2003, the numbers of lung cancer deaths exceeded those of breast cancer for the first time. However, the age-standardised mortality rate in 2003 was 29.3 per 100,000, which was still slightly higher than the rate for lung cancer at 28.5 per 100,000. As for incidence, age-specific mortality increased steeply above age 40, reaching a peak in those aged 85 and over.

Mortality from breast cancer rose gradually from 1950 but by the late 1990s, the rate in females aged 55–69 had fallen dramatically, by over 20 per cent, from its peak in the mid-

1980s. About a third of this was due directly to the effect of the introduction of breast screening. The rest was due to improved treatment, including chemotherapy and increasingly widespread use of adjuvant tamoxifen, and to the indirect effects of screening, including raised awareness leading to earlier presentation and diagnosis outside the screening programme.[16]

Breast cancer is unusual in that the relative survival curve continues to decline for up to 20 years after diagnosis;[17, 18] for most cancers, the curve is virtually flat after five years. This suggests that the disease has an adverse effect on mortality well beyond five years. Five-year survival from breast cancer rose from 52 per cent for women diagnosed in England during 1971–75 to 66 per cent for those diagnosed during 1986–90. During the 1990s, five-year survival increased markedly: for women diagnosed in 1998–2001, five-year survival was 80 per cent. This improvement was partly due to earlier diagnosis as a result of breast screening, although much of the increase was due to improved treatment – as indicated by the sharp reductions in mortality despite the increases in incidence.[9]

Patterns of survival by age for cancers of the breast and prostate are unusual: five-year survival is higher in middle age, lower in younger and older patients (Figure 8.8). The reasons for generally lower survival in elderly cancer patients may include the use of less aggressive treatment in these patients.

Figure **8.8**

Five-year relative survival from breast and prostate[1] cancers: by age at diagnosis, for patients diagnosed during 1998–2001

England

Percentages

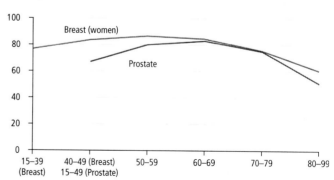

1   Numbers of diagnosed cases of prostate cancer are extremely low below the age of 40.

Source: Office for National Statistics

Prostate

Prostate cancer overtook lung cancer as the most common type of cancer in males in 1999. There were almost 28,000 newly diagnosed cases of prostate cancer in 2001 and the age-standardised incidence rate was around 90 per 100,000 (Figure 8.9). Rates increased gradually from 29 per 100,000 to 48 per 100,000 between 1971 and 1990, after which there were two periods of rapid increases – from 1991 to 1994 and again from 1997 to 2001. These recent increases are due to the increasingly widespread use of the prostate-specific antigen (PSA) test. PSA testing commonly detects asymptomatic prostate cancers in older men, which would otherwise have gone undetected and has no impact on the patient's life expectancy. Due to this and other limitations of PSA testing,[19] nation-wide screening programme has not been introduced and the test is used on an ad hoc basis.

Figure **8.9**

Prostate cancer incidence and mortality (age-standardised), 1950–2003

England & Wales

Rate per 100,000

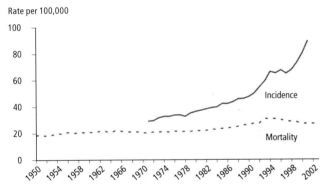

Source: Office for National Statistics

The steep increases in incidence since the early 1990s are evident in all age groups, but especially so in elderly men. The earlier underlying upward trend in prostate cancer seen throughout the 1970s and 1980s could have been due to a gradual improvement in the diagnosis of this cancer, prior to the introduction of PSA testing. Another possibility is the increasing prevalence of some risk factor(s), although too little is currently understood about the aetiology of prostate cancer to pinpoint these.

In 2003, prostate cancer accounted for 13 per cent of all cancer deaths in males, in whom it was the second most common cause of cancer death after lung cancer. There were 9,200 deaths[3] and the corresponding age-standardised rate was 27 per 100,000.

The age-standardised mortality rates have been much more stable over time compared with those for incidence, although a steady rise from the early 1980s (in parallel with incidence) resulted in deaths from prostate cancer overtaking those from colorectal cancer in the early 1990s.

Five-year survival for men diagnosed in England with prostate cancer during 1971–75 was 31 per cent. There has been a large increase in survival of 40 percentage points since the early 1970s. In comparison with most other cancers, survival from prostate cancer is relatively high, with five-year survival of 71 per cent for patients diagnosed during 1998–2001. The estimated survival rates are highly sensitive to the inclusion of localised cancer, detected by PSA testing during the 1990s. These cases tend to have a good prognosis, which has the effect of increasing the survival estimates.

Lung

Lung cancer is much more common in males than in females – in 2001, there were around 20,000 newly diagnosed cases in males and 13,000 in females. Up to the early 1990s, lung cancer was by far the most common cancer in males, with age-standardised rates of around 110 per 100,000 throughout the 1970s and early 1980s (Figure 8.10). From the mid-1980s incidence began to fall steadily, and continued to do so throughout the 1990s, reaching a rate of 65 per 100,000 in 2001 – a decrease of around 40 per cent from the level in the mid-1970s. Rates of lung cancer in females were always considerably lower than those in males, but the pattern of incidence over time is quite different to that for males; changes in the incidence lag around 20 years behind those in males, and only reached a plateau in the mid-1990s. Incidence rose from 19 per 100,000 in 1971 to around 34 per 100,000 in the early 1990s – an increase of nearly 80 per cent – and remained close to this level up to 2001.

Figure **8.10**

Lung cancer incidence and mortality (age-standardised): by sex, 1950–2003

England & Wales

Rate per 100,000

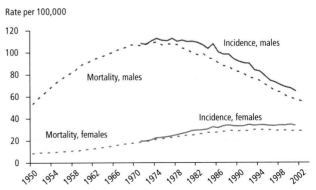

Source: Office for National Statistics

By far the greatest risk factor for lung cancer is tobacco smoking,[20] and the differences in the patterns of incidence between the sexes reflect historical differences in smoking habits. Cigarette smoking became popular in males about 20 years earlier than in females, reaching a peak in males in the late 1940s. Smoking levels declined from this point, but in females levels remained fairly constant for the following 20 years,[21] and only started to decline after 1970. The peaks in the incidence of lung cancer for males and females, in the early 1970s and mid-1990s, respectively, were around 20 years later than the peaks in the prevalence of smoking, reflecting the long period between exposure and onset for lung cancers attributable to smoking.

In 2003, 17,200 males and 11,600 females died from lung cancer.[3] It was the most common cause of cancer death in both males and females, accounting for nearly a quarter of all cancer deaths in males and about a sixth of all cancer deaths in females. In males, the age-standardised rate was 54 per 100,000, and in females, 29 per 100,000, a male-to-female ratio of nearly 2:1. Following the pattern of incidence, mortality rose steeply with age to peak in males aged 85 and over and in females aged 75–84.

Trends in mortality from lung cancer over time are closely similar to those for incidence, due to the very low survival rates. In males, the age-standardised rate doubled from 53 per 100,000 in 1950 to a peak of almost 110 per 100,000 in 1974. The rate began to decline in the early 1980s reaching levels similar to those in the early 1950s by 2003. In females, changes in the mortality rate lag around 20 years behind those in males, and only reached a plateau of around 30 per 100,000 in the mid-1990s, declining slightly thereafter.[1]

Lung cancer has one of the lowest survival rates of any cancer and improvements in survival have been very small. In both men and women, five-year survival rates from lung cancer improved by less than one percentage point on average every five years between 1971–75 and 1986–90, with this trend continuing during the 1990s. For lung cancer patients diagnosed in England during 1998–2001, five-year survival was 6 per cent in men and 7 per cent in women. The low rates of survival are explained by the frequently advanced stage of the disease at diagnosis, the aggressiveness of the disease and the large number of patients for whom surgery is not appropriate. Five-year survival falls from 28 and 36 per cent at the youngest ages for males and females respectively, to around only 2 per cent for the most elderly (Figure 8.11).

Figure **8.11**

Five-year relative survival from lung cancer: by age at diagnosis and sex, for patients diagnosed during 1998–2001

England

Percentages

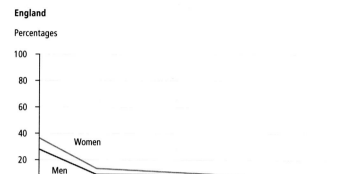

Source: Office for National Statistics

Colorectal (colon and rectum combined)

In 2001, there were similar numbers of colorectal cancer cases in males and females, close to 16,000 and 14,000, respectively, but the age-standardised rate was considerably higher in males – 53 per 100,000 compared with 35 per 100,000 in females, a ratio of 1.5 to 1 (Figure 8.12). Colorectal cancer was the second most common cancer in males up to the early 1990s, when it was overtaken by prostate cancer. There was a gradually increasing trend from the early 1970s with rates increasing from 43 per 100,000 in 1971 to around 56 per 100,000 by the late 1990s. In females, rates of colorectal cancer remained remarkably constant over the period, varying by only about 10 per cent. Although the incidence of colorectal cancer was over 70 per cent higher than that of lung cancer in females in 1971,

Figure **8.12**

Colorectal cancer incidence and mortality (age-standardised): by sex, 1950–2003

England & Wales

Rate per 100,000

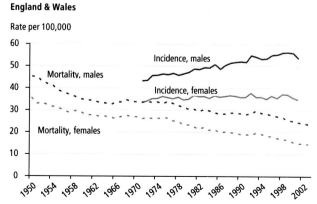

Source: Office for National Statistics

the increasing incidence of lung cancer has resulted in a narrowing of the difference to only about 10 per cent since the late 1980s.

Around a third of colorectal cancers are thought to be caused by inheritable genetic factors.[22] The main 'environmental' risk factors are poor diet,[23] obesity[24] and smoking.[23] In particular, there is evidence that a diet high in vegetables decreases the risk of colorectal cancer, and although the role of dietary fibre intake is unclear,[26] recently published results from the EPIC study (the European Prospective Investigation into Cancer and Nutrition) suggest that dietary fibre is protective.[27]

About 7,500 males and 6,600 females died from colorectal cancer in 2003,[3] accounting for around a tenth of all cancer deaths in both sexes. The age-standardised mortality rates were 24 and 14 per 100,000 in males and females, respectively. The age-specific mortality rates followed a similar pattern to those for incidence, with rates rising steeply in both males and females from about age 50.

Despite an increase in incidence in males and little change in females, there have been declines in the age-standardised mortality rates from colorectal cancer in both sexes over time. The mortality rates fell by nearly 50 per cent in males and nearly 60 per cent in females between 1950 and 2003. Consequently, mortality from colorectal cancer in males was exceeded by that from prostate cancer in the early 1990s, and in females by lung cancer deaths in the late 1970s.

There were clear and substantial improvements in five-year survival from cancers of the colon and rectum between the late 1970s and early 1980s. These were followed by further increases in survival in the 1990s. Overall, five-year survival from both colon and rectal cancer increased by just over 25 percentage points between the early 1970s and the late 1990s. For patients diagnosed in England during 1998 to 2001, five-year survival from colon cancer was around 50 per cent for both men and women; and from rectal cancer, was 50 per cent for men and 54 per cent for women. These trends suggest that improvements in survival may be attributable both to earlier diagnosis and to improved treatment,[28] the latter by improvements in surgery[29] and reductions in operative mortality.[30] Survival from cancer of the colon varied much less across the age groups than for most cancers (Figure 8.13).

Figure **8.13**

Five-year relative survival from colon cancer: by age at diagnosis and sex, for patients diagnosed during 1998–2001

England

Percentages

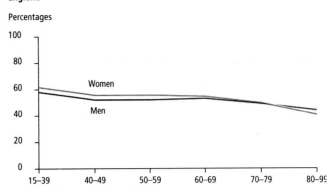

Source: Office for National Statistics

Bladder

Bladder cancer was the fourth most common cancer in males in 2001, with 7,000 cases registered and an age-standardised incidence rate of 22.7 per 100,000. In females, it was a less common cancer with 2,800 newly diagnosed cases in 2001 and a rate of 6.4 per 100,000. Trends in the incidence of this cancer over time have been similar in both sexes, but with rates in females always around a quarter of those in males. In both males and females, incidence increased steadily through the 1970s, up to the late 1980s, levelled off, and then began to decline around the mid-1990s.

By 2001, the rates in both sexes had returned to around the levels seen in 1971. However, there are well-recognised differences in the classification and registration of some bladder tumours, which are recorded as malignant by some cancer registries and as non-malignant (benign) by others.[31] For the period 1995–99, in England, over 90 per cent of bladder cancers were recorded as malignant in five of the nine regional cancer registries. The remaining four registries – Northern and Yorkshire, North Western, East Anglia and Thames – classified between 60 and 77 per cent of their bladder tumours as malignant.[31]

Cigarette smoking is an established risk factor for bladder cancer, but the time trends in incidence do not resemble those of lung cancer, which suggests they cannot be explained by changes in the prevalence of smoking. Bladder cancer is also strongly linked to occupational exposure to chemicals in the dye and rubber industries.[32, 33] Several chemicals were banned in the 1950s and 1960s, which may have contributed to the decline in incidence.

Age-standardised mortality rates in males increased gradually from around 10 per 100,000 in the 1950s, to a peak of about 12–13 per 100,000 in the 1970s and fell thereafter to rates of around 9 per 100,000 by the 2000s. For females, trends over time were more stable with mortality rates between 3 and 4 per 100,000 over the period 1950–2003.

Bladder cancer is one of the few cancers in which men have a substantial survival advantage over women; for adults diagnosed in England during 1998–2001 the difference was seven percentage points at five years after diagnosis. Differences in the proportions of small papillomas could underlie at least part of the observed differences in survival between men and women.[9] The advantage for men is most marked in those aged 15–49 or 70–99 at diagnosis; this may be due to the registration of more transitional cell papillomas in these age groups. Age is also an important factor. Five-year survival from bladder cancer for men diagnosed during 1998–2001 aged 15–49 was 84 per cent, but was just 46 per cent for men aged 80–99 at diagnosis (Figure 8.14).

Overall, relative survival at five years after diagnosis was 60 per cent in men and 53 per cent in women, for patients diagnosed during 1998 to 2001. Survival had improved similarly in both men and women, by approximately four and six percentage points, respectively, every five years during the 1970s and early 1980s, but there was less improvement in survival thereafter.

Figure **8.14**

Five-year relative survival from bladder cancer: by age at diagnosis and sex, for patients diagnosed during 1998–2001

England

Percentages

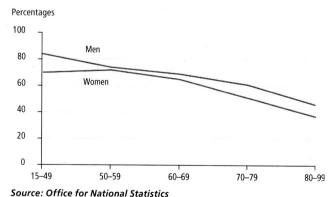

Source: Office for National Statistics

Stomach and oesophagus

In 1971, stomach cancer was the third most common type of cancer in males and the fourth most common in females, but by 2001 these ranks had fallen to fifth and ninth, respectively. The incidence rate in males has always been around double that in females. Over the last three decades of the 20th century

the rates in both sexes declined steadily, by almost 50 per cent in males and about 55 per cent in females to 16.6 and 6.6 per 100,000, respectively, in 2001.

Dietary factors are strongly related to stomach cancer. High intake of salt and nitrates (in preserved foods) increases the risk,[34] whereas high intake of fresh fruit and vegetables and vitamin C has a protective effect.[35]

Mortality from stomach cancer has been declining steadily in both sexes since 1950 and more quickly than for incidence. In 2003, the age-standardised mortality rates in males and females were 10.1 and 4.2 per 100,000, respectively, compared with 43.9 and 26.5 per 100,000, respectively, in 1950.

Survival from stomach cancer for patients diagnosed in England during 1998–2001 was quite low – only around 13 per cent after five years in men and 15 per cent in women. However, this is still an improvement on patients diagnosed in the early 1970s when five-year survival was around 5 per cent. The frequently advanced stage of the disease at diagnosis and the small numbers of patients who are suitable for curative surgery explain the low rates of survival from stomach cancer.

Around 4,100 males and 2,400 females were diagnosed with oesophageal cancer in 2001. Incidence rates have increased gradually in both sexes from 7.7 and 4.2 per 100,000 in 1971 for males and females, respectively, to 13.7 and 5.7 in 2001.

There are two main types of oesophageal cancer; squamous cell carcinoma (SCC) and adenocarcinoma. For SCC, the main risk factors are excessive alcohol consumption and tobacco smoking, which in combination have an effect that is greater than additive.[36] Smoking is also associated with an increased risk of adenocarcinoma and overall, over 70 per cent of deaths from cancer of the oesophagus in England in 1998–2002 were estimated to be attributable to smoking.[37] Poor diet is also associated with adenocarcinoma, but the main risk factor is obesity and the increasing prevalence of obesity in the UK population may have contributed to the increasing incidence of this type of oesophageal cancer.[15]

Around 4,100 males and 2,300 females died from oesophageal cancer in 2003.[3] The age-standardised mortality rate was 13.4 per 100,000 for males – in whom it was the fourth most common cause of cancer death – and 5.0 per 100,000 for females, a male-to-female ratio of 2.7:1. Trends in mortality closely followed those of incidence because of the low survival rates from oesophageal cancer.

Survival from cancer of the oesophagus is low in both sexes. In England, over the period 1971–2001, five-year survival increased by around only five percentage points to 8 per cent in men and 11 per cent in women, for patients diagnosed during 1998–2001. Survival decreased with age and was considerably better than average in the younger patients (aged 15–39).

Although survival rates for cancers of the oesophagus and stomach are broadly similar, the mortality-to-incidence ratio (the age-standardised mortality rate for a cancer divided by the age-standardised incidence rate) is much higher than would be expected for cancer of the oesophagus, and lower than would be expected for stomach cancer, especially for males. This suggests some misclassification of deaths from stomach cancer to cancer of the oesophagus[38] although it is not clear why this occurs more in males than females.

Ovary and uterus

Cancers of the ovary and uterus were the fourth and fifth most common cancers, respectively, in females in 2001. The incidence of both these cancers has increased gradually: rates per 100,000 for ovarian cancer from around 15 in 1971 to 18 in 2001 (27 per cent increase), and uterine cancer from 11 to 15 over the same period (39 per cent increase).

The main risk factors for these cancers are the same as those for breast cancer: early onset of menstrual periods, low number of children and late menopause. Cancer of the uterus is also strongly associated with obesity, so the increasing prevalence of obesity[15] may have contributed to the increase in the incidence of this cancer. As with breast cancer, the increase in incidence could be related to the decline in birth rates since the 1960s. However, unlike breast cancer, prolonged use of oral contraceptives is associated with a reduced risk from both ovarian[39] and uterine[40] cancers.

In 2003, about 4,100 females died from ovarian cancer, making it the fourth most common cause of cancer death in females, accounting for more deaths than all the other gynaecological cancers combined.[3] Over the period 1950–2003, the age-standardised mortality rate remained relatively stable at around 11–13 per 100,000. However, this rate disguises rises and falls in the different age groups. For females aged 75 and over, there was a doubling of the age-specific rate over the period, as well as a 50 per cent increase for those aged 65–74, whereas rates fell in the 20–59 age range.

Ovarian cancer has the lowest survival of the gynaecological cancers, essentially because it is often at an advanced stage when diagnosed. Symptoms of ovarian cancer are frequently vague and are difficult to distinguish from other conditions. The improvements in survival occurred for women diagnosed between the late 1970s and early 1980s, and during the mid-1990s, with increases of around five percentage points in five-

year survival during both periods. In England, relative survival for women diagnosed during 1998–2001 was 38 per cent at five years after diagnosis.

Over the period 1950 to 2003, the age-standardised mortality rate from cancer of the uterus fell gradually from 6.2 per 100,000 in 1950, to 3.3 per 100,000 in 2003.

Cancer of the uterus has a higher survival rate than for many other cancers because it can be diagnosed at an early stage. Early diagnosis is aided by its early presentation with post-menopausal bleeding or particularly irregular or heavy bleeding around the menopause. If detected at an early stage, both cancer of the uterus and pre-cancerous changes that carry a high risk of progressing to cancers are curable in most cases. Five-year survival improved on average by almost three percentage points every five years for women diagnosed during 1971–2001. Five-year survival for women diagnosed in England during 1998–2001 was 76 per cent.

Cervix

In 1971, the incidence of cervical cancer was higher than that of both ovarian and uterine cancers, at around 16 per 100,000. There was a small decline in incidence through the 1970s, followed by a sharp increase in the mid-1980s. Then, following the introduction of the national cervical screening programme in 1988, there was a sharp decline in incidence levels, which fell to around 9 per 100,000 in 2001.

Between 1950 and the early 1990s, the mortality rate for cervical cancer fell steadily from 11.2 to under 5.0 per 100,000. This long-term decline in mortality predates the introduction of screening in 1988 and may be attributable to improvements in hygiene and nutrition, smaller family sizes, delayed childbearing and a decline in sexually transmitted diseases.[41] The downward trend steepened following the introduction of the national cervical screening programme, and mortality was 2.7 per 100,000 in 2003 – just under 1,000 deaths.

For patients diagnosed in 1986–1990, survival from cervical cancer was fairly high: five-year survival was 61 per cent. Survival declined steeply with age. In 1998–2001, five-year survival was 86 per cent in the youngest age group (under 40) but just over 30 per cent in the elderly (80 and over). From the early 1970s to the late 1980s, there was an improvement in five-year survival of nine percentage points. Although the revised screening programme was highly successful in reducing incidence and mortality,[42–44] there was no significant improvement in the treatment of cervical cancer in the period, and five-year survival for women diagnosed during 1998–2001 in England was only marginally higher at 63 per cent.

Pancreas

Almost as many people died from, as were diagnosed with, pancreatic cancer each year: around 3,100 deaths in males and 3,200 in females in 2003.[3] This reflects the extremely low survival from this cancer, which is rarely diagnosed early enough for effective treatment. The age-standardised incidence and mortality rates were roughly 10 per 100,000 in males and 7–8 per 100,000 in females in the early 2000s.

Despite the importance of pancreatic cancer as a major cause of cancer mortality, remarkably little is known about its aetiology.[45] Tobacco smoking is the most consistently established risk factor, at least doubling a person's risk of developing pancreatic cancer, but is estimated to account for less than 30 per cent of cases.[37, 45, 46] Dietary factors are also considered likely to be involved, with the strongest evidence relating to a probable protective effect of vegetable and fruit consumption.[26]

The mortality rates in both males and females increased between 1950 and the late 1970s. For males, the rates subsequently fell, while in females, the rates levelled off and remained stable thereafter. By 2003, the age-standardised mortality rate was 9.9 per 100,000 for males and 7.2 per 100,000 for females.

Survival rates from cancer of the pancreas are lower than for any other major cancer, reflecting the advanced stage of disease and limited opportunities for effective treatment of most patients. Survival improved only marginally since the 1970s, with the five-year survival rate not significantly better than for patients diagnosed a decade or so earlier. In England, relative survival for patients diagnosed with pancreatic cancer during 1998 to 2001 was 3 per cent in men and 2 per cent in women at five years after diagnosis. Five-year survival varies with age, from 8–10 per cent at the youngest ages to one per cent for the most elderly.

Conclusion

One in three people develop cancer during their lives. The four most common cancers – breast, lung, colorectal and prostate – accounted for over half the total number of new cases (240,000) of malignant cancer registered in England and Wales in 2001. Just over half (120,400) of the total were in males and just under half (119,500) in females. Between 1971 and 2001, the age-standardised incidence of cancer increased by around 21 per cent in males and 39 per cent in females.

One in four people die from cancer. The four most common cancers accounted for just under half of the 135,500 deaths from cancer in England and Wales in 2003. Around 70,600 of the total were in males and 65,000 in females. Cancer accounted for 28 per cent of all deaths in males and 23 per cent in females. Between 1950 and 2003, age-standardised cancer mortality changed very little.

Five-year relative survival is very low for cancers of the pancreas, lung, oesophagus and stomach, in the range 2–15 per cent for patients diagnosed in England in 1998–2001; survival from colon cancer was around 50 per cent, from cancers of the bladder, cervix and prostate 53–71 per cent, and from breast cancer 80 per cent.

For the majority of cancers, a higher proportion of women than men survived for at least five years after diagnosis. Among adults, the younger the age at diagnosis, the higher the survival for almost every cancer. Survival improved for most cancers in both sexes during the 1990s.

Acknowledgements

The National Cancer Intelligence Centre (NCIC) at the Office for National Statistics acknowledges with gratitude the directors and all the staff of the regional cancer registries in England and of the Welsh Cancer Intelligence and Surveillance Unit for their continued co-operation with the NCIC at ONS in the processing of the extremely large numbers of cancer registrations and death records.

Notes and references

1. Quinn M J, Babb P J, Brock A, Kirby L and Jones J (2001) *Cancer Trends in England and Wales 1950–1999,* TSO: London.

2. Swerdlow A J (1986) Cancer regstration in England and Wales: some aspects relevant to interpretation of the data. *The Journal of the Royal Statistical Society Series A (Statistics in Society)* **149**, 146–160.

3. ONS (2004) *Mortality statistics 2003: cause, England and Wales,* ONS: London.

4. Rooney C and Devis T (1996) Mortality trends by cause of death in England and Wales 1980-94: the impact of introducing automated cause coding and related changes in 1993. *Population Trends* **86**, 29–35.

5. Office for National Statistics (2002) Report: Results of the ICD-10 bridge coding study, England & Wales, 1999. *Health Statistics Quarterly* **14**, 75–83.

6. Brock A, Griffiths C and Rooney C (2004) The effect of the introduction of ICD-10 on cancer mortality trends in England and Wales. *Health Statistics Quarterly* **23**, 7–17.

7. Rooney C, Griffiths C and Cook L (2002) The implementation of ICD10 for cause of death - some preliminary results from the bridge coding study. *Health Statistics Quarterly* **13**, 31–41.

8. Coleman M P, Babb P J, Stockton D, Forman D and Moller H (2000) Trends in breast cancer incidence, survival and mortality in England and Wales. *Lancet* **356**, 590–591.

9. Coleman M P, Babb P, Damiecki P, Grosclaude P, Honjo S, Jones J, Knerer G, Pitard A, Quinn M, Sloggett A and De Stavola B (1999) *Cancer Survival Trends in England and Wales, 1971–1995: Deprivation and NHS Region,* TSO: London.

10. Berrino F, Capocaccia R, Coleman M P, Esteve J, Gatta G, Hakulinen T, Micheli A, Sant M and Verdecchia A (2003) Survival of Cancer Patients in Europe: the EUROCARE-3 Study. *Annals of Oncology* **14, Suppl 5,**

11. ONS has been advised, both by expert epidemiologists and by members of the former Steering Committee on Cancer Registration, that non-melanoma skin cancer (ICD-10 C44) was greatly under-registered. Registration varied widely depending on a cancer registry's degree of access to outpatient records and general practitioners. It also frequently happens that a person has more than one tumour of this type, and registries had adopted different practices in recording these 'multiple' tumours.

12. Quinn M, Wood H, Cooper N, Rowan S (eds) (2005) Chapter 2, Figures 2.3 and 2.4 in *Cancer Atlas of the UK and Ireland 1991–2000,* SMPS No 6. Palgrave Macmillan: Basingstoke. www.statistics.gov.uk/StatBase/Product.asp?vlnk=14059&Pos=&ColRank=1&Rank=272.

13. Department of Health and Social Security (1986) *Breast cancer screening: report to the health ministers of England, Wales, Scotland and Northern Ireland (Forrest report),* HMSO: London.

14. Beral V (2003) Breast cancer and hormone-replacement therapy in the Million Women Study. *Lancet* **362**, 419–427.

15. Seidell J C and Flegal K M (1997) Assessing obesity: classification and epidemiology. *British Medical Bulletin* **53**, 238–252.

16. Blanks R G, Moss S M, McGahan C E, Quinn M J and Babb P J (2000) Effect of NHS breast screening programme on mortality from breast cancer in England and Wales, 1990-8: comparison of observed with predicted mortality. *British Medical Journal* **321**, 665–669.

17. Langlands A O, Pocock S J, Kerr G K and Gore S M (1979) Long-term survival of patients with breast cancer: a study of the curability of the disease. *British Medical Journal,* 1247.

18. Zahl P-H and Tretli S (1997) Long-term survival of breast cancer in Norway by age and clinical stage. *Statistics in Medicine* **16**, 1435–1449.

19. Quinn M and Babb P (2002) Patterns and trends in prostate cancer incidence, survival, prevalence and mortality. Part II: individual countries. *BJU International* **90**, 174–184.

20. Blot W J and Fraumeni J F, Jr (1996) Cancers of the Lung and Pleura, in Schottenfeld D and Fraumeni J F, Jr. (eds.) *Cancer Epidemiology and Prevention,* second edition, Oxford University Press: New York, 637–665.

21. Wald N, and Nicolaides-Bouman A (1991) UK *Smoking Statistics,* second edition. Oxford University Press: Oxford.

22. Lichtenstein P, Holm N V, Verkasalo P K, Iliadou A, Kaprio J, Koskenvuo M, Pukkala E, Skytthe A and Hemminki K (2000) Environmental and heritable factors in the causation of cancer - analyses of cohorts of twins from Sweden, Denmark, and Finland. *New England Journal of Medicine* **343**, 78–85.

23. Higginson J, Muir C S and Munoz N (1992) *Human Cancer: Epidemiology and Environmental Causes.* Cambridge University Press: Cambridge.

24. Bergstrom A, Pisani P, Tenet V, Wolk A and Adami H O (2001) Overweight as an avoidable cause of cancer in Europe. *International Journal of Cancer* **91**, 421–430.

25. Giovannucci E (2001) An updated review of the epidemiological evidence that cigarette smoking increases risk of colorectal cancer. *Cancer Epidemiology Biomarkers and Prevention* **10**, 725–731.

26. Potter J D (1997) *Food, Nutrition and the Prevention of Cancer: a Global Perspective*, World Cancer Research Fund in association with American Institute for Cancer Research: Washington.

27. Bingham S A, Day N E, Luben R, Ferrari P, Slimani N, Norat T, Clavel-Chapelon F, Kesse E, Nieters A, Boeing H, Tjonneland A, Overvad K, Martinez C, Dorronsoro M, Gonzalez C A, Key T J, Trichopoulou A, Naska A, Vineis P, Tumino R, Krogh V, Bueno-De-Mesquita H B, Peeters P H, Berglund G, Hallmans G, Lund E, Skeie G, Kaaks R and Riboli E (2003) Dietary fibre in food and protection against colorectal cancer in the European Prospective Investigation into Cancer and Nutrition (EPIC): an observational study. *Lancet* **361**, 1496–1501.

28. Coleman M P, Rachet B, Woods L M, Mitry E, Riga M, Cooper N, Quinn M J, Brenner H and Esteve J (2004) Trends and socioeconomic inequalities in cancer survival in England and Wales up to 2001. *British Journal of Cancer* **90**, 1367–1373.

29. McArdle C S and Hole D J (2002) Outcome following surgery for colorectal cancer. *British Medical Bulletin* **64**, 119–125.

30. Mitry E, Bouvier A M, Esteve J and Faivre J (2002) Benefit of operative mortality reduction on colorectal cancer survival. *British Journal of Surgery* **89**, 1557–1562.

31. Anderson O and Stephenson J (2004) *UKACR comparison of cancer registrations. Report number 3. Bladder tumours.* Internal report. Differences in the coding of non-invasive transitional cell papillomas in the bladder will be resolved through the implementation by all registries of the recommendations made by the European Network of Cancer Registries. Registries with a high percentage of all bladder tumours recorded as malignant will have defined transitional cell papillomas as malignant tumours.

32. Case R A, Hosker M E, McDonald D B and Pearson J T (1954) Tumours of the urinary bladder in workmen engaged in the manufacture and use of certain dyestuff intermediates in the British chemical industry. I. The role of aniline, benzidine, alpha-naphthylamine, and beta-naphthylamine. *British Journal of Industrial Medicine* **11**, 75–104.

33. Case R A and Hosker M E (1954) Tumour of the urinary bladder as an occupational disease in the rubber industry in England and Wales. *British Journal of Preventative and Social Medicine* **8**, 39–50.

34. Forman D (1987) Dietary exposure to N-nitroso compounds and the risk of human cancer. *Cancer Surveys* **6**, 719–738.

35. Department of Health (1998) *Nutritional aspects of the development of cancer. Report of the working group on diet and cancer of the Committee on Medical Aspects of Food and Nutrition Policy,* TSO: London.

36. Tuyns A J, Pequignot G and Jensen O M (1977) Oesophageal cancer in Ille et Villaine in relation to alcohol and tobacco consumption. Multiplicative risks (in French). *Bulletins du Cancer* **64**, 45–60.

37. Twigg L, Moon G and Walker S (2004) *The Smoking Epidemic in England,* Health Development Agency: London

38. Newnham A, Quinn M J, Babb P, Kang J Y and Majeed A (2003) Trends in the subsite and morphology of oesophageal and gastric cancer in England and Wales 1971–1998. *Alimentary Pharmacology and Therapeutics* **17**, 665–676.

39. Weiss N S, Cook L S, Farrow DC, Rosenblatt KA (1996) Ovarian Cancer, in Schottenfeld D and Fraumeni JF, Jr. (eds) *Cancer Epidemiology and Prevention,* second edition, Oxford University Press: New York, 1040–1057.

40. No authors listed (1988) Endometrial cancer and combined oral contraceptives. The Who Collaborative Study of Neoplasia and Steroid Contraceptives. *International Journal of Epidemiology* **17**, 263–269.

41. Woodman C B J, Rollason T, Ellis J, Tierney R, Wilson S and Young L (1996) Human papillomavirus infection and risk of progression of epithelial abnormalities of the cervix. *British Journal of Cancer* **73**, 553–556.

42. Quinn M, Babb P, Jones J and Allen E (1999) Effect of screening on incidence of and mortality from cancer of cervix in England: evaluation based on routinely collected statistics. *British Medical Journal* **318**, 904–908.

43. Sasieni P and Adams J (2000) Analysis of cervical cancer mortality and incidence data from England and Wales: evidence of a beneficial effect of screening. *Journal of the Royal Statistical Society Series A* **163**, 191–209.

44. Sasieni P and Adams J (1999) Effect of screening on cervical cancer mortality in England and Wales: analysis of trends with an age period cohort model. *British Medical Journal* **318**, 1244–1245.

45. Anderson K E, Potter J D and Mack T M (1996) Pancreatic Cancer, in Schottenfeld D, Fraumeni J F, Jr. (eds) *Cancer Epidemiology and Prevention,* second edition, Oxford University Press: New York, 725–771.

46. Kuper H, Boffetta P and Adami H O (2002) Tobacco use and cancer causation: association by tumour type. *Journal of Internal Medicine* **252**, 206–224.

Appendix Table 8A

Incidence of selected major cancers (age-standardised*): males, 1971–2001

England & Wales — Rate per 100,000

Year of diagnosis	All cancers (x nmsc)†	Bladder	Brain	Colorectal	Kidney	Larynx	Leukaemia	Lip, mouth & pharynx	Lung	Melanoma of skin	Multiple myeloma	Non-Hodgkin's lymphoma	Oesophagus	Pancreas	Prostate	Stomach	Testis
1971	332.1	23.5	5.8	43.3	5.8	5.5	8.3	8.7	108.3	1.7	2.9	5.2	7.7	11.7	29.2	32.0	2.9
1972	335.1	24.5	5.7	43.5	6.0	5.7	8.7	9.1	107.2	2.0	3.0	5.6	7.9	11.7	29.6	31.9	2.9
1973	343.2	24.3	5.2	45.7	6.2	5.8	8.9	8.3	110.4	2.1	3.1	5.9	8.0	11.7	31.7	32.1	3.1
1974	350.2	23.5	5.2	45.8	6.5	6.1	9.7	8.5	112.7	2.3	3.4	6.0	8.2	12.2	32.8	31.0	3.3
1975	350.9	24.0	5.3	46.4	7.1	5.8	9.5	8.6	111.0	2.4	3.5	6.4	8.6	12.3	32.8	31.5	3.3
1976	348.4	23.8	5.2	46.1	6.6	5.9	9.3	8.1	110.5	2.5	3.6	6.6	8.9	11.9	33.8	30.3	3.2
1977	356.2	25.1	5.4	46.7	7.2	5.8	9.3	7.8	112.7	2.5	3.9	6.9	8.6	12.2	33.9	30.3	3.3
1978	353.4	25.6	5.4	45.8	6.9	5.9	9.7	7.3	110.0	2.6	4.1	7.1	9.0	12.5	32.8	29.8	3.6
1979	359.0	26.4	6.1	46.5	7.0	5.8	9.9	7.8	111.0	2.8	4.1	7.7	8.2	13.0	35.3	28.9	3.3
1980	363.1	27.1	6.2	47.2	7.1	5.8	9.6	7.8	109.7	3.0	4.2	7.9	8.9	12.2	36.5	30.1	3.7
1981	370.8	28.0	6.4	48.7	7.7	6.0	10.1	7.7	110.0	3.2	4.3	8.4	9.1	12.3	37.4	29.3	3.9
1982	370.8	27.8	6.2	48.5	8.1	6.1	10.2	8.1	109.0	3.3	4.2	8.7	9.4	12.1	38.4	28.5	3.7
1983	372.0	28.4	6.5	49.3	8.2	5.8	10.3	8.0	106.8	3.6	4.8	9.1	9.2	12.1	39.3	28.9	3.7
1984	370.8	28.8	6.7	49.2	8.4	6.2	10.3	7.9	103.4	3.5	4.6	9.6	9.6	11.9	39.8	27.3	4.2
1985	388.3	30.2	7.0	50.8	8.6	6.3	11.1	8.0	107.6	4.6	5.3	10.4	10.1	12.0	42.4	27.8	4.4
1986	374.9	29.1	6.8	48.6	8.4	6.2	10.0	7.8	100.2	4.7	5.1	10.8	10.5	11.6	42.3	27.1	4.6
1987	381.7	29.9	7.3	50.4	8.9	6.2	10.5	7.9	98.2	5.4	5.3	11.9	11.0	11.3	43.7	25.5	4.8
1988	392.3	31.5	7.2	51.4	9.2	6.8	11.4	8.3	98.2	6.3	5.5	12.5	11.5	11.6	45.9	25.9	5.0
1989	384.8	30.4	7.4	51.8	10.1	6.3	10.9	7.9	94.0	5.7	5.1	12.5	11.2	11.0	46.1	24.8	5.1
1990	385.7	30.9	7.3	52.0	10.0	6.3	10.9	8.1	91.7	6.0	5.1	13.2	11.6	11.3	47.6	23.6	4.9
1991	388.2	30.5	7.5	51.8	9.9	6.1	11.5	8.5	90.3	5.9	5.4	13.6	11.8	11.2	50.1	22.6	5.2
1992	400.0	30.9	8.1	54.8	10.5	6.4	11.0	9.0	89.9	6.5	5.6	14.2	12.4	11.1	54.8	23.0	5.4
1993	396.0	30.8	7.7	54.1	10.8	6.0	11.1	8.6	84.0	7.5	5.4	14.1	12.5	10.8	59.2	21.3	5.5
1994	402.7	30.3	7.7	53.2	11.1	6.4	11.2	9.1	82.9	7.4	5.2	14.8	12.9	10.3	66.4	21.6	5.3
1995	395.9	30.2	7.8	53.4	10.7	5.8	11.6	8.7	78.9	7.3	5.6	14.0	12.6	10.3	65.3	20.7	6.1
1996	392.9	28.7	7.7	55.0	10.8	5.9	10.6	8.9	74.5	7.3	5.5	14.1	12.6	10.2	67.6	19.8	5.9
1997	390.0	27.0	8.2	55.2	11.6	5.8	10.8	9.2	72.9	7.8	5.3	14.2	13.0	10.0	65.1	19.9	5.8
1998	393.0	27.5	7.8	56.1	11.3	5.6	11.3	9.4	70.5	8.4	6.2	14.7	12.8	10.0	67.9	19.0	6.3
1999	397.3	27.1	8.1	56.2	11.3	5.5	11.2	10.1	68.6	8.1	5.8	15.3	13.0	10.3	73.5	18.8	6.7
2000	402.7	23.8	8.2	55.9	11.8	6.0	11.9	10.2	67.5	9.7	6.2	15.4	13.5	10.4	80.6	17.8	6.6
2001	401.4	22.7	7.9	53.5	11.7	5.5	11.4	10.1	64.7	10.1	6.1	15.7	13.7	9.9	89.8	16.6	6.6

* Directly age-standardised using the European standard population.
† All cancers excluding non-melanoma skin cancer.

Source: Office for National Statistics

Appendix Table **8B**

Incidence of selected major cancers (age-standardised*): females, 1971–2001

England & Wales

Rate per 100,000

Year of diagnosis	All cancers (x nmsc)†	Bladder	Brain	Breast	Cervix	Colorectal	Kidney	Larynx	Leukaemia	Lip, mouth & pharynx	Lung	Melanoma of skin	Multiple myeloma	Non-Hodgkin's lymphoma	Oesophagus	Ovary	Pancreas	Stomach	Uterus
1971	243.3	5.7	3.8	66.9	15.9	33.2	2.9	4.9	4.0	19.1	3.1	2.1	3.5	4.2	14.5	6.9	15.1	10.9
1972	249.5	5.8	3.6	71.9	15.1	33.9	2.8	5.3	3.9	19.4	3.4	2.2	3.7	4.2	14.6	7.0	14.9	11.0
1973	254.1	6.0	3.4	73.0	15.3	35.0	3.0	5.7	3.8	20.3	3.7	2.2	4.0	4.4	14.0	7.0	14.7	11.4
1974	266.0	6.2	3.7	77.6	15.0	35.1	2.9	5.8	4.2	22.2	3.9	2.7	4.2	4.5	14.9	7.5	14.6	11.5
1975	263.8	5.9	3.4	74.6	15.0	36.0	3.0	5.9	4.2	22.5	3.9	2.6	4.7	4.7	14.6	7.4	14.9	11.7
1976	262.1	6.1	3.5	73.0	14.6	35.5	3.1	6.0	3.8	23.1	4.2	2.5	4.5	4.6	14.8	7.7	13.9	12.2
1977	266.8	6.5	3.7	74.7	15.0	35.0	3.2	6.2	3.8	23.9	4.2	2.8	4.7	4.8	15.4	7.6	13.8	11.9
1978	267.5	6.3	3.5	76.2	14.4	35.7	3.3	5.8	3.6	24.9	4.4	2.7	4.6	4.8	14.9	7.5	13.7	11.6
1979	268.9	6.9	4.1	74.4	14.7	34.5	3.3	5.8	3.6	26.0	4.8	2.8	5.0	4.6	15.1	7.8	13.2	11.7
1980	276.3	6.9	4.1	77.8	15.3	34.8	3.4	5.8	3.4	27.1	5.0	2.9	5.3	4.6	15.8	7.6	12.6	11.8
1981	282.6	7.6	4.2	77.5	15.4	36.5	3.5	6.1	3.7	28.6	5.4	2.9	5.7	5.0	15.8	7.7	12.8	11.9
1982	284.8	7.4	4.2	79.6	14.7	36.0	3.6	6.1	3.5	29.1	5.7	3.1	5.9	5.0	15.8	7.9	12.3	11.9
1983	284.6	7.6	4.4	78.0	14.8	36.1	3.8	6.7	3.6	29.3	6.1	3.0	6.3	4.9	16.3	7.8	11.9	11.9
1984	286.9	7.6	4.6	78.6	15.4	35.2	3.9	6.4	3.7	30.0	6.1	3.2	6.5	5.0	16.2	7.7	11.7	12.0
1985	305.0	8.2	4.6	85.8	16.4	36.4	4.0	6.8	3.6	32.0	7.6	3.6	7.4	5.1	16.9	8.2	11.5	12.4
1986	298.0	8.3	4.5	85.2	16.1	35.8	4.0	6.3	3.3	31.2	7.4	3.2	7.3	4.9	16.6	7.9	10.6	12.0
1987	309.5	8.1	4.6	88.4	15.8	36.1	4.2	6.8	3.6	32.9	8.4	3.6	7.9	5.2	17.5	8.2	11.2	11.7
1988	315.1	8.8	5.0	90.1	16.5	36.5	4.4	6.9	3.6	33.5	9.0	3.6	8.7	5.3	17.2	8.0	10.2	12.3
1989	317.0	8.9	5.0	95.4	15.1	36.2	4.5	6.8	3.5	32.9	8.4	3.5	8.6	5.5	17.2	8.4	10.1	12.2
1990	317.5	8.2	4.8	98.6	15.4	35.7	4.7	6.6	3.7	32.7	7.5	3.5	8.4	5.4	16.7	8.0	9.3	12.3
1991	323.8	8.2	4.8	105.3	12.9	35.8	4.9	6.5	3.5	32.9	7.7	3.4	9.1	5.5	17.5	8.0	9.3	12.6
1992	332.7	8.8	5.4	107.8	12.0	37.6	4.9	6.7	4.0	34.0	8.4	3.5	9.5	5.8	17.5	7.9	9.0	12.5
1993	322.9	8.7	5.3	101.6	11.6	35.8	4.8	6.8	3.7	33.3	9.6	3.6	9.5	5.6	17.1	7.8	8.4	12.7
1994	327.8	8.0	5.1	104.8	11.0	35.8	5.3	7.0	3.8	33.7	9.4	3.7	9.9	5.9	17.0	7.8	8.4	12.8
1995	325.6	8.4	5.4	104.0	10.3	34.9	5.1	7.0	3.9	33.7	9.6	4.0	9.3	5.7	18.2	7.7	8.1	12.9
1996	325.8	7.9	5.3	105.1	10.1	36.3	5.4	6.7	4.1	33.1	9.2	3.6	9.4	5.5	18.4	7.6	7.7	13.0
1997	330.5	8.0	5.1	108.3	9.5	35.3	5.7	6.7	4.5	33.0	9.3	3.5	9.7	5.6	18.8	7.4	7.9	13.5
1998	336.4	7.8	5.5	112.1	9.4	37.1	5.5	7.2	4.4	33.6	9.8	3.9	10.3	5.7	19.1	7.2	7.3	13.4
1999	343.4	8.0	5.1	116.8	9.4	36.9	5.9	7.3	4.6	33.5	9.6	3.9	10.9	5.9	18.6	8.0	6.8	14.3
2000	339.2	6.8	5.4	113.6	8.7	35.5	5.8	7.0	4.7	34.1	11.1	4.3	10.9	5.8	18.1	7.8	7.0	15.4
2001	337.2	6.4	5.2	114.2	8.6	34.6	5.7	6.9	4.7	33.3	11.7	3.8	11.0	5.7	18.4	7.5	6.6	15.2

* Directly age-standardised using the European standard population.
† All cancers excluding non-melanoma skin cancer.

Source: Office for National Statistics

Appendix Table 8C

Mortality from selected major cancers (age-standardised*†): males, 1950–2003

England & Wales

Rate per 100,000

Year of death	All cancers (x nmsc)**	Bladder	Brain	Colorectal	Kidney	Larynx	Leukaemia	Lip, mouth & pharynx	Lung	Melanoma of skin	Multiple myeloma	Non-Hodgkin's lymphoma	Oesophagus	Pancreas	Prostate	Stomach	Testis
1950	238.4	9.4	3.3	45.2	3.2	4.7	5.3	9.1	53.1	0.5	0.6	2.2	8.4	8.6	18.7	43.9	1.0
1951	246.7	10.2	3.6	44.9	3.1	4.8	5.2	8.9	58.0	0.6	0.9	2.6	8.4	8.9	18.8	45.2	0.9
1952	248.4	10.6	4.1	43.0	3.4	4.4	5.8	8.2	61.8	0.6	0.9	2.8	8.4	9.4	18.3	44.1	1.0
1953	249.5	10.2	3.9	41.9	3.5	4.2	5.9	7.8	65.8	0.6	1.1	2.8	7.5	9.4	19.0	43.8	0.9
1954	254.1	10.2	4.0	41.2	3.5	3.8	6.0	8.4	70.6	0.7	1.2	2.8	7.3	9.5	20.0	42.2	1.0
1955	256.1	10.6	4.3	39.0	3.7	4.0	6.3	7.7	74.2	0.8	1.2	2.7	7.4	9.7	19.8	42.7	0.8
1956	258.0	11.0	4.2	38.1	3.6	3.8	6.5	6.8	77.4	0.8	1.4	2.7	7.5	9.6	21.0	41.0	1.0
1957	260.0	11.0	4.2	37.2	3.6	3.7	6.8	6.8	80.5	0.7	1.5	2.8	7.0	9.7	20.1	41.8	0.8
1958	261.8	10.6	4.6	36.4	3.9	3.7	6.6	6.7	82.7	0.6	1.6	3.1	6.8	10.2	20.9	41.2	1.0
1959	265.0	10.4	4.5	35.3	3.5	3.5	6.7	6.6	87.4	0.7	1.6	3.1	7.3	10.7	20.8	40.8	0.9
1960	266.5	11.0	4.8	34.7	3.5	3.7	7.5	5.8	89.8	0.8	1.8	3.3	6.8	10.5	21.0	39.7	1.0
1961	267.9	11.1	4.8	34.5	3.7	3.5	7.0	5.6	91.5	0.7	1.7	3.2	7.0	10.4	20.9	39.3	0.9
1962	271.1	12.0	4.7	34.1	4.1	3.3	6.9	5.5	94.0	0.8	1.8	3.4	7.2	10.3	21.7	38.4	0.9
1963	271.2	11.4	4.6	33.3	4.0	3.2	7.4	5.0	95.3	0.8	2.0	3.5	7.0	10.9	21.7	38.1	1.0
1964	272.4	11.9	4.8	33.2	4.1	2.9	7.7	5.2	97.3	0.9	2.0	3.9	6.7	11.3	20.8	36.4	1.0
1965	274.0	11.5	4.8	32.5	4.1	3.1	7.0	4.8	99.2	0.9	2.2	3.6	6.9	11.3	22.3	36.0	1.0
1966	278.9	12.1	4.6	33.6	4.2	3.0	7.6	4.7	100.8	1.0	2.1	3.8	7.3	11.7	21.7	36.0	1.0
1967	280.0	12.1	4.7	33.7	4.3	2.9	7.4	4.6	103.6	1.0	2.2	4.0	7.3	11.4	21.3	35.1	0.9
1968	283.9	12.6	4.0	34.7	4.2	2.7	7.9	4.9	104.4	1.0	2.4	4.2	7.9	12.0	21.1	33.7	1.1
1969	284.9	12.5	4.3	33.9	4.3	2.9	7.8	4.6	106.8	1.1	2.5	3.9	7.3	12.1	21.2	33.7	0.9
1970	284.7	12.6	4.2	33.8	4.1	3.1	7.6	4.6	106.6	1.1	2.5	4.0	7.7	12.0	20.4	33.1	1.1
1971	282.3	12.5	4.5	33.6	4.2	2.8	7.6	4.4	106.2	1.0	2.5	3.9	7.7	12.2	20.6	32.4	1.1
1972	286.1	12.8	4.7	34.0	4.2	2.6	7.4	4.4	107.9	1.1	2.7	3.9	7.9	12.2	21.0	31.9	1.1
1973	285.6	12.6	4.3	33.5	4.4	2.8	7.7	4.1	108.2	1.1	2.8	4.0	7.8	12.0	21.1	31.3	1.1
1974	287.7	12.7	4.9	33.7	4.2	2.9	7.5	3.8	109.6	1.2	3.0	4.2	8.1	11.9	21.2	30.4	1.0
1975	284.3	12.4	4.5	33.0	4.5	2.6	7.8	4.2	106.8	1.2	3.1	4.1	8.1	12.6	21.0	30.1	1.0
1976	288.3	12.7	4.7	34.0	4.9	2.9	7.6	4.2	107.7	1.4	3.1	4.1	8.3	12.0	21.6	29.4	1.2
1977	284.7	12.6	4.8	33.0	5.0	2.6	7.5	3.9	107.3	1.3	3.1	4.2	8.4	12.1	21.3	27.9	1.1
1978	286.6	12.4	5.4	32.1	4.6	2.7	8.0	3.8	107.1	1.4	3.5	4.9	8.7	12.5	21.4	28.1	0.9
1979	286.7	12.2	4.5	31.4	4.6	2.8	7.7	4.1	103.9	1.6	3.6	4.7	8.5	12.6	21.4	26.9	0.7
1980	284.4	12.2	4.6	30.4	4.4	2.6	7.9	3.9	102.4	1.6	3.5	5.0	8.9	12.5	21.9	25.8	0.8
1981	283.1	12.1	4.4	30.5	4.7	2.8	7.6	4.1	99.6	1.7	3.6	4.5	9.0	11.8	22.0	25.2	0.6
1982	280.2	12.0	4.0	29.5	5.0	2.7	7.7	3.9	97.8	1.7	3.4	5.1	9.2	11.3	22.2	23.8	0.5
1983	285.1	12.3	4.6	30.5	5.2	2.5	7.8	4.2	99.1	1.7	3.8	5.5	9.6	11.5	23.1	25.1	0.6
1984	277.1	11.3	4.9	29.7	5.3	2.2	7.3	4.1	94.9	1.9	3.6	5.5	9.1	11.3	22.8	23.1	0.6

* Directly age-standardised using the European standard population.
† Rates have been adjusted for coding and classification changes over the period 1950–2003.
** All cancers excluding non-melanoma skin cancer.

Source: Office for National Statistics

Appendix Table **8C** continued

Mortality from selected major cancers (age-standardised*†): males, 1950–2003

England & Wales

Rate per 100,000

Year of death	All cancers (x nmsc)**	Bladder	Brain	Colorectal	Kidney	Larynx	Leukaemia	Lip, mouth & pharynx	Lung	Melanoma of skin	Multiple myeloma	Non-Hodgkin's lymphoma	Oesophagus	Pancreas	Prostate	Stomach	Testis
1985	275.4	11.5	4.9	28.9	5.0	2.4	7.3	3.7	93.9	1.9	3.9	5.4	10.1	11.2	23.6	22.0	0.4
1986	270.5	11.0	4.5	28.3	5.2	2.4	7.2	3.7	90.4	1.8	3.8	5.8	9.7	10.8	24.0	21.7	0.4
1987	270.4	10.7	4.9	28.4	5.2	2.5	7.2	3.7	87.8	1.9	4.2	6.2	10.4	10.8	24.4	20.9	0.5
1988	272.1	11.2	5.0	28.8	5.1	2.4	7.2	3.9	87.2	1.9	4.0	6.6	10.8	10.4	25.1	20.2	0.5
1989	269.0	10.7	5.1	28.8	5.5	2.5	7.1	3.9	83.3	2.0	4.1	6.6	10.6	10.5	26.1	19.6	0.4
1990	267.3	11.0	5.0	28.5	5.6	2.3	6.8	3.7	82.4	2.2	3.8	6.8	11.3	10.6	26.3	18.5	0.5
1991	265.9	11.0	4.9	28.1	5.4	2.4	7.2	3.9	80.2	2.3	3.8	6.6	11.3	10.3	27.5	17.9	0.4
1992	264.2	11.3	5.4	28.6	5.8	2.4	6.9	3.8	77.2	2.2	3.8	6.8	11.5	10.2	27.6	17.3	0.4
1993	269.8	11.5	5.7	29.8	6.0	2.6	7.2	3.8	76.5	2.5	4.3	7.6	12.4	10.4	30.9	16.5	0.4
1994	265.0	11.0	5.7	28.7	6.0	2.4	7.1	4.2	74.3	2.3	4.2	7.4	12.9	9.9	30.7	16.5	0.3
1995	260.2	11.2	5.7	28.4	6.0	2.4	7.3	3.8	71.1	2.5	4.3	7.8	12.7	9.9	30.8	15.1	0.3
1996	254.0	10.6	5.8	27.8	5.9	2.4	6.8	3.9	68.3	2.4	4.1	7.6	12.8	10.0	30.1	14.9	0.4
1997	246.6	10.2	6.1	27.2	5.8	2.4	6.9	3.9	64.7	2.4	4.0	7.5	12.7	9.7	29.0	14.0	0.2
1998	245.7	9.9	5.9	26.7	6.0	2.2	6.9	3.9	64.0	2.5	4.1	7.6	13.0	9.7	28.7	13.5	0.3
1999	238.2	9.4	6.0	25.5	6.1	2.2	7.0	3.9	60.8	2.6	4.1	8.0	12.9	9.6	28.3	13.0	0.3
2000	232.2	9.3	6.1	25.1	5.8	2.1	7.0	3.5	59.0	2.7	3.6	7.3	12.9	10.1	26.9	12.0	0.3
2001	228.4	9.3	6.2	24.4	5.8	2.1	7.0	3.9	57.0	2.6	3.8	7.2	12.9	9.5	27.4	11.1	0.2
2002	226.6	9.0	6.0	24.1	6.2	1.9	6.7	3.8	55.9	2.7	4.0	7.5	13.1	9.6	27.1	10.9	0.2
2003	222.1	8.7	6.0	23.5	5.9	1.8	7.1	3.4	53.8	2.8	4.0	7.2	13.4	9.9	27.2	10.1	0.3

* Directly age-standardised using the European standard population.
† Rates have been adjusted for coding and classification changes over the period 1950–2003.
** All cancers excluding non-melanoma skin cancer.

Source: Office for National Statistics

Appendix Table **8D**

Mortality from selected major cancers (age-standardised*†): females, 1950–2003

England & Wales

Rate per 100,000

Year of death	All cancers (x nmsc)**	Bladder	Brain	Breast	Cervix	Colorectal	Kidney	Larynx	Leukaemia	Lip, mouth & pharynx	Lung	Melanoma of skin	Multiple myeloma	Non-Hodgkin's lymphoma	Oesophagus	Ovary	Pancreas	Stomach	Uterus
1950	176.6	3.2	2.3	34.5	11.2	35.4	1.5	3.8	2.5	8.2	0.5	0.5	1.2	3.5	10.7	5.9	26.5	6.2
1951	173.0	3.0	2.2	34.3	10.7	32.7	1.8	4.1	2.5	8.4	0.5	0.7	1.5	3.4	10.7	5.6	26.2	5.9
1952	173.3	3.0	2.3	34.8	10.4	32.9	1.9	4.1	2.5	9.0	0.7	0.8	1.4	3.4	10.5	6.2	25.2	6.0
1953	170.4	3.2	2.6	34.0	10.1	32.3	1.8	4.4	2.2	8.9	0.7	0.7	1.5	3.4	10.6	5.8	24.3	5.7
1954	171.1	3.3	2.7	34.5	9.7	31.4	1.8	4.4	2.4	9.2	0.7	0.9	1.6	3.6	10.7	5.9	24.0	5.6
1955	170.3	3.2	2.6	34.5	9.8	30.8	1.7	4.3	2.4	9.5	0.8	1.1	1.8	3.6	11.3	6.2	23.3	5.4
1956	170.3	3.3	2.8	34.4	9.8	30.0	1.8	4.6	2.4	9.8	0.7	1.2	1.7	3.6	11.2	5.8	22.9	5.5
1957	167.9	3.2	2.8	34.0	9.6	28.8	1.6	4.5	2.4	10.1	0.9	1.3	1.8	3.5	11.3	6.3	21.8	5.4
1958	170.6	3.1	3.1	35.1	10.4	29.3	1.9	4.4	2.4	10.4	0.8	1.2	2.0	3.6	11.1	6.3	22.0	5.2
1959	169.5	3.3	3.1	33.8	9.8	29.5	1.7	5.0	2.2	10.6	0.8	1.3	1.9	3.4	11.2	6.6	21.6	5.3
1960	169.1	3.1	3.0	34.6	9.9	28.1	1.9	4.9	2.3	11.3	0.8	1.4	2.0	3.5	11.1	6.5	21.1	5.3
1961	169.0	3.1	3.2	35.1	9.4	27.6	1.9	4.9	2.2	12.0	0.9	1.4	2.3	3.6	11.4	6.5	20.4	5.3
1962	168.9	3.2	3.0	35.2	9.4	27.4	1.8	5.2	2.1	12.4	0.9	1.4	2.0	3.6	11.3	6.8	19.7	5.3
1963	168.2	3.0	3.1	35.3	9.2	27.0	1.9	5.1	2.0	13.0	0.9	1.4	2.1	3.5	11.2	6.6	19.7	5.2
1964	170.3	3.2	3.0	36.5	9.6	27.1	1.9	4.9	2.2	13.6	1.0	1.6	2.2	3.9	11.5	6.6	18.1	4.8
1965	169.3	3.4	2.9	35.4	9.1	26.6	1.8	5.2	2.1	14.3	1.1	1.6	2.4	3.7	11.7	6.9	17.7	5.1
1966	170.0	3.2	3.0	35.7	9.0	25.9	2.0	4.9	2.1	15.0	1.0	1.8	2.5	3.8	11.9	7.1	17.8	4.9
1967	171.2	3.2	3.0	36.7	8.9	26.8	1.9	4.9	1.9	15.9	1.0	1.7	2.6	3.8	11.7	7.1	17.0	4.6
1968	173.3	3.4	2.7	36.5	8.9	27.4	2.0	5.2	2.0	16.5	1.1	1.8	2.3	3.8	12.1	7.1	16.8	5.1
1969	175.4	3.3	2.8	37.7	8.7	27.1	2.1	4.9	2.0	16.9	1.0	1.9	2.6	4.1	12.5	7.1	16.2	5.1
1970	175.1	3.4	2.8	38.0	8.4	26.8	2.0	4.7	2.0	17.6	1.1	1.9	2.4	3.9	12.8	7.2	16.1	4.9
1971	175.0	3.3	2.9	38.9	8.3	25.9	2.0	4.7	1.9	18.2	1.3	2.0	2.6	4.1	12.8	7.2	15.0	4.9
1972	175.4	3.4	2.9	38.6	7.8	26.3	1.9	5.1	1.8	19.0	1.2	1.9	2.8	3.9	12.5	7.2	15.0	4.5
1973	176.3	3.3	3.0	39.5	7.9	26.1	2.1	4.4	1.7	19.5	1.2	1.9	2.8	4.1	11.8	7.4	14.3	4.9
1974	177.5	3.5	3.2	38.7	7.1	26.1	2.1	4.8	1.8	20.9	1.3	2.2	2.5	4.3	12.0	7.7	14.0	4.9
1975	178.0	3.4	3.0	40.0	7.5	26.2	2.1	4.7	1.8	21.3	1.3	2.2	2.8	4.2	12.3	7.4	13.6	4.4
1976	181.0	3.5	3.0	40.0	7.7	26.3	2.1	4.8	1.9	21.7	1.6	2.2	2.7	4.3	12.6	7.8	13.5	4.5
1977	179.3	3.5	3.4	39.9	7.4	24.9	2.0	4.8	1.8	22.5	1.4	2.4	2.9	4.4	12.2	7.7	12.7	4.5
1978	180.4	3.6	3.3	40.1	7.4	24.7	2.1	4.9	1.6	23.3	1.4	2.3	2.9	4.5	12.7	7.4	12.7	4.6
1979	182.0	3.4	3.0	39.9	6.8	23.2	2.1	4.8	1.9	23.6	1.6	2.5	3.1	4.3	11.9	7.6	12.4	4.4
1980	182.3	3.4	2.9	40.1	6.7	23.2	2.2	4.6	1.7	24.5	1.6	2.5	3.1	4.3	11.8	7.6	11.5	4.4
1981	182.6	3.5	2.7	41.1	6.6	22.3	2.0	4.7	1.9	24.4	1.6	2.5	3.2	4.2	11.8	7.2	10.9	4.4
1982	182.5	3.2	2.7	40.6	6.3	21.2	2.2	4.8	1.7	25.6	1.9	2.5	3.2	4.4	11.2	7.4	10.5	4.5
1983	183.0	3.4	3.1	40.9	6.3	22.0	2.3	4.7	1.6	25.8	1.5	2.4	3.5	4.4	11.6	7.3	10.1	4.3
1984	181.4	3.2	3.1	40.1	5.9	20.7	2.3	4.4	1.7	26.9	1.7	2.4	3.4	4.5	12.0	7.5	9.7	3.8

* Directly age-standardised using the European standard population.
† Rates have been adjusted for coding and classification changes over the period 1950–2003.
** All cancers excluding non-melanoma skin cancer.

Source: Office for National Statistics

Appendix Table **8D** continued

Mortality from selected major cancers (age-standardised*†): females, 1950–2003

England & Wales

Rate per 100,000

Year of death	All cancers (x nmsc)**	Bladder	Brain	Breast	Cervix	Colorectal	Kidney	Larynx	Leukaemia	Lip, mouth & pharynx	Lung	Melanoma of skin	Multiple myeloma	Non-Hodgkin's lymphoma	Oesophagus	Ovary	Pancreas	Stomach	Uterus
1985	181.6	3.2	3.1	40.0	6.0	21.1	2.3	4.5	1.7	26.7	1.7	2.5	3.7	4.4	11.5	7.4	9.2	3.9
1986	180.1	3.3	3.0	40.3	6.3	19.8	2.3	4.4	1.6	27.2	1.9	2.4	3.6	4.5	11.5	7.5	8.4	3.6
1987	181.3	3.2	3.1	40.1	5.9	19.9	2.5	4.6	1.7	27.7	1.8	2.6	3.9	4.5	11.7	7.5	8.5	3.7
1988	181.9	3.1	3.2	39.9	5.9	19.7	2.5	4.4	1.5	28.7	1.9	2.6	4.2	4.4	11.3	7.5	8.4	3.6
1989	182.1	3.3	3.2	40.1	5.5	19.4	2.5	4.5	1.6	28.6	1.8	2.8	4.2	4.7	11.6	7.6	7.8	3.6
1990	178.7	3.3	3.2	38.9	5.3	18.9	2.4	4.0	1.5	28.2	1.8	2.6	4.1	4.8	11.7	7.5	7.5	3.5
1991	177.7	3.1	3.1	38.4	5.0	18.8	2.8	4.1	1.5	28.6	1.7	2.7	4.4	4.7	11.2	7.1	7.1	3.6
1992	176.4	3.2	3.2	37.8	4.8	18.7	2.7	4.0	1.5	28.4	1.7	2.5	4.6	4.7	11.2	7.3	6.9	3.3
1993	180.7	3.5	3.8	38.7	4.7	19.4	2.8	4.4	1.5	29.4	2.1	3.0	4.7	5.2	11.7	7.5	6.6	3.4
1994	178.5	3.5	3.7	37.9	4.2	19.0	2.7	4.3	1.6	29.5	2.1	2.8	4.9	5.1	11.5	7.3	6.6	3.2
1995	176.1	3.3	3.8	36.8	4.1	18.2	2.8	4.2	1.4	29.3	1.9	3.0	4.9	5.2	11.7	7.4	6.2	3.4
1996	173.2	3.2	3.9	35.4	4.1	17.9	2.7	4.2	1.4	29.3	1.9	2.9	5.0	5.2	12.4	7.2	5.5	3.3
1997	170.5	3.2	3.8	34.5	3.7	17.2	2.9	4.4	1.5	28.4	1.9	2.7	4.8	5.2	11.6	7.2	5.7	3.3
1998	168.1	3.2	4.0	33.6	3.5	16.6	2.9	4.2	1.5	28.9	2.0	2.9	4.7	4.9	11.8	7.0	5.4	3.3
1999	166.1	3.1	3.8	32.8	3.3	16.4	2.7	4.7	1.5	28.8	1.9	2.8	5.0	5.2	11.3	7.4	5.1	3.1
2000	163.3	3.2	3.7	32.0	3.3	15.4	2.8	4.1	1.5	28.4	2.0	2.7	4.9	5.1	11.1	7.4	4.8	3.4
2001	160.3	2.9	3.8	30.8	3.1	14.7	2.7	4.1	1.6	28.3	2.0	2.5	4.8	4.8	11.4	7.3	4.6	3.4
2002	159.4	3.0	3.9	30.2	2.9	14.7	2.7	4.3	1.5	28.4	1.9	2.6	4.8	5.1	11.4	7.4	4.4	3.2
2003	156.4	3.0	3.8	29.3	2.7	14.4	2.9	3.9	1.5	28.5	2.0	2.6	4.5	5.0	11.0	7.2	4.2	3.3

* Directly age-standardised using the European standard population.
† Rates have been adjusted for coding and classification changes over the period 1950–2003.
** All cancers excluding non-melanoma skin cancer.

Source: Office for National Statistics

Appendix 8E Technical terms

Adenocarcinoma – a malignant epithelial tumour derived from glandular tissue (tissue which produces a secretion).

Adjuvant – in terms of treating cancer, a second form of treatment that is given in addition to the main form. For example, adjuvant radiotherapy before or after surgery, adjuvant chemotherapy after surgery or radiotherapy.

Aetiology – the cause(s) of a disease.

Ascertainment (level) – the proportion of all newly diagnosed cases of cancer that are registered by a cancer registry.

Benign – tumours which are usually slow growing, in which the cells resemble those of their tissue of origin, which do not invade surrounding tissue or spread to distant sites, and which are not usually fatal.

Carcinoma – a malignant tumour derived from epithelial tissue (tissue covering the internal organs and other internal surfaces of the body; also forms glands).

Chemotherapy – the use of drugs to treat cancer by killing tumour cells (chemotherapeutic drugs).

Leukaemia - a group of cancers of the white blood cells in the bone marrow and/or the lymph nodes.

Male-to-female ratio – the number of cases or deaths (or the age-standardised rate) in males divided by that in females.

Malignant – tumours which grow by invasion into surrounding tissues and have the ability to spread to distant sites.

Papilloma – a small benign epithelial tumour.

Squamous cell – type of epithelial cell found in many parts of the body, for example lungs, kidneys, mouth, oesophagus, and skin.

Stage – a measure of the size and extent of a tumour at the time of diagnosis.

Transitional cell – type of epithelial cell which forms the lining of the bladder and urinary tract.

Tumour – a mass of abnormal tissue, the growth of which exceeds and is uncoordinated with the normal tissue from which it originates, and which persists in the same excessive manner after the stimuli which evoked the change have ceased (also known as a neoplasm).

Mental health

Claudia Cooper and Paul Bebbington

Chapter 9

Introduction

About a tenth of adults worldwide, an estimated 450 million people, are affected by mental disorders at any one time.[1] The World Health Organisation's *Global Burden of Disease Study* (2001) reported that depression, schizophrenia, alcohol-related disorders and bipolar affective disorder (manic depression) were all among the 10 disorders accounting for most years lived with disability.[2] Considering disability alone without the impact of premature death, 43 per cent of the total European burden of disability results from mental disorders.[1]

Mental health was established as a key priority in the NHS Plan.[3] *The National Service Framework for Mental Health*,[4] published in 1999, provides a structure for the development of mental health services in England. There is a focus on management of mental disorders in primary care and in the community rather than in hospital where possible, and Crisis Resolution Teams have been introduced to try and prevent the need for hospital admission by responding quickly to people in crisis. The Scottish Executive[5] and the Welsh Assembly Government[6] have also produced documents outlining plans for their national mental health services development.

In this chapter, information is presented about the prevalence and factors associated with the main types of mental disorder and non-fatal suicidal behaviours in the Great British population. The primary source of data is the surveys of psychiatric morbidity among adults and children in Great Britain.[7–10] Provision and uptake of treatment and services are also discussed.

Mental disorders

Mental disorders can be divided into neurotic disorders, a category comprising depression, anxiety disorders and obsessive compulsive disorder; psychoses, which are severe mental disorders characterised by loss of contact with reality; and personality disorders, in which there are severe disturbances of a person's character, thought patterns and behaviour from late childhood or adolescence and continuing into adulthood which cause distress to the person or to those around them. The prevalence and risk factors for each of these categories of mental disorder, and for suicidal behaviours are discussed.

Neurotic disorders

Symptoms of neurotic disorders include depression, anxiety, and sometimes obsessions (intrusive, and unwelcome thoughts, impulses or images), compulsions (repetitive behaviours performed reluctantly in response to obsessions) and panic attacks. They can result in physical impairments and problems

with social functioning as severe as those associated with chronic physical disorders[11] and are also associated with increased mortality compared with the general population.[12] Although they are usually less disabling than 'major' psychiatric disorders, such as schizophrenia, due to their high prevalence they place more of a burden on services,[2] and people with mental disorders miss three to four times more work days per year than those without mental disorders.[13]

In 2000, over 8,000 adults living in private households were interviewed for the National Psychiatric Morbidity Survey (NPMS).[7] Prevalence of neurotic disorders in the week prior to interview was assessed, using the revised version of the Clinical Interview Schedule (CIS-R).[14] The CIS-R covers 14 types of neurotic symptoms, such as sleep problems, depression and anxiety, and produces a total score that reflects the overall severity of the symptoms. A score above 11 indicates a clinically significant level of symptoms, at which a neurotic disorder is diagnosed. The CIS-R allows for specific diagnoses to be made using a computer algorithm.

In the NPMS, one in six (15 per cent) adults interviewed scored above 11 and were hence diagnosed with a neurotic disorder.[7] One in 14 people scored above 17 indicating the presence of a more severe neurotic disorder likely to require treatment and usually associated with referral to secondary care. Figure 9.1 shows the prevalence rates for the six neurotic disorders studied. The most prevalent, Mixed Anxiety and Depressive disorder, is a 'catch-all' category that includes people scoring above 11 on the CIS-R who do not meet the criteria for the other five disorders. Generalised Anxiety Disorder was the next

Figure **9.1**

Weekly prevalence of neurotic disorders: by sex, 2000

Great Britain

Rate per 1,000 adults

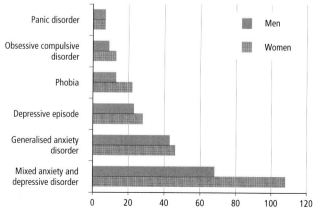

Source: Survey of Psychiatric Morbidity among Adults in Great Britain, Office for National Statistics

most common. The remaining disorders (depressive episode, phobias, obsessive compulsive and panic disorder) were less prevalent. Overall rates of neurotic disorder did not change significantly between the 1993 and 2000 NPMS.

All neurotic disorders were more common in women, except for panic disorder which is equally common in men and women (Figure 9.1). They were most likely to occur in middle age, and were less common in young men and older people (Figure 9.2). Table 9.3 shows how people with neurotic disorders differed from the general population in a number of sociodemographic characteristics. They were more likely to have an unskilled occupation Registrar General's Social Class (RGSC) V, to lack formal qualifications, to be economically inactive and to rent accommodation from a local authority or housing association. They were also more likely to be living alone, acting as single parents, separated or divorced, and less likely to be married or cohabiting. Greater socio-economic adversity probably explains many of these associations; for example, 21 per cent of single parents fell into the lowest income category, compared with only 1 per cent of married parents.[15] Adversities such as unemployment, poverty and poor housing can be important aetiological factors in mental disorders, and impede recovery. Conversely, mental disorders may bring about financial and social hardship by decreasing the person's ability to continue in work, and maintain relationships.

In the Ethnic Minority Psychiatric Illness Rates in the Community (EMPIRIC) study,[16] carried out in 2000 to investigate ethnic differences in mental health in England, 4,281 people were interviewed, from White, Irish, Black Caribbean, Bangladeshi, Indian and Pakistani ethnic groups.

Figure **9.2**

Weekly prevalence of neurotic disorders: by age and sex, 2000

Great Britain

Percentages

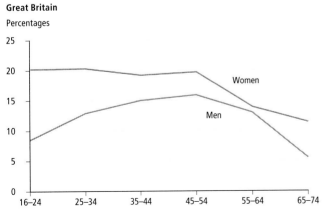

Source: Survey of Psychiatric Morbidity among Adults in Great Britain, Office for National Statistics

Table **9.3**

Sociodemographic characteristics of people with and without a neurotic disorder, 2000

Great Britain   Percentages

	People with neurotic disorder	People without neurotic disorder
Marital status		
Married / cohabiting	62	67
Single	21	23
Separated / divorced	14	7
Widowed	4	4
Family unit type		
Living as a couple	62	67
Single parent	9	4
One person only	20	16
Adult living with parent(s)	9	13
Highest qualification		
Degree	13	15
Teaching, HND, nursing	7	7
A Level	14	15
GCSE	35	36
No qualifications	31	27
Social Class		
I Professional	3	5
II Intermediate	27	29
IIINM Skilled non-manual	25	24
IIIM Skilled manual	19	19
IV Partly skilled	18	16
V Unskilled	7	5
Employment status		
Employed	58	69
Unemployed	4	3
Economically inactive	39	28
Tenure		
Owned	62	74
Rented from LA/HA	26	15
Rented from other source	12	10

Source: Survey of Psychiatric Morbidity among Adults in Great Britain, Office for National Statistics

Rates of neurotic disorders were higher in Irish men and Pakistani women, and lower in Bangladeshi women. There were few differences when people from White, Black Caribbean and South Asian ethnicities were compared (Figure 9.4 – see overleaf).

Figure **9.4**

Prevalence of psychiatric morbidity and suicidal thoughts and attempts: by ethnic group and sex, 2000

England

Percentages

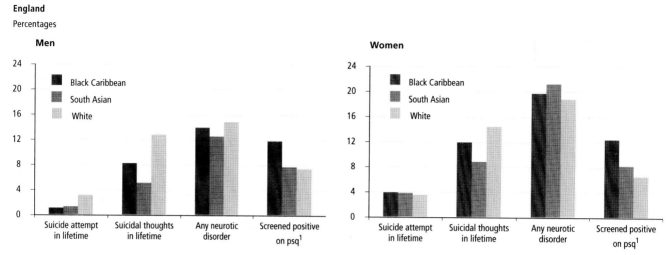

1 Psychosis screening questionnaire.

Source: Ethnic Minority Psychiatric Illness Rates in the Community, Department of Health

Psychotic disorders

Psychotic disorders produce disturbances in thinking and perception sufficiently severe to distort the person's perception of the world and the relationship of events within it. They include schizophrenia and other delusional disorders, and are relatively infrequent. The 2000 NPMS reported an annual prevalence of around one person in 200,[7] which is comparable to the rates reported in the 1993 NPMS.

Psychotic disorders were most common between the ages of 30 and 54. People with psychosis were much more likely than the general population to experience socio-economic disadvantages (Table 9.5). They had fewer educational qualifications, were much less likely to be in work, more likely to be renting accommodation from a local authority or housing association and more likely to have an unskilled or partly skilled occupation (RGSC IV or V). They were also more likely to be separated or divorced, and to be living alone. The reasons for these associations are likely to be similar to those for neurotic disorders.

The EMPIRIC[16] study found that although there was a two-fold greater estimated prevalence in the Black Caribbean group, this was not statistically significant, and there were no major differences in the rate of psychotic disorders between ethnic groups. Considering women only, Black Caribbean women were more likely to give affirmative answers[16] on the Psychosis Screening Questionnaire[17] than white women (Figure 9.4). This screens for any psychotic experiences and symptoms rather than an actual psychotic disorder. There were marked excesses in prevalence of psychosis in African and African-Caribbean groups in the two NPMS,[7, 18] but the difference between

prevalences in White and Black groups, which had been adjusted for other sociodemographic variables, were not significant in either survey. Brugha and colleagues[19] showed, using the 1993 data, that the result was non-significant in the published report precisely because the difference between the groups could be accounted for in terms of sociodemographic disadvantage. Reported rates of psychosis for those in contact with treatment services have consistently shown elevated rates of schizophrenia in Black Caribbean people.[20] Such consistency indicates a strong possibility that the increased rates are real, and likely to reflect the social circumstances of Black Britons. However, some have argued that these higher rates are accounted for by factors influencing the likelihood of receiving a diagnosis or treatment, rather than a higher prevalence. Proposed explanations for this have included clinicians mistaking cultural expressions of distress for psychosis, racism by psychiatrists and in the community, and differential responses by police, social and treatment services to Black people compared with other ethnic groups.[16]

Personality disorder

People with 'personality disorders' have patterns of behaviour or experience resulting from their particular personality characteristics that differ from those expected by society, and lead to distress or suffering for them or others. In the 2000 NPMS, the Structured Clinical Interview for DSM-IV was used to diagnose personality disorder, in a process comprising a self-completion screening questionnaire and subsequent second stage interview by trained psychologists. Just over one in 20 men and one in 30 women[7] had a personality disorder (Figure 9.6). The overall prevalence of personality disorder, 4.4

Table 9.5

Sociodemographic characteristics of people with and without a psychotic disorder, 2000

Great Britain   Percentages

	People with psychotic disorder	People without psychotic disorder
Marital status		
Married / cohabiting	39	66
Single	29	23
Separated / divorced	30	7
Widowed	3	4
Family unit type		
Living as a couple	39	66
Single parent	7	5
One person only	43	16
Adult living with parent(s)	12	13
Highest qualification		
Degree	2	15
Teaching, HND, nursing	7	7
A Level	7	15
GCSE	44	36
No qualifications	40	27
Social Class		
I Professional	1	5
II Intermediate	18	29
IIINM Skilled non-manual	21	25
IIIM Skilled manual	21	19
IV Partly skilled	21	16
V Unskilled	19	6
Employment status		
Employed	28	67
Unemployed	2	3
Economically inactive	70	30
Tenure		
Owned	38	73
Rented from LA/HA	49	17
Rented from other source	13	10

Source: Survey of Psychiatric Morbidity among Adults in Great Britain, Office for National Statistics

per cent, was somewhat lower than in a USA study using similar methods but a smaller sample size, which reported a prevalence of around 10 per cent.[21] Because individual personality disorders are relatively rare, there is a high risk of sampling errors even in large studies. In the 2000 NPMS, obsessive compulsive personality disorder was the most prevalent, but this has not been replicated elsewhere, and

Figure 9.6

Prevalence of personality disorders:[1] by sex, 2000

Great Britain

Rate per 1,000 adults

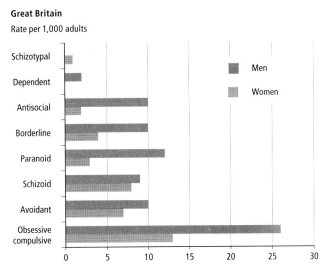

1 *From clinical interviews.*

Source: Survey of Psychiatric Morbidity among Adults in Great Britain, Office for National Statistics

there is a lack of consensus currently about which personality disorders are most prevalent in the community.[7, 21,22] All large studies have found that personality disorders are more common in men, and in the NPMS 2000 this was found for the individual disorders. Others have found that borderline personality disorder[23] is more common in women.

Suicidal thoughts and attempts

About one in seven (14.9 per cent)[8] people interviewed in the 2000 NPMS had considered suicide at some point in their lives. This is similar to rates reported in the USA[24] and Australia.[25] An estimated 4.4 per cent of people in Great Britain had attempted suicide at some time (Figure 9.7 – see overleaf). Thinking about and attempting suicide are far more common than completed suicide. The age-standardised annual suicide rate in England has been falling since 1998;[26] in 2003 it was 8.5 per 100,000 population. Non-fatal suicidal behaviours are more common in women, even though there are approximately three times more completed suicides deaths among men.[26] Among people with psychosis, attempting suicide is equally common in men and women.[9]

Younger people are much more likely than older people to report thinking at some time about attempting suicide.[8] It seems unlikely that this represents an increase in the rate of suicidal behaviour, because the completed suicide rate is falling.[26] It may result from a greater willingness in younger people to report suicidal behaviour. Nearly one in 40 people reported that they had deliberately harmed themselves without wanting to die.[8] Reasons most commonly given were to draw

Figure **9.7**

Prevalence of ever attempting suicide: by age and sex, 2000

Great Britain

Percentages

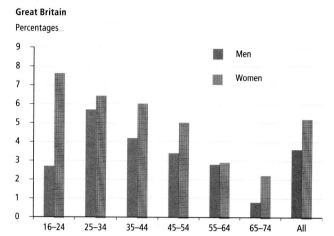

Source: Survey of Psychiatric Morbidity among Adults in Great Britain, Office for National Statistics

attention to themselves or acting in anger. Self-cutting was the most prevalent method used. Young women have the highest rates of deliberate self-harm without suicidal intent.

People with a mental illness or who have substance misuse problems are much more likely to attempt suicide in their lifetime (Figure 9.8). Those who have a psychotic disorder have the highest reported rates (45 per cent).[9] People with neurotic disorders were also more likely to attempt suicide.[8] The neurotic disorders for which the highest rates (between 25 and

Figure **9.8**

Prevalence of ever attempting suicide in people with psychiatric disorder or substance misuse problems: by sex, 2000

Great Britain

Percentages

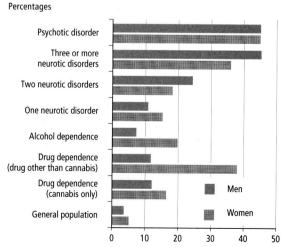

Source: Survey of Psychiatric Morbidity among Adults in Great Britain, Office for National Statistics

30 per cent) were reported are phobias, Obsessive Compulsive Disorder and depressive disorder.

Because suicidal attempts are strongly associated with mental illness, it is not surprising that they share many socio-economic associations (Table 9.9). While similar numbers of people in all social classes report having thought about suicide, people in manual occupations are more likely to have actually attempted suicide. Compared to those who have not, people who have attempted suicide are more likely to be single or divorced, living alone, and renting accommodation from a local authority or housing association and they are more likely to be economically inactive. Unemployment is strongly related to suicidal thoughts, attempts and deliberate self-harm, particularly in women. Unemployed women are four times as likely to attempt suicide, and over four times as likely deliberately to harm themselves as those in employment. More white people reported suicidal thoughts, and in men, suicidal attempts, in the EMPIRIC study (Figure 9.4).

Comorbidity

'Comorbidity' is the presence of two or more mental or substance misuse disorders together, for example alcohol dependence and depression. A study based on the General Practice Research database (GPRD), which collects information from primary care practices covering approximately 2.6 per cent of the population (in 1998), estimated that between 1993 and 1998 there were 3.5 million GP consultations involving comorbid patients in England and Wales, that they consume far more health services than people with either condition alone, and the incidence of cases of comorbidity seems to be increasing.[27] The relationship between substance misuse and psychiatric illness is complicated. They share an association with socio-economic disadvantages. Substance misuse can also cause psychiatric symptoms, for example, depressed mood[28] and sometimes psychosis in vulnerable individuals.[29] Certain psychiatric symptoms, such as impulsivity or anxiety, may exacerbate drug and alcohol misuse.

The NPMS reported the proportion of people who were dependent on any illicit substance, and assessed the physical, social and psychological effects of alcohol use using the Alcohol Use Disorders Identification Test (AUDIT)[30] (Figure 9.10). People who score eight or more on the AUDIT are regarded as drinking at hazardous levels, which means an established pattern of drinking that brings the risk of physical or psychological harm. Those who scored 16 and over are regarded as drinking at harmful levels. Further assessment of people scoring more than 10 on the AUDIT determined whether they were dependent on alcohol. People with antisocial personality disorder (ASPD) were more than four

Table **9.9**

Sociodemographic characteristics of people who have ever made a suicide attempt and those who have not, 2000

Great Britain   Percentages

	People who have made a suicide attempt in their lifetime	People who have not made a suicide attempt in their lifetime
Marital status		
Married / cohabiting	36	57
Single	38	11
Separated / divorced	25	29
Widowed	3	4
Family unit type		
Living as a couple	48	66
Single parent	12	5
One person only	26	16
Adult living with parent(s)	13	13
Highest qualification		
Degree	10	15
Teaching, HND, nursing	4	7
A Level	12	15
GCSE	43	36
No qualifications	31	27
Social Class		
I Professional	2	5
II Intermediate	19	30
IIINM Skilled non-manual	25	25
IIIM Skilled manual	20	19
IV Partly skilled	22	16
V Unskilled	12	5
Employment status		
Employed	53	68
Unemployed	6	3
Economically inactive	40	30
Tenure		
Owned	47	74
Rented from LA/HA	42	16
Rented from other source	12	10

Source: Survey of Psychiatric Morbidity among Adults in Great Britain, Office for National Statistics

times as likely to be dependent on a drug, and more likely to drink hazardous and harmful amounts of alcohol than the general population.[10] This was not true of people with other personality disorders. It must be taken into account that some

of the behaviours associated with illegal drug use, such as criminal acts, can score as criteria for ASPD. People with neurotic disorders were no more likely to drink hazardously than the general population, but they were more likely to drink harmful amounts of alcohol, which may indicate that those with neurotic disorders who drank regularly were less able to control their consumption. Compared with people who scored under six on the CIS-R indicating few neurotic symptoms, they were twice as likely to be dependent on drugs, and in those with more severe neurotic disorders (CIS-R 18 and over), rates of drug dependence were quadrupled. People with OCD had particularly high rates of alcohol and drug dependence.

Figure **9.10**

Prevalence of alcohol and drug misuse: by psychiatric disorder, 2000

Great Britain

Percentages

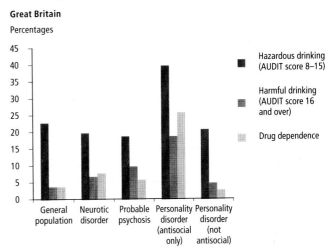

Source: Survey of Psychiatric Morbidity among Adults in Great Britain, Office for National Statistics

Rates of alcohol misuse or drug dependence were not significantly different in people with psychotic disorders compared with the general population, even though high rates of substance misuse have been reported in people with psychosis using psychiatric services.[31] This may be because the NPMS failed to demonstrate truly greater prevalence because of the small numbers of people with psychotic disorder included, or because those who are comorbid make more demands on services. A study in 2001 found that 44 per cent of Community Mental Health Team (CMHT) patients reported problem use of drugs and alcohol within the last year, while 75 per cent of drug service and 85 per cent of alcohol service patients had a past-year psychiatric disorder.[31]

Mental health status of key groups

Children and adolescents

Of the 5- to 15-year-olds interviewed in the 1999 National survey of mental health of children and adolescents in Great Britain[15] almost one in 10 had emotional or behavioural problems which impacted on their lives and placed a burden on their families. Figures 9.11 and 9.12 show the prevalences reported for the main categories of psychiatric disorders. Boys were more likely to have a mental disorder, and in particular a conduct or hyperkinetic disorder (such as Attention Deficit Hyperactivity Disorder). There was less differences between the sexes in the prevalence of emotional disorders. With the exception of hyperkinetic disorders, prevalences increased from childhood to adolescence. Children with mental disorders were much more likely to have special educational needs than those without.

There is a strong association between child and parent mental health. Children with a mental disorder were twice as likely to have a parent who also screened positive for mental illness, and the parents of children with more than one mental disorder were the most likely to have mental disorders themselves.[32] Childhood psychiatric disorders were highly associated with socio-economic deprivation. Children whose parents had unskilled occupations (RGSC V) were about three times more likely to have a mental illness than children whose parents had professional occupations (RGSC I). Children from single parent, step families, larger families (four or five children) and families with high levels of discord, and children who had experienced more stressful events, were also more likely to have a mental disorder.[15]

Suicide is the second leading cause of death among young people in most developed countries, including the UK. Youth suicide rates have been markedly higher in Scotland and Northern Ireland, compared with England and Wales in recent years. In the 1999 survey, rates of self-harm, as reported by parents, were low in children without mental disorders, but rose substantially in those diagnosed with a disorder. In 5- to 10-year-olds, 6 per cent of children with anxiety disorders and 7.5 per cent with conduct, hyperkinetic or less common mental disorders had harmed themselves. In 11- to 15-year-olds, 19 per cent of children with depression and 13 per cent who had a conduct disorder had done so.[33]

Mental health of other groups

Recent surveys have reported on rates of mental disorder in vulnerable groups, including prisoners;[34] homeless adults living in hostels, night shelters, private sector leased accommodation or roofless people using day centres;[35] and residents of institutions specifically catering for people with mental health problems, including hospitals, nursing and residential care homes, hostels, group homes and supported accommodation.[36]

Services

Use of medication and other treatment

In the 1993 NPMS, fewer than 14 per cent of people with current neurotic disorder were receiving any treatment; 9 per cent were receiving psychotropic medication and 8 per cent some kind of 'talking therapy' (psychological treatment).[37] In the 2000 NPMS, the proportion receiving treatment had risen to nearly a quarter[7] due to an increase in the use of

Figure **9.11**

Prevalence of mental disorders: by age for boys, 1999

Great Britain
Percentages

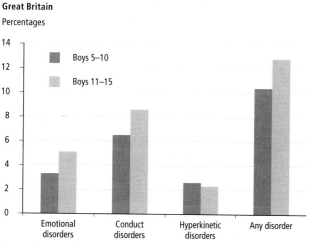

Source: Survey of Psychiatric Morbidity among Adults in Great Britain, Office for National Statistics

Figure **9.12**

Prevalence of mental disorders: by age for girls, 1999

Great Britain
Percentages

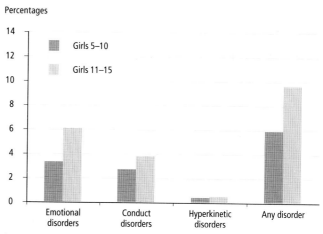

Source: Survey of Psychiatric Morbidity among Adults in Great Britain, Office for National Statistics

antidepressants (two-fold in women, and three-fold in men).[38] Reports from the GPRD (1994–1998) (Table 9.13)[39] and Department of Health statistics for prescriptions dispensed between 1993 and 2003[40] also reported that antidepressant prescribing increased. The GPRD found an increase in the proportion of antidepressants prescriptions from the Selective Serotonin Reuptake Inhibitor (SSRI) class. These antidepressants, introduced in the late 1980s, have fewer side effects than earlier drugs. This may have led to doctors being more willing to prescribe them for less severe depression,[38] and it has also been suggested that in some cases people have been labelled as having depression and prescribed antidepressants inappropriately, when in fact they are experiencing 'ordinary social unhappiness'.[41]

Alternatively, efforts to promote treatment of depression over the past decade, for example in the Royal College of Psychiatrists' 'Defeat Depression' campaign, might have increased appropriate use of medication for neurotic disorders.[38] Since the 2000 NPMS, concerns that SSRIs may cause severe withdrawal syndromes and an increase in suicidal thoughts have been reported in the media[42] and the psychiatric literature.[43] National Institute for Clinical Excellence (NICE) guidelines (2004)[44] recommend that antidepressants should not be used for the initial treatment of mild depression. The impact of these events on future prescribing remains to be seen.

The value of psychological treatments for treating neurotic disorder is now well established.[45] NICE recommends their use as first line treatments for mild depression and anxiety disorders. However, only one in 12 people with neurotic disorders receive any psychological treatment,[7] and this proportion did not change significantly between the 1993 and 2000 NPMS.[38] Not everyone identified as having a neurotic disorder on the CIS-R will need treatment. In a sub-study of the 2000 NPMS that investigated treatment needs for neurotic disorders,[46] clinicians found that 15 per cent of people who scored 12–17 on the CIS-R, and 24 per cent of people scoring over 18 were not receiving treatment from which they could benefit. Most of these unmet needs were for support and cognitive therapy rather than medication. Nearly two-thirds of people with depression judged to need medication were receiving it, but a lesser proportion (10 per cent) judged likely to benefit were receiving Cognitive Behaviour Therapy (CBT). For less specific psychological treatment in the form of general support and counselling, the equivalent figure was 55 per cent. Thus, it seems that the majority of people who might benefit from psychotropic medication now receive it, whereas psychological therapies represent a very significant unmet need. The greater resources required for psychological therapies in terms of professional training and time may be an important factor in this.

In the 2000 NPMS of people with psychosis, 91 per cent were receiving some kind of treatment – 88 per cent were receiving psychotropic medication, and 29 per cent psychological treatment[9] (Figure 9.14 – see overleaf). Compared to the reference categories (in brackets), men (women) and people who were not working due to a long-term illness or disability (economically active e.g. employed) were more likely to be taking medication for psychosis; whereas people with a comorbid neurotic disorder (no neurotic disorder) and those with long standing physical complaints (no physical complaints) were less likely.[9] It is probable that those not working were more ill, and hence more likely to be taking medication, while those on medication may have had fewer neurotic symptoms due to the treatment they were receiving. It is not clear why women should be less likely to receive drug treatment for psychosis.

New types of antipsychotic medication introduced in the last decade, the atypical antipsychotics, have fewer side effects than conventional antipsychotics. In 2002, NICE recommended they should be considered as first-line options for people with

Table 9.13

Prevalence of treated mental disorders (age-standardised): by sex, 1994–1998

England and Wales   Rate per 1,000 patients

	Males			Females		
	Depression	Anxiety	Schizophrenia	Depression	Anxiety	Schizophrenia
1994	19.9	17.8	1.9	50.5	41.7	1.7
1995	22.3	19.2	2.0	55.9	44.6	1.7
1996	25.0	20.9	2.0	60.8	47.4	1.7
1997	27.2	22.2	2.0	67.0	51.4	1.6
1998	29.0	23.8	2.0	70.1	54.4	1.7

Source: Key Health Statistics from General Practice 1998, Office for National Statistics

Figure **9.14**

Treatment received by people with psychosis and neurotic disorders,[1] 2000

Great Britain

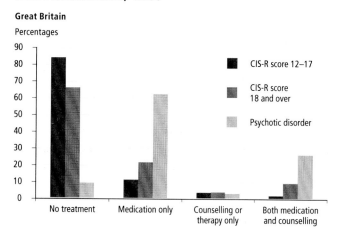

1 CIS-R score of 12–17 represents mild to moderate neurotic disorders and CIS-R score of 18 and over represents more severe neurotic disorders.

Source: Survey of Psychiatric Morbidity among Adults in Great Britain, Office for National Statistics

newly diagnosed schizophrenia.[47] The proportion of people with schizophrenia prescribed atypical antipsychotics more than quadrupled in men and women from 1994 to 1998, according to the GPRD.[39] Greater prescription of these more expensive drugs explains why spending on antipsychotics increased by 19 per cent between 2002 and 2003, while the total number of prescriptions increased by only 7 per cent.[40] Fewer people in 2000 than in 1993 (one in 10) took their antipsychotic medication in injected depot form rather than as tablets,[9] perhaps because atypical antipsychotics were not initially available as injections. People over 45 were nearly 10 times as likely to be receiving their antipsychotics as a depot injection; this would be expected if they were continuing to take medication prescribed before the introduction of atypical antipsychotics. The other main classes of psychotropic medication prescribed to people with psychosis were antidepressants, taken by about a third of people in the survey, and sedative drugs, taken by just over a fifth.

Use of inpatient services

Most psychiatric treatment now takes place in the community. Only 1 per cent of people with neurotic disorders,[7] and 3 per cent of people with psychotic disorders[9] interviewed in the 2000 NPMS had been inpatients for the treatment of mental and emotional problems in the last three months. Hospital Episode Statistics (April 1999 – March 2000) indicate that 3.2 per 1,000 of the general population in England are admitted to psychiatric hospital annually,[48] with similar rates in Scotland.

Men and people aged 25–44 were most commonly admitted. Depression and anxiety were the most likely reason for English hospital admission, although in London, schizophrenia and related psychoses accounted for the greatest proportion of admissions. Psychosis was the most common diagnosis in people staying in hospital for more than 90 days. In England and Wales, about a third of psychiatric inpatients are formally detained under the Mental Health Acts.[49]

Use of GP services

Most mental disorders are managed in primary care. In the 2000 NPMS, 39 per cent of people with neurotic disorder had spoken to their GP about mental or emotional problems in the last year.[7] This was a small if significant increase from 35 per cent in 1993.[38] Nevertheless, it appears that most people with neurotic disorders have not consulted their GP about their symptoms in the last year. The EMPIRIC study found that in England, Bangladeshi women were least likely, and Irish women most likely, to consult their GP for an emotional problem.[16] Three-fifths of people with a psychotic disorder had consulted their GP about their mental health in the last year,[9] suggesting that in this group too, many people were not in regular contact with their primary care physician.

Use of Community services

Most psychiatric services are now delivered by CMHTs, composed of psychiatrists, community psychiatric nurses, clinical psychologists, social workers, occupational therapists and other mental health workers. People may also see psychiatrists in outpatients, or attend day care services as part of their treatment. Table 9.15 shows the proportion of people with mental illnesses who reported contact with these services. People with psychotic disorders used most services; 40 per cent had seen a psychiatrist or psychiatric nurse,[9] 40 per cent had used a community care service, and 20 per cent a day care service in the last three months. People with neurotic disorders were less likely to have been in contact with services in the same period; 4 per cent had seen a psychiatrist[7] and 8 per cent had used a community care service.

Receipt of any service

Taking data for services received in the 2000 survey and the follow-up survey 18 months later together, about half of people with neurotic disorders reported some contact with primary or secondary services or treatment at either time point.[46] According to NHS principles of equity and proportionality, it would be expected that the only determinant of service receipt would be illness severity.[37] Higher severity of neurotic symptoms was indeed an important predictor of

Table **9.15**

Use of psychiatric outpatients, community and day services by people with mental illness in the last three months, 2000

Great Britain   Percentages

	Psychotic disorder	Neurotic disorder
Psychiatrist (Community Mental Health Team)	18	2
Psychologist	2	1
Community psychiatric nurse	23	1
Other nursing services	2	3
Social worker	10	2
Self help group	7	1
Home help / care worker	4	1
Outreach worker	2	1
Any community care service	40	8
Community mental health centre	10	1
Day activity centre	10	1
Any day care service	20	2
Psychiatric outpatients	22	2
Any psychiatrist	40	4

Source: Survey of Psychiatric Morbidity among Adults in Great Britain, Office for National Statistics

receiving treatment. More services were also received by women, people who were widowed, divorced, or living alone, single parents, the long term sick or disabled, and those who had a household weekly income of under £100.[46] These factors were also associated with greater risk of mental disorders, so the results do not necessarily indicate inequality of service provision. The higher rate of consultation in White people is potentially more concerning, as it could indicate that people from ethnic minorities face barriers in accessing services for mental health problems. This requires further attention, as the number of non-White people interviewed was very small. People with psychosis were much more likely to be in contact with services. Only a quarter had not had any contact with mental health services in the last three months or spoken to their GP about their mental health in the last year.[9]

Refusing services

In the 2000 NPMS, 16 per cent of people with psychotic disorders had not sought help in the last year from a doctor or another mental health professional when they (or others) thought they should have done, but only 8 per cent had refused help that was offered.[9] The main reasons people with psychosis gave for not seeking help were that they did not think anyone could help, or they were afraid of possible

treatment or tests. A similar proportion (9 per cent) of people with a neurotic disorder reported turning down health services that were offered, compared with only 3 per cent of the general population.[7] Counselling was the service people most commonly rejected, accounting for half the services refused. In the 2000 NPMS sub-study of treatment needs, 20 per cent of people with depression or anxiety did not want medication, and 24 per cent of people with anxiety and 14 per cent of people with depression did not want CBT, while 27 per cent of people with anxiety and 19 per cent of those with depression did not want more general support, reassurance or counselling.[46] These findings indicate that most people, around eight out of 10, would accept drug or psychological treatment if it was offered.

Treatment outcomes

Clinical recovery

Half of people found to have a neurotic disorder in the 2000 NPMS, still met the criteria for the disorder 18 months later.[46] Greater severity of disorder was associated with a lesser chance of recovery. Many of the socio-economic factors associated with prevalence of neurotic disorders were also associated with a reduced chance of clinical recovery in 18 months. These were manual occupations, earning less, unemployment and long-term sickness or disability; less social support and more adverse life events. These factors could directly impair recovery, or they may represent a general lack of support and opportunity to improve circumstances. Once these factors were taken into account, people who had received treatment over the 18 months were twice as likely to have recovered. Psychotic disorders usually have a more prolonged course, with relapses followed by periods of remission over many years.

When the children who had emotional disorders in the 1999 study were interviewed three years later, approximately a quarter were still unwell.[50] Comorbid physical illness, more stressful life events, and poor maternal mental health in 1999 predicted poor recovery. Conduct and hyperkinetic disorders were more persistent, with 43 per cent of children with conduct disorders remaining unwell three years later. The disorder was more likely to persist if the child had special education needs, or was shouted at frequently, and if their mother had poor mental health. It has now been shown that childhood mental and behavioural disorders can predict emotional and behaviour problems in later life. For example, adolescent self-reported emotional problems predict emotional disorders 10 years later,[51] and children who have behaviour problems at age three are more likely to be convicted of a criminal offence as an adult.[52]

Chapter 9: Mental health

Focus on Health: 2006

Quality of life

It is clearly important to consider the impact of mental illness on peoples' lives as well as the level of symptoms they experience. Questionnaires have been developed that attempt to measure 'quality of life', by asking about people's own perceptions and about some objective measures of their life, in areas such as work, finance, leisure, health and relationships. Figure 9.16 shows how people interviewed in the 2000 NPMS rated their 'quality of life' 18 months later. It compares people with no neurotic disorder, those with a persistent neurotic disorder, and those who developed or recovered from a neurotic disorder over the time period.

Figure **9.16**

Reported poor quality of life for people with and without neurotic disorders, 2000

Great Britain

Percentages

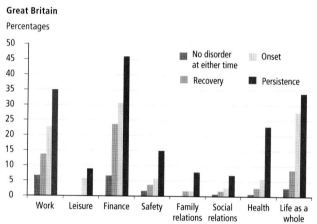

Source: Survey of Psychiatric Morbidity among Adults in Great Britain, Office for National Statistics

Only 3 per cent of people without a neurotic disorder at either time rated their overall quality of life as poor, compared with 34 per cent of people with a persistent disorder.[46] People with mental illness will probably experience a deterioration in their quality of life because they feel worse, and it can be difficult when unwell to sustain work and leisure activities, as well as relationships with family and friends. Socio-economic adversity, a strong associate of developing (and poor recovery from) a mental illness, is also likely to be associated with poor quality of life.

Conclusion

One in six adults has a neurotic disorder, and one in seven has considered suicide at some point in their lives. Psychosis is less common, but causes considerable distress and disability in those affected. Mental disorders are related to socio-economic adversity. Rates of mental illness in the community have not changed significantly in recent years, but more people are

being treated with psychotropic medication, while psychological therapies remain a significant unmet need. Despite the increase in the overall level of treatment, about half of people with neurotic disorders, and a quarter of people with psychosis are not in regular contact with health services, including many likely to benefit from treatment.

References

1. Thornicroft G and Maingay S (2002) The global response to mental illness. *BMJ* **325**, 608–609.

2. World Health Organization (2001) *World Health Report 2001*, Geneva: WHO.
    www.who.int/whr/2001/en/whr01_ch2_en.pdf

3. Department of Health (2000) *The NHS Plan: a plan for investment, a plan for reform*, TSO: London.

4. Department of Health (1999) *National service framework for mental health: modern standards and service models*, TSO: London.

5. The Scottish Executive (2003) *The National Programme for Improving Mental Health and Well-Being* at:
    www.scotland.gov.uk/library5/health/npmh-00.asp

6. Welsh Assembly Government (2002) *Adult Mental Health Services, A National Service Framework for Wales* at:
    www.wales.nhs.uk/sites/documents/334/adult-mental-nsf-e.pdf

7. Singleton N, Bumpstead R, O'Brien M, Lee A and Meltzer H (2001) *Psychiatric morbidity among adults living in private households*, TSO: London.
    www.statistics.gov.uk/downloads/theme_health/psychmorb.pdf

8. Meltzer H, Lader D, Corbin T, Singleton N, Jenkins R, Brugha T (2002) *Non-fatal suicidal behaviour among adults aged 16 to 74 in Great Britain*, TSO: London.
    www.dh.gov.uk/assetRoot/04/06/07/66/04060766.pdf

9. O'Brien M, Singleton N, Sparks J, Meltzer H and Brugha T (2000) *Adults with a psychotic disorder living in private households*, TSO: London.
    www.statistics.gov.uk/downloads/theme_health/PMA_Psycho_v2.pdf

10. Coulthard M, Farrell M, Singleton N and Meltzer H (2002) *Tobacco, alcohol and drug use and mental health*, TSO: London.
    www.statistics.gov.uk/downloads/theme_health/Tobacco_etc_v2.pdf

11. Wells K B, Golding J M, Burnam MA (1988) Psychiatric disorder and limitations in physical functioning in a sample of the Los Angeles general population. *American Journal of Geriatric Psychiatry* **145**, 712–717.

120

12. Murphy J M, Monson R R, Olivier D C, Sobol A M and Leighton A H (1987) Affective disorders and mortality, a general population study. *Archives of General Psychiatry* **44**, 473–480.

13. Alonso J, Angermeyer M C, Bernert S *et al* (2004) Disability and quality of life impact of mental disorders in Europe: Results from the European Study of the Epidemiology of Mental disorders (ESEMeD) project. *Acta Psychiatrica Scandinavica, Supplement*, **109(420)**, 38–46.

14. Lewis G, Pelosi A J, Araya R C and Dunn G (1992) Measuring psychiatric disorder in the community: a standard assessment for use by lay interviewers. *Psychological Medicine* **22(2)**, 465–486.

15. Maughan B, Brock A and Ladva G (2004) Chapter 12 Mental health in *The Health of Children and Young People* at: www.statistics.gov.uk/Children/downloads/mental_health.pdf

16. Nazroo J and Sproston K (eds) (2002) *Ethnic minority psychiatric illness rates in the community (EMPIRIC)*, TSO: London. www.dh.gov.uk/assetRoot/04/02/40/34/04024034.pdf

17. Bebbington P E and Nayani T (1995) The Psychosis Screening Questionnaire. *International Journal of Methods in Psychiatric Research* **5**, 11–19.

18. Meltzer H, Gill B, Petticrew M and Hinds K (1995) *The prevalence of psychiatric morbidity among adults living in private households*, HMSO: London.

19. Brugha T, Jenkins R, Bebbington P, Meltzer H, Lewis G and Farrell M (2004) Risk factors and the prevalence of neurosis and psychosis in ethnic groups in Great Britain. *Soc Psychiatry Psychiatr Epidemiol* **39**, 939–946.

20. Bhugra D and Bhui K (2001) African-Caribbeans and schizophrenia: contributing factors. *Advances in Psychiatric Treatment* **7**, 283–293.

21. Samuels J F, Nestadt G, Romanoski A J, Folstein M F and McHugh P R (1994) DSM-III personality disorders in the community. *Am J Psychiatry* **151**, 1055–1062.

22. Michael Gelder *et al* (eds) (2000) *Oxford Textbook of Psychiatry*, Oxford University Press: Oxford.

23. Swartz M, Blazer D, George L and Winfield I (1990) Estimating the prevalence of borderline personality disorder in the community. *Journal of Personality Disorders* **4**, 257–272.

24. Kessler R C, Borges G and Walters E E (1999) Prevalence and risk factors for lifetime suicide attempts in the National Comorbidity study. *Arch Gen Psychiatry* **56**, 617–626.

25. Pirkis J, Burgess P and Dunt D (2000) Suicidal ideation and suicide attempts among Australian adults. *Crisis* **21(1)**, 16–25.

26. National Institute for Mental Health in England (2005) *National suicide prevention strategy for England: annual report 2004*, TSO: London. www.dh.gov.uk/assetRoot/04/10/16/69/04101669.pdf

27. Frischer M, Crome I, Croft P, Millson D, Collins J and Conolly C (2002) *A national epidemiological study of comorbid substance abuse and psychiatric illness in primary care between 1993–1998 using the General Practice Research Database* at: www.mdx.ac.uk/www/drugsmisuse/frischer_exec.doc

28. McIntosh C and Ritson B (2001) Treating depression complicated by substance misuse. *Advances in Psychiatric Treatment* **7**, 357–364.

29. Henquet C, Krabbendam L, Spauwen J, Kaplan C, Lieb R, Wittchen H U and van Os J (2005) Prospective cohort study of cannabis use, predisposition for psychosis, and psychotic symptoms in young people. *BMJ* **330**,11–13.

30. Saunders J B, Aasland O G, Babor T F, de la PuenteJ R and Grant M (1993) Development of the Alcohol Use Disorders Screening Test (AUDIT). WHO collaborative project on early detection of persons with harmful alcohol consumption. II. *Addiction* **88**,791–804.

31. Weaver T, Madden P, Charles V, Stimson G, Renton A, Tyrer P, Barnes T, Bench C, Middleton H, Wright N, Paterson S, Shanahan W, Seivewright N, and Ford C (2002) *Co-morbidity of substance misuse and mental illness Collaborative study (COSMIC): A study of the prevalence and management of co-morbidity amongst adult substance misuse and mental health treatment populations* at: www.nta.nhs.uk/publications/docs/COSMIC_briefing.pdf

32. Meltzer H, Gatward R, Goodman R and Ford T (2000) The mental health of children and adolescents in Great Britain, TSO: London. www.statistics.gov.uk/downloads/theme_health/ChildAdol_Mental_Health_v1.pdf

33. Meltzer H, Harrington R, Goodman R and Jenkins R (2001) *Children and adolescents who try to harm, hurt or kill themselves: a report of further analysis from the National Survey of Mental Health of children and adolescents in Great Britain in 1999*, TSO: London. www.statistics.gov.uk/downloads/theme_health/Childselfabuse_v1.pdf

34. Singleton N, Meltzer H, Gatward R, Coid J and Deasy D (1997) *Psychiatric morbidity among prisoners in England and Wales*, TSO: London.

35. Gill B, Meltzer H, Hinds K and Petticrew M (1996) *Psychiatric morbidity among homeless people*, OPCS Surveys of Psychiatric Morbidity in Great Britain Report 7, HMSO: London.

36. Meltzer H, Gill B, Petticrew M and Hinds K (1996) *The prevalence of psychiatric morbidity among adults living in institutions*, OPCS Surveys of Psychiatric Morbidity in Great Britain Report 4, HMSO: London.

37. Bebbington P E, Brugha T S, Meltzer H, Jenkins R, Ceresa C, Farrell M and Lewis M (2000) Neurotic disorders and the receipt of psychiatric treatment. *Psychological medicine* **30**, 1369–1376.

38. Brugha T S, Bebbington P E, Singleton N, Melzer D, Jenkins R, Lewis G, Farrell M, Bhugra D, Lee A and Meltzer H (2004) Trends in service use and treatment for mental disorders in adults throughout Great Britain. *British Journal of Psychiatry* **185**, 378–384.

39. Office of National Statistics (2000) *Key Health Statistics from General Practice 1998*, (Series MB6 No.2), TSO: London. www.statistics.gov.uk/downloads/theme_health/Key_Health_Stats_ 1998.pdf

40. Department of Health (2004) *Prescriptions dispensed in the community: Statistics for 1993 to 2003*, England, TSO: London. www.dh.gov.uk/assetRoot/04/09/40/68/04094068.PDF

41. Shooter M (2005) Dancing with the Devil? A personal view of psychiatry's relationships with the pharmaceutical industry. *Psychiatric Bulletin* **29**, 81–83.

42. BBC Panorama: The secrets of seroxat www.bbc.co.uk/go/search/int/all/n/allbbc/panorama%2520seroxat/ -/http://news.bbc.co.uk/1/hi/programmes/panorama/2310197.stm

43. Fergusson D, Doucette S, Glass KC, Shapiro S, Healy D, Hebert P and Hutton B (2005) Association between suicide attempts and selective serotonin reuptake inhibitors: systematic review of randomised controlled trials. *BMJ* **330**, 396.

44. National Institute for Clinical Excellence (2004) *CG 23 Depression: management of depression in primary and secondary care*. www.nice.org.uk/pdf/CG023NICEguideline.pdf

45. Roth A and Fonagy P (1996) *What works for whom?: a critical review of psychotherapy research*, Guilford Press: New York, 364– 366.

46. Singleton N and Lewis G (eds) (2003) *Better or worse: a longitudinal study of the mental health of adults living in private households in Great Britain*, TSO: London. www.statistics.gov.uk/downloads/theme_health/PMA- AdultFollowup.pdf

47. National Institute for Clinical Excellence (2002) *CG 43: Full guidance on the use of newer (atypical) antipsychotic drugs for the treatment of schizophrenia*, TSO: London. www.nice.org.uk/page.aspx?o=32923

48. Thompson A, Shaw M, Harrison G, Verne J, Ho D and Gunnell D (2004) Patterns of hospital admission for adult psychiatric illness in England: analysis of Hospital Episode Statistics data. *British Journal of Psychiatry* **185(4)**, 334–341.

49. Ford R, Durcan G, Warner L, Hardy P and Muijen M (1998) One day survey by the Mental Health Act Commission of acute adult psychiatric inpatient wards in England and Wales. *BMJ* **317**,1279– 1283.

50. Meltzer H, Gatward R, Corbin T, Goodman R and Ford T (2003) *Persistence, onset, risk factors and outcomes of childhood mental disorders*, TSO: London. www.statistics.gov.uk/downloads/theme_health/PMA ChildPersist.pdf

51. Hofstra M B, van der Ende J and Verhulst FC (2001) Adolescents' self-reported problems as predictors of psychopathology in adulthood: 10-year follow-up study. *BJPsych* **179**, 203–209.

52. Stevenson J and Goodman R (2001) Association between behaviour at age 3 years and adult criminality. *BJPsych* **179**, 197– 202.

Preventive healthcare

David Dix

Chapter 10

Introduction

Preventive healthcare programmes and changes in personal health behaviours have the potential to improve both the quality and length of life. Factors contributing to otherwise avoidable morbidity and mortality are smoking, diet, lack of exercise, alcohol, high-risk sexual behaviour, and drug-taking. These are examined in other chapters covering individual health behaviours. This chapter will focus on aspects of preventive healthcare that involve national intervention programmes aimed at health protection and early detection of diseases, and some health promotion related behaviours (for example, breastfeeding and dental care).

Immunisation

Introduction

Since the mid-1800s, improvements in sanitation, living conditions, nutrition, and hygiene have reduced the incidence and severity of a range of infectious diseases. Together with these factors, immunisation has been at the forefront of preventing the spread of infection. The importance of immunisation is demonstrated by the impact it has had on the incidence of diseases that were formerly major causes of serious illness and of death, particularly among children.

Childhood immunisation programme

In line with Department of Health and World Health Organisation recommendations, children in the UK are immunised in several stages.[1] To protect against diphtheria, tetanus, pertussis (whooping cough), and polio, infants are given a combination vaccine (DTaP/IPV/Hib) in three successive injections at two, three and four months of age to ensure the development of a good primary immune response. The vaccination also includes protection against haemophilus influenzae type B (Hib). As immunity wanes over time, a further dose of a combination vaccine (dTaP/IPV or DTaP/IPV) against diphtheria, tetanus, pertussis and polio is given before going to school, usually at between three years and four months to five years of age. A further booster, single injection (Td/IPV) is given between 13 and 18 years of age for diphtheria, tetanus and polio (Table 10.1).

Protection against meningitis C is given by a separate course of injections at two, three and four months old at the same time as the DTaP/IPV/Hib vaccine. The Meningitis C conjugate vaccine (MenC), introduced in 1999, does not protect against other types of meningococcal organism.

Since 1988, a combination vaccine (MMR) has been used to protect against measles, mumps and rubella, given in a single dose at around 13 months of age. In 1996 a second dose was introduced for children aged between three and five years to provide long-term protection.

Until recently, all children between 10 and 14 years of age were routinely tested for tuberculosis protection and given Bacillus Calmette-Guérin (BCG) vaccine where they were known not to be protected. From September 2005 an improved, targeted,

Table **10.1**

Full immunisation schedule[1]

United Kingdom

When to immunise	What is given
At or soon after birth, to 'at risk' infants	Tuberculosis (BCG)
2, 3 and 4 months old	Diphtheria, tetanus, pertussis (whooping cough), polio and Hib (DTaP/IPV/Hib) MenC
Around 13 months old	Measles, mumps and rubella (MMR)
3 years and 4 months to 5 years old	Diphtheria, tetanus, pertussis (whooping cough) and polio (dTaP/IPV or DTaP/IPV) Measles, mumps and rubella (MMR)
13 to 18 years old	Diphtheria, tetanus, polio (Td/IPV)

1 Each vaccination is given by single injection.

Source: Department of Health

neonatal and other at-risk based programme has replaced the schools' BCG programme for older children in the UK.

Diphtheria, tetanus, pertussis (whooping cough)

Diphtheria is an acute, communicable respiratory disease with initial symptoms of sore throat, low fever and swollen neck glands, progressing to more severe illness (breathing difficulties, and symptoms of shock such as low blood pressure and rapid heartbeat) and possibly death. Until immunisation for the disease was introduced in the 1940s, diphtheria was widespread in Britain and was a leading cause of death among children. By the end of the 1950s it had almost disappeared, falling from over 46,000 notified cases in England and Wales in 1940 to about 50 in 1960. Incidence continued to decline during the rest of the century and diphtheria is now a very rare disease. Of the few cases that are confirmed, most are associated with importations from countries where the disease is still endemic. In 2004 there were ten notified cases[2] and there were no deaths in 2003.[3]

Tetanus is caused by a bacterium usually found in soil or animal manure, and gains entry to the body through infecting a wound from, for example, a garden tool. It causes painful muscle spasms and can be fatal. In 1961, when vaccination was introduced, there were 24 tetanus deaths in England and Wales. Since then, the disease has been almost eliminated among children (the last case in a child under five years old was in 1981) and incidence has declined so that between 1990 and 2003 there were less than ten notified cases a year. In 2004 there were 12 cases, and there were no deaths in 2003.

Pertussis, or whooping cough, is a highly infectious bacterial disease transmitted by droplet spread (through saliva or mucus, which may be coughed up). The condition usually produces an irritating cough that develops into fits, and may last for two or three months. Serious illness and deaths occur chiefly among infants under six months old.

Notifications of pertussis were almost 158,000 in England and Wales in 1950, resulting in 394 deaths in that year. Cases declined with the introduction of immunisation in the 1950s to less than 17,000 in 1970 (Figure 10.2). A large drop in vaccine uptake in the 1970s led to epidemics in the late 1970s and early 1980s but with the restoration of widespread coverage in the 1990s incidence fell considerably. In 2004, there were 504 notified cases, and there was one death in 2003.

As diphtheria, tetanus and pertussis are now generally protected against using a combination vaccine, immunisation rates (coverage) for these diseases are almost identical. For example, in 2004/05, 90 per cent of children in England had been immunised against diphtheria by their first birthday. By 24

Figure **10.2**

Pertussis (whooping cough) notifications, 1950–2004

England & Wales

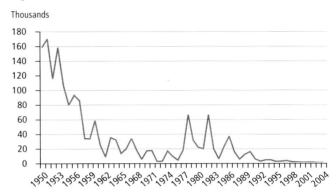

Source: Office for National Statistics (to 1993); Health Protection Agency

months of age, coverage reached 94 per cent for England and for the UK as a whole. The levels of coverage in Wales, Scotland and Northern Ireland were 96, 98 and 97 per cent respectively.[4]

Polio

Polio (or poliomyelitis), an acute illness often causing severe paralysis, was widespread in Britain at the beginning of the twentieth century, affecting young children especially. Immunisation was introduced in the 1950s using the Salk vaccine (inactivated polio vaccine, IPV), given by injection, and in the 1960s the Sabin oral vaccine (OPV) was also introduced. Polio is now generally protected against using IPV as a component of the combination vaccine for the previously mentioned diseases. The result of routine immunisation was a rapid decline in notified cases from 7,760 in England and Wales in 1950 to just six in 1970. In 2004 there were no cases notified.

Haemophilus influenzae type B (Hib)

Haemophilus influenzae type B (Hib) is a bacterium carried in the nose or throat, spread through coughing or sneezing or close contact with an infected person. It gives rise to a range of diseases such as meningitis, pneumonia and osteomyelitis, and may cause septicaemia (bacterial poisoning of the blood). Children under the age of five are most affected. Most frequently it results in meningitis, often creating serious complications such as hearing disorders, learning disabilities or seizures. One child in 20 with Hib meningitis will die.

The impact of immunisation for Hib, as for the other diseases, is very striking. In 1992, when immunisation for the disease was widely introduced nationally, there were 875 laboratory-confirmed reports of Hib infection in England and Wales. The following year reports had fallen to 294, declining to 37 in 1998. Reported cases at all ages have generally risen since, reaching 266 in 2003 (provisional data).[5] Most of this rise has been among children less than four years of age, and to prevent this rise continuing a Hib booster campaign was implemented in May 2003.The impact of immunisation is still very marked, particularly at the youngest ages. In 1992 there were 760 reported cases among children under five years old, which fell to 118 by 2003.

Immunisation with Hib became established quickly after its introduction (initially as a single vaccine), and coverage reached 92 per cent in England for children aged 24 months by 1994/95. Hib vaccine is now normally included in combination with the DTaP/IPV injection. In 2004/05 overall coverage in the UK was 94 per cent, comprising 93 per cent in England, 96 per cent in Wales and 97 per cent in both Scotland and Northern Ireland.

Meningitis C

Meningococcal group C is a bacterial infection that can cause meningitis and septicaemia. It is transmitted by droplet spread or direct contact with a carrier. Children under one year old are most at risk, followed by those aged up to five. There is also a significant risk among young people aged 15–24 years.

In 1998, the year before the MenC vaccine was introduced, there were 811 laboratory-confirmed cases of meningitis C in England and Wales. In 2000, following the introduction of the vaccine, the number of confirmed cases dropped to 711, further declining to 97 in 2003.

The MenC vaccine is now well established. In 2004/05, coverage for children aged 24 months was 93 per cent in England and in the UK overall. In Wales and Scotland it was 96 per cent and in Northern Ireland it was 97 per cent.

Measles, mumps, rubella

Measles is a highly infectious viral illness spread by droplet infection. It can cause fever and complications ranging from ear infections (otitis media) to encephalitis. Routine immunisation for measles was begun in the UK in 1968. In that year in England and Wales there were over 236,000 notified cases and 51 deaths, including 40 deaths to children aged under five. Following the introduction of the vaccine the number of notifications fell by about two-thirds to an average of 90,000 a year in the early 1980s, though cases continued to fluctuate as measles epidemics tend towards a two-year cycle. A combined injection for measles, mumps and rubella (MMR) was introduced in 1988, achieving a higher uptake than the previous single vaccine. Notifications continued to fall, from

over 26,000 in 1989, when there were three deaths, to less than 2,400 in 2004. In 2003 there were no deaths from the disease.

Mumps is another acute viral illness spread by droplet infection, transmitted through coughing or sneezing and through direct contact with saliva. Symptoms include fever, headache, and painful swollen glands, and in more severe cases complications such as swelling of the testes (orchitis) or of the ovaries (oophoritis), deafness, or meningitis may occur. Immunisation for mumps was introduced as part of the combination MMR vaccine in 1988, with an almost immediate effect on the incidence of the disease. Consultations with general practitioners for the illness fell from 2.2 per thousand in that year to 0.6 per thousand in 1990 in England and Wales. There was also a steep decline in notified cases from nearly 21,000 in 1989 to about 2,400 in 1992, as the MMR vaccine became established, with coverage in England, for example, reaching 92 per cent in 1992/93.

The number of cases remained low during the 1990s for all ages (Figure 10.3). However there was an increase in notified cases for children under 15 at the turn of the century. Although 2002 showed some remission, the number of cases for this age group had risen to over 2,800 by 2004, the greatest number since 1990.

Incidence for those aged 15 and over showed an even clearer and more dramatic pattern of increase during this time. Notifications went up almost threefold between 2002 and 2003 and more than fivefold between the next successive years, reaching well over 13,000 in 2004. The increase largely reflects lower immunity among older teenagers and young adults in their early 20s, particularly those born between 1983 and 1986 immediately before the introduction of routine

Figure **10.3**

Mumps notifications:[1] by age, 1989–2004

England & Wales

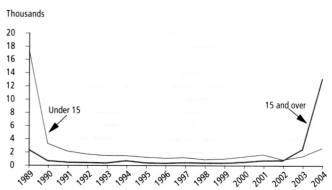

1 *Excludes a small number of cases where the age is not known.*

Source: Health Protection Agency

vaccination in 1988. These young people would not have been exposed to mumps in childhood because of the swift success of the MMR vaccine in controlling the disease. Older adults were more likely to have had mumps when it was still a common childhood infection.[6]

Rubella is normally a mild infectious disease, causing a rash, swollen glands, and occasionally pain or inflammation of the joints. However, if it is caught by a woman who is pregnant it can cause severe defects in the unborn child, such as mental impairment, deafness, cataracts and blindness, or heart problems. Immunisation for the disease was introduced in the UK in 1970, initially targeting schoolgirls and non-immune women of childbearing age. The programme did reduce the number of births of malformed children, but as it did not successfully eliminate infection of susceptible pregnant women (often infected by their own children or children of friends), routine immunisation of all children against rubella was introduced with the MMR vaccine in 1988.

Incidence of rubella, following the introduction of MMR, has declined very markedly. In 1989 there were nearly 24,600 notified cases in England and Wales, a rate of 0.5 cases per thousand. In 1990 the rate had more than halved to 0.2 per thousand. Cases generally continued to fall (although there were brief peaks in incidence in 1993 and 1996) reaching just under 1,300 in 2004, a rate of 0.02 per thousand.

In the UK as a whole, MMR vaccination coverage reached 92 per cent by 1996/97, but in 1997/98 it began to fall, declining to 81 per cent in 2003/04. There was a slight improvement, to 82 per cent, in 2004/05. However, there is substantial variation between countries. In 2004/05 England had the lowest coverage (81 per cent), followed by Wales (82 per cent), whereas coverage in both Scotland and Northern Ireland was 88 per cent. The World Health Organisation (WHO) recommends immunity levels of around 95 per cent to prevent outbreaks of disease.

The impact of public concerns following the publication in 1998 of the *Lancet* paper by Wakefield and others[7] questioning the safety of MMR is thus very noticeable. Further studies have allayed some of the public's anxieties about the vaccine, in particular a recent (2005) publication concerning the incidence of autism following the 1993 withdrawal of MMR in Japan.[8, 9]

Tuberculosis

Tuberculosis (TB) is a disease caused by one of three types of mycobacterium, transmitted by droplet infection through coughs or sneezes. It generally requires prolonged contact with the infected individual at close quarters in order to spread. In about three-quarters of cases the lungs and respiratory system

Figure 10.4

Completed diphtheria and MMR immunisations,[1] 1995/96–2004/05

United Kingdom

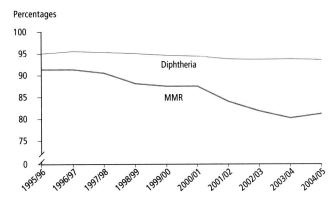

1   *Vaccination courses completed by age 24 months.*
Source: Health Protection Agency

are affected, although TB may also take a non-respiratory form affecting other parts of the body. Symptoms include coughing, weight loss, fever and severe fatigue, requiring treatment with a combination of special antibiotics for a period of at least six months. It is particularly associated with circumstances that give rise to the weakening of the immune system such as poor living conditions, homelessness, drug use, alcoholism, or old age.

TB was extremely prevalent in Great Britain in the 19th century and during the first half of the 20th. The disease first became notifiable in 1912, and in the following year there were almost 120,000 cases recorded in England and Wales, of both respiratory and non-respiratory types. Incidence declined with the steady improvement in living conditions so that by 1950 the number of cases had dropped to around 50,000. Following the introduction of the BCG vaccine in 1953 and other advances such as specific chemotherapy in the same decade, overall incidence continued to fall so that in 1987 there were a little over 5,000 cases. Since then, incidence has remained low but has nevertheless increased in recent years so that in 2004 there were over 6,700 cases notified, and just under 400 deaths. The increase is concentrated within the inner cities, particularly London, and among ethnic minority groups. Incidence in Scotland declined from just over 500 cases in 1996 to less than 400 in 2004.[10]

BCG vaccination is just one important aspect of TB prevention. It gives substantial, but limited, protection and cannot by itself control the spread of TB for which other measures such as effective surveillance and early treatment are also vital. Recognising this, a programme targeting those groups most at risk, replacing the schools-based programme for older children, has been introduced. Among those still recommended for BCG vaccination are infants living in areas with high incidence of TB, previously unvaccinated new immigrants from countries with a high prevalence of the disease, and children for whom, after screening for TB risk factors, vaccination is considered appropriate.

Immunisation programmes for older people

Influenza

The influenza (flu) virus is transmitted by droplet infection through coughing or sneezing, causing fever, sore throat, coughs and aching, lasting usually for about a week. People whose immune systems are less able to cope, such as the elderly, may suffer more serious illness. The weakened state produced by the virus can give rise to complications involving other conditions, particularly pneumonia, which can be fatal.

Influenza incidence rises during the winter months, and in years when cases are widespread, it can be responsible for a large proportion of the additional deaths usually observed over the winter period compared with the rest of the year. For example, it is estimated that in the 1999/2000 influenza season (October–May), influenza caused over 17,000 excess deaths in England and Wales. There may be far fewer deaths in other years when the infection is less prevalent. The comparable number of excess influenza deaths during the 2003/04 season was about 2,000.[11]

Because of the dangers of an outbreak affecting the more vulnerable members of the population, particularly the aged, the UK Health Departments' policy is that influenza immunisation is offered to all persons aged 65 and over. It is also offered to other at-risk groups such as those with chronic respiratory or heart disease, or in long-stay residential care homes. Annual vaccination is required as the prevalent strains of the influenza virus are constantly changing, requiring corresponding changes to the vaccines used to counter the infection.

In 2000, the Department of Health in England recommended that influenza vaccination for the elderly risk group would begin at 65, the initial age having previously been set at 75.[12] At the same time as extending the target population, a national rapid reporting scheme was put in place to monitor the programme so that detailed observation of coverage for particular groups such as the elderly became possible. Before these changes, it is estimated that in 1999/2000, some 44 per cent of people aged 65 or over in Great Britain were vaccinated. In 2003/04, coverage for this age group reached 71 per cent in England, exceeding the target of 70 per cent. The equivalent coverage in Wales was 63 per cent and in both Scotland and Northern Ireland it was 73 per cent.

Pneumococcal disease

Alongside influenza immunisation for older people, a further programme of vaccination against pneumococcal disease was introduced throughout the UK in 2003. Pneumococcal infection is caused by a bacterium (streptococcus pneumoniae or the pneumococcus) which may affect the lungs and is the most common cause of serious pneumonia. The bacterium can also infect the blood stream, causing invasive pneumococcal disease (IPD). About 5,000 cases of IPD are recorded in England and Wales each year. Young children and people with compromised immune systems are particularly vulnerable. Unimmunised older people are among the groups most at risk, and the vaccine (a single, separate injection) is therefore usually offered at the same time as that for influenza.[13] Immunisation is additionally recommended for those at younger ages who are considered to be at risk. One injection will provide protection for some years.

In Scotland and Northern Ireland the vaccine has been offered to those aged 65 and over since the introduction of the programme in 2003, while in England and Wales it has been brought in by stages, from an initial starting age of 80 in 2003 rising to the target age range of 65 and over in 2005.

Cancer screening

Introduction

More than one in three people will develop cancer during their lifetime.[14] Accordingly, cancer is a major focus of attention in preventive health. Alongside the progress made in reducing lung cancer incidence by action taken against smoking, the well-established screening programmes for breast and cervical cancers are an important means of early detection to reduce cancer morbidity and mortality. A national bowel cancer screening programme for older people is also to be introduced across the UK, beginning in England in 2006.

One in nine women will develop breast cancer in her lifetime. The aim of breast screening is to detect already developing cancer in its early stages, enabling earlier and more effective treatment. Alongside improvements in treatment and the development of new drugs such as tamoxifen, screening has significantly contributed to the reduction in mortality rates for breast cancer.[15, 16]

It is generally accepted that cervical screening has been largely responsible for the reduction in morbidity and mortality from this disease, the incidence of which has halved since the introduction of a national screening programme throughout the UK in the late 1980s.[17] In England and Wales, the age-standardised incidence of invasive cervical cancer fell from 16.5 cases per 100,000 to 8.6 per 100,000 between 1988 and 2001 (Figure 10.5).

Figure **10.5**

Incidence of invasive cervical cancer (age-standardised), 1971–2001

England & Wales

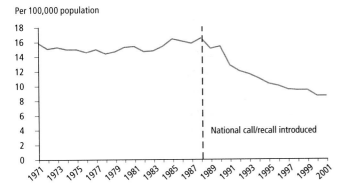

Per 100,000 population

Source: Office for National Statistics

Breast screening

Breast cancer screening programmes were begun across the UK in 1988. Since that time, the national programmes have sought to invite all eligible women aged between 50 and 64 for screening once every three years. The screening process involves the use of a low dose X-ray (a mammogram) to examine both breasts and show up any cancerous growth.

In 2003/04 in England, over 1.5 million women aged 50–64 were invited for breast screening, of whom just under 76 per cent (1.2 million) were screened. Five per cent of those screened (just over 60,000) were referred for assessment. A total of almost 8,400 cases of cancer were detected, some 7.1 cancers per thousand women screened. As well as those invited for screening under the programme, a further 117,500 women of all ages were screened following self-referral or referral by a GP. The total number of cancers detected for all ages screened (45 and over) was just over 11,200 (7.9 cancers per thousand women screened overall).[18]

The **coverage** of the breast screening programme comprises the proportion of women eligible to be screened who have had a test with a recorded result at least once in the previous three years. As women may receive their first invitation at any time between their 50th and 53rd birthdays, a good assessment of the effectiveness of the programme is provided by measuring coverage for women aged 53–64; in 2003/04 this was 75 per cent. A further 13 per cent had never been screened. These largely comprised women who were not registered with a general practitioner, together with those who had declined to enter the programme. The remaining 12 per cent comprised those women who were screened more than three years previously.

In the year ending March 1992, **uptake** (the proportion of women aged 50–64 invited for screening for whom a test result has subsequently been recorded) was 72 per cent in England. It remained at about the same level until 1994/95 when it increased to 77 per cent. Uptake for the 50–64 age group dipped slightly in the following year but has since remained stable at between 75 and 76 per cent. In 2003/04 it was 76 per cent (77 per cent in Wales).

In accordance with the recommendations of the NHS Cancer Plan in 2000,[19] the upper age limit for invitation for breast screening was increased from 64 to 70 in England in 2004. The other countries of the UK are also raising the upper age limit routinely covered by their screening programmes following similar recommendations. In addition, two-view mammography (where two X-ray views are taken of each breast from different angles) has been introduced across the UK for first and subsequent screening rounds (in Scotland it is used for the first screening round only). It is expected that this will significantly increase the detection of small cancers.

Cervical screening

Screening for cervical cancer was introduced into Great Britain in the 1960s, but this had only limited coverage and follow-up until the UK-wide call and recall programme was put in place in 1988. Routine screening is now offered under the programme to all eligible women aged between 25 and 64 in England, the lower limit for first invitation having been raised from 20 in October 2003. The target populations for routine screening in Wales, Scotland and Northern Ireland comprise women aged 20–64, 20–60 and 20–65 respectively.

Women are invited for screening at three-year intervals up to the age of 49. From age 50, in England, invitations are sent at five-year intervals up to age 64. In the rest of the UK invitations for screening remain at three-year intervals.

The aim of cervical screening is to detect cell abnormalities that can lead to the development of cancer, so that with appropriate treatment the cells can be removed or destroyed before a cancer can occur. The method of screening is the smear test, by which a sample of cells is collected, smeared onto a slide and examined under a laboratory microscope. Liquid based cytology (LBC), an improved means of preparing samples for examination, is increasingly being used. LBC will normally yield clearer results than the conventional smear test, so that it should greatly reduce the number of occasions when women are recalled because the smear could not be read.

In England about 4.7 million women were invited for cervical screening in 2004/05, almost all of whom (4.1 million) were within the target range of 25–64 years old.[20]

The coverage of the cervical screening programme comprises the proportion of eligible women (i.e., excluding those ineligible for clinical reasons such as hysterectomy), who have been screened in the previous five years and for whom an adequate test result has been obtained. Total coverage in England in 2004/05 for the age range of 25–64, was 80 per cent (coverage in Wales for these ages was very similar, at 79 per cent). There has been little change in overall coverage since 1994/95, when the proportion was 82 per cent.

Health promotion

Introduction

In addition to the national intervention programmes for immunisation and screening, health promotion programmes, which encourage people individually to change their health behaviour for the better, are an important aspect of preventive healthcare. This section examines patterns of breastfeeding together with smoking and drinking in pregnancy, and the national stop smoking programme.

Breastfeeding

Breastfeeding brings benefits to both mother and child.[21] It provides the most appropriate nutrition for a baby's first six months and the transmission of antibodies from the mother guards the baby against chest and other infections, gastroenteritis, asthma, eczema and allergies; protection which is not available through the use of bottled milk. The mother also benefits. Breastfeeding helps the womb to return to normal after childbirth, it reduces the risk of pre-menopausal breast and ovarian cancer, and even helps her to regain shape, as the production of breast milk uses up 500 calories per day. In addition to the physical benefits, breastfeeding helps to develop a strong emotional bond between mother and child. Recognising these advantages of breastfeeding for the earliest stages of a child's life, and in line with guidance from the World Health Organisation, the Department of Health recommends exclusive breastfeeding for a baby's first six months.[22]

The Infant Feeding Survey, carried out every five years, shows that the age, educational level and social status of mothers are all strongly associated with breastfeeding, and that there are noticeable differences in breastfeeding patterns between the countries of the UK.

Prevalence of breastfeeding

The Infant Feeding Survey found that 69 per cent of babies born in the UK in 2000 were initially breastfed (even if only on one occasion). Breastfeeding rates drop substantially over time, however. At six weeks, 42 per cent of mothers were still breastfeeding, and at six months the proportion was 21 per cent.[23]

There was some further variation between countries. In England and Wales, 71 per cent of babies were initially breastfed, compared with 63 per cent in Scotland and 54 per cent in Northern Ireland. Scottish mothers were found to breastfeed the longest, with 40 per cent of those who initially breastfed still breastfeeding at six months, compared with 34 per cent in England and Wales and 21 per cent in Northern Ireland.

Older mothers are more likely to breastfeed their babies. In 2000, among mothers under 20 years of age, 46 per cent initially breastfed their child compared with 58 per cent of those aged 20–24, 67 per cent of mothers aged 25–29, and 78 per cent of those aged 30 or over. Higher breastfeeding rates were found among older mothers in all the countries.

The 2000 survey found that in all countries of the UK, mothers who left full-time education at age 16 were least likely to breastfeed. Among those mothers who completed full-time education after the age of 18, a total of 88 per cent initially breastfed compared with 54 per cent who left school at 16. This was consistent with findings from previous years. For example, the 1995 survey reported similar proportions, at 88 per cent and 51 per cent respectively.

For all stages of a baby's life up to nine months, the survey found that mothers in the managerial and professional occupations are the most likely to breastfeed. Some 85 per cent of mothers in these occupations initially breastfed their baby, compared with 73 per cent of those in intermediate occupations and 59 per cent in routine and manual occupations. Among mothers who had never worked or who were long term unemployed, the proportion was 52 per cent. At six months, 31 per cent of women in the managerial and professional occupations were breastfeeding, compared with 13 per cent of those who were in routine occupations or were unemployed.

Smoking and drinking in pregnancy

Smoking in pregnancy

Smoking in pregnancy can harm the unborn child.[24] It creates an increased risk of reduced birth weight, miscarriage, and perinatal death compared with not smoking. Continued smoking during pregnancy also raises the likelihood of sudden infant death syndrome. It is therefore monitored as an important aspect of public health promotion.

In 2000, according to the Infant Feeding Survey, 35 per cent of mothers smoked in the twelve months before their pregnancy or during it. Three per cent gave up less than a year before their pregnancy was confirmed, and 11 per cent gave up on confirmation. Two per cent gave up smoking later in their pregnancy.

Twenty per cent of mothers in the UK smoked throughout their pregnancy, although the majority of these did cut down. Only two per cent of mothers did not reduce their smoking. As Table 10.6 shows, there was little variation between countries.

Smoking before and during pregnancy was more prevalent among younger women. A large majority (65 per cent) of young mothers under 20 smoked before or during their pregnancy. Some 40 per cent at this age smoked throughout. Smoking in pregnancy declined with age so that among those aged 30 and over, 13 per cent continued to smoke throughout. Socio-economic status was also found to be associated with smoking in pregnancy, so that although only eight per cent of women in managerial and professional occupations smoked throughout their pregnancy, about a third of women (36 per cent) who had never worked or who were long-term unemployed smoked throughout.

Drinking in pregnancy

The Infant Feeding Survey also found that in 2000, 87 per cent of mothers who had recently given birth had sometimes drunk alcohol before pregnancy. Of all mothers, 61 per cent drank while pregnant, down from 66 per cent in 1995. Of those who drank before they became pregnant, 65 per cent cut down

drinking, while 30 per cent gave up. The remaining five per cent did not reduce their alcohol intake.

Older mothers were more likely to drink at all during pregnancy. A little more than half of younger mothers drank during pregnancy (53 per cent of those aged under 20) whereas more than two-thirds of mothers aged 35 or over (71 per cent) had drunk while pregnant. Nevertheless, the level of drinking was low. Only 3 per cent of those who drank during pregnancy drank more than seven units per week, or one unit a day on average.

In England and Wales, 87 per cent of mothers drank before pregnancy and 62 per cent during it, while in Scotland the proportions were similar, at 89 per cent and 59 per cent respectively. In Northern Ireland the proportions were lower, at 82 per cent and 52 per cent.

The survey found that receiving advice about the effects of alcohol[25] was not related to whether women gave up drinking during pregnancy. However, women who received advice (in the majority of cases, from a midwife, printed information, or a doctor) were more likely to have reduced the amount they drank during pregnancy (67 per cent compared with 59 per cent of those not given advice).

Smoking cessation

Smoking is responsible for about nine out of 10 deaths from lung cancer, and makes a significant contribution to morbidity

Table **10.6**

Mothers' smoking behaviour: by country, 2000

United Kingdom

Percentages

	United Kingdom	England and Wales	Scotland	Northern Ireland
Non-smokers	65	65	64	64
Never smoked	52	52	53	54
Gave up over a year before pregnancy	13	13	11	10
All smokers	35	35	36	36
Smoked before pregnancy but gave up	16	16	14	14
Gave up less than a year before pregnancy	3	3	3	3
Gave up on confirmation of pregnancy	11	11	9	10
Gave up later in pregnancy, stayed quit	2	2	2	1
Smoked throughout pregnancy	20	19	22	23
Gave up, but started again	4	4	5	4
Cut down	14	14	15	16
Did not cut down	2	2	2	3

Source: Infant Feeding Survey, Office for National Statistics

and mortality from other cancers such as bladder cancer. It is also responsible for a large part of the burden of illness and mortality caused by heart disease, respiratory diseases such as chronic bronchitis and emphysema, and other conditions.[26]

Two-thirds of smokers would like to give up smoking altogether.[27] To help them to do this, and recognising the burden of illness and death caused by smoking, the 1998 White Paper *Smoking Kills* announced a programme of NHS Stop Smoking Services in England.[28] Similar programmes were also initiated in the other countries of the UK. In its Public Service Agreement in July 2004, the Department of Health set a target to reduce the proportion of adult smokers to 21 per cent or less by 2010.[29]

Stop smoking services provide advice to smokers from health professionals on the dangers of smoking and on ways to quit. Practical assistance is also given. Courses of nicotine replacement therapy (NRT) enable smokers in the process of giving up to overcome withdrawal symptoms. NRT provides the body with nicotine (normally in the form of a patch, although chewing gum or nasal spray may be used) in decreasing doses until the craving becomes manageable. An alternative to NRT, a short course of bupropion (Zyban) is also available. This drug, which does not itself contain nicotine, can help limit the symptoms of withdrawal and reduce cravings for nicotine. These treatments assist a smoker in the early stages of adjusting to doing without cigarettes, so that they can become established as a non-smoker with a much lower risk of taking up the habit again.

In England in 2004/05, according to provisional data, almost 530,000 people accessing NHS Stop Smoking services set a date to quit smoking. This was a very large increase on 2000/01, when about 132,500 smokers set a quit date during the early stages of the programme. In each year of the programme, significantly more women than men have set a date to quit smoking (57 per cent compared with 43 per cent in 2004/05). This is despite the fact that men and women are almost equally likely to smoke. Upon follow up at four weeks from the quit date, 58 per cent of men and 55 per cent of women reported successfully having given up.[30]

Recognising the health dangers posed by smoking among pregnant women, the White Paper on Tobacco set a target to reduce the proportion of women smoking throughout pregnancy in England from 23 per cent (the level recorded by the Infant Feeding Survey in 1995) to 15 per cent in England by 2010. Towards this goal, NHS Stop Smoking Services in England in 2004/05 helped over 15,000 pregnant women to set a quit date. At the four-week follow-up, the proportion who reported having successfully quit was 51 per cent.[30]

Oral health

Introduction

Good oral health is the result of a variety of factors. Better diet, close attention to oral hygiene (such as regular brushing with a flouride toothpaste), fluoridation of the water supply (where this has taken place) and effective dental care all play a part. Recognising these factors, the NHS Plan in 2000 included recommendations for oral health within England.[31] The plan particularly focused on the dental health of children, with the target that by 2003, 70 per cent of five-year-old children should have no experience of tooth decay. In 1994 the Health of the Nation oral health plan set a target that on average 12-year-old children in England should have no more than one decayed, missing or filled permanent tooth by 2003.[32]

Children

The importance of safeguarding children's oral health has long been recognised by the government's provision that a child attending a state funded school should receive an oral health check at least three times in their school life. In addition, NHS dental care is free for children up to the age of sixteen or eighteen if they remain in full-time education. More generally, regular visits to the dentist have an important role to play. This is noticeable in the results from the UK Children's Dental Health surveys carried out in 1983, 1993 and 2003.[33-35]

Dental attendance

Most children have visited the dentist at least once by the age of five. Between 1983 and 2003 among five-year-old children, the proportion who had never visited the dentist fell markedly, from 14 per cent to 6 per cent, while for eight-year-olds, it dropped from 4 per cent to 2 per cent.

The UK Children's Dental Health Survey in 2003 found that the majority of children of all ages visited the dentist regularly. More than half of five-year-olds were regular attenders, although about a third only attended the dentist when they were having problems. A little under two-thirds of older children attended regularly (Table 10.7).

The survey also found that about three-quarters of children from ages five to 15 last visited the dentist for a check-up rather than as a result of having trouble with their teeth, so it appears that the importance of oral health care is widely appreciated.

Across all ages studied, significantly fewer children who attended regularly were reported as having oral health problems over the previous 12 months compared with those who visited the dentist only in response to a problem with their teeth.

Table **10.7**

Children's reported dental attendance: by age, 2003

United Kingdom   Percentages

	Regular attender	Only attends with trouble	Occasional attender
5 years	56	34	10
8 years	62	26	12
12 years	63	23	14
15 years	63	21	16

Source: Children's Dental Health Survey, Office for National Statistics

Dental health in younger children

Experience of dental decay among younger children substantially improved between 1983 and 1993, although little improvement occurred in the following ten years. Among five-year-olds in 2003, 57 per cent had no obvious decay experience compared with 50 per cent in 1983. This falls short of the target set in the NHS Plan that 70 per cent of five-year-olds in England should have no decay experience by 2003.

Dental health in older children

Among older children, substantially more of those surveyed in 2003 were found to be free from obvious decay experience

Table **10.8**

Tooth condition in permanent teeth:[1] by age, 1983–2003

United Kingdom   Percentages

	1983	1993	2003
12-year-olds			
No decay	19	48	62
Obvious decay experience	81	52	38
Teeth with obvious decay:			
decay into dentine	32	24	12
filled decay (otherwise sound)	69	39	26
missing due to decay	14	7	3
15-year-olds			
No decay	7	37	50
Obvious decay experience	93	63	50
Teeth with obvious decay:			
decay into dentine	42	30	13
filled decay (otherwise sound)	85	52	42
missing due to decay	24	7	6

1 *Percentages add to more than 100 as children may have more than one type of decay.*

Source: Children's Dental Health Survey, Office for National Statistics

compared with twenty years earlier. In 2003, 62 per cent of 12-year-olds and 50 per cent of 15-year-olds were found to be free from decay experience (Table 10.8). This is a considerable improvement on 1983, when 19 per cent of 12-year-olds and seven per cent of 15-year-olds were found to be free from obvious decay experience. As was the case with younger children, most of the improvement occurred in the ten years to 1993, although there was also a significant reduction in decay experience between 1993 and 2003.

The proportion of 12-year-olds with at least one tooth with decay into dentine (dentine is the hard tissue that makes up the bulk of a tooth) reduced by more than half between 1983 and 2003, while that for 15-year-olds decreased by over two-thirds. The proportion of 12- and 15-year-old children with filled permanent teeth also more than halved over the period. The 2003 survey found that 12-year-olds in England had an average of 0.7 teeth with obvious decay experience, so that the target for reducing decay experience among older children was met.

Adults

Dental attendance

According to the UK Adult Dental Health Survey, in 1998 twice as many adults who were dentate (retained some natural teeth) reported attending for regular check-ups (59 per cent) compared with those who only attended when they had trouble with their teeth (30 per cent). Women were more likely to report attending for regular check-ups than men, 66 per cent compared with 52 per cent (Table 10.9).[36]

Table **10.9**

Regular dental attendance:[1] by age and sex, 1978–1998

United Kingdom   Percentages

	1978	1988	1998
16–24	44	45	48
25–34	47	48	53
35–44	47	59	62
45–54	40	54	64
55 and over	32	45	66
Men	36	42	52
Women	50	58	66
All	43	50	59

1 *Dentate adults.*

Source: Adult Dental Health Survey, Office for National Statistics

Young people, particularly young men aged 16–34, were the least likely to report seeking regular check-ups. Across almost all age groups, women were more likely to report attending the dentist regularly than men, with the exception of those aged 75 and over (Table 10.10).

Figure 10.10

Regular dental attendance:[1] by age and sex, 1998

United Kingdom

Percentages

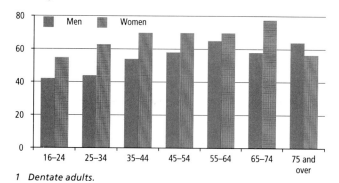

1 Dentate adults.

Source: Adult Dental Health Survey, Office for National Statistics

There was a large rise between 1978 and 1998 in the overall proportion of dentate adults who reported attending for regular check-ups. Most of this increase was concentrated among people aged 35 and over. In 1998, those who reported visiting the dentist only when they had trouble had on average twice as many decayed or unsound teeth as those who attended regularly for check-ups.

In 1998, across all ages, a greater proportion of both men and women in the non-manual classes (comprising the professional, intermediate and skilled non-manual classes grouped according to the Registrar General's Social Class used in the survey) reported attending the dentist regularly. Among the non-manual classes 58 per cent of dentate men attended for regular check-ups, compared with 50 per cent in the skilled manual group and 42 per cent of men in the unskilled manual, partly skilled and unskilled groups. For women, the proportions were 71 per cent, 66 per cent and 55 per cent respectively.

Condition and loss of teeth

An important measure of dental health is the proportion of the population who still retain some natural teeth. Among those aged 16 or over in 1998, 90 per cent of men and 85 per cent of women were dentate. This is a considerable improvement compared with 1978, when the proportions were 75 per cent for men and 67 per cent for women.

The proportion of the population retaining some natural teeth has markedly improved for all the countries of the UK over the lifetime of the survey, although some differences still remain (Table 10.11). In England and in Northern Ireland, 88 per cent of those aged 16 or over still retained some teeth in 1998, while the proportion was somewhat lower in Wales (84 per cent) and in Scotland (83 per cent).

In 1998, less than one per cent of the population aged under 45 were found to have no natural teeth, but tooth loss increased significantly with age so that among those 75 and

Table 10.11

Dentate adults aged 35 and over: by age, sex, country and social class,[1] 1998

United Kingdom

Percentages

	35–44	45–54	55–64	65–74	75 and over
Men	99	93	82	69	48
Women	99	94	79	60	40
England	99	95	82	66	44
Wales	100	86	75	62	37
Scotland	97	88	66	51	36
Northern Ireland	100	94	79	54	43
Non-manual	100	97	93	73	56
Skilled manual	98	90	72	60	38
Partly skilled, unskilled manual	98	90	65	50	30

1 Using the Registrar General's Social Class based on occupation of head of household.

Source: Adult Dental Health Survey, Office for National Statistics

Table **10.12**

Adults with any decayed or unsound teeth:[1] by social class[2] and age, 1998

United Kingdom   Percentages

	16–24	25–34	35–44	45–54	55–64	65 and over	All
Non-manual	44	54	43	55	53	49	50
Skilled manual	56	64	58	58	44	58	57
Partly skilled, unskilled manual	58	70	62	55	68	59	62
All[3]	51	60	51	57	54	54	55

1   Base is all dentate adults.
2   Using the Registrar General's Social Class based on occupation of head of household.
3   Includes those for whom social class was not known and armed forces.

Source: Adult Dental Health Survey, Office for National Statistics

over, 52 per cent of men and 60 per cent of women had lost all their teeth. However, there are other factors involved besides age, for example changes in the practice of dentistry, and the use of fluoride toothpaste.

Men and women from non-manual backgrounds were found to be significantly more likely to have some natural teeth remaining than those from skilled and unskilled manual backgrounds (Table 10.11).

It was also found that a lower proportion of those from non-manual backgrounds were likely to have any decayed or unsound teeth compared with those from skilled and unskilled manual backgrounds: 50 per cent of dentate adults compared with 57 per cent and 62 per cent respectively, (Table 10.12).

Conclusion

Preventive health measures, put into practice through health promotion and public health programmes, are of great importance for the wellbeing of the population, reducing the burden (physical and social) of illness and premature mortality. Some of the major public health intervention programmes have existed in some form for a long enough time to demonstrate a considerable, and ongoing, impact on health. The success of vaccination in reducing childhood mortality is an important example. Other UK-wide programmes, such as screening for breast and cervical cancers, have developed more recently but have in turn had a significant effect in reducing morbidity. These successes are sufficient to encourage the extension of existing programmes and the introduction of further initiatives. The recent changes in the ages routinely covered by the breast and cervical screening programmes are examples, together with the introduction of vaccination for pneumococcal disease.

Health promotion designed to affect individual health behaviours has also influenced some aspects of public health significantly, and there has been an increase in awareness of

some of the factors necessary for improved health. The rise in public response to the help given by smoking cessation services is one example of this; the decrease in drinking among pregnant women, and the improvements in oral health among adults and to some extent among children, are others.

Notes and references

1.   Full details of the UK immunisation schedule are available at: www.immunisation.nhs.uk

2.   Health Protection Agency (2005) Statutory notifications of infectious diseases: *Final totals for 2004, England and Wales*, at: www.hpa.org.uk/infections

3.   Office for National Statistics (2004) *Mortality Statistics 2003: cause, England and Wales*. ONS: London.

4.   Health and Social Care Information Centre (2005) *NHS Immunisation Statistics, England: 2004–05*. Bulletin 2005/05/HSCIC/. Department of Health at: www.dh.gov.uk

5.   Health Protection Agency (2005) Epidemiological data - Haemophilus Influenzae Type B (Hib) at: www.hpa.org.uk/infections

6.   Savage E, Ramsay M et al (2005) Mumps outbreaks across England and Wales in 2004: observational study. *BMJ* **330**, 1119–1120.

7.   Wakefield A J et al (1998) Ileal-lymphoid-modular hypoplasia, non-specific colitis, and pervasive developmental disorder in children. *The Lancet* **351**, 637–641.

8.   Honda H, Shumizu Y and Rutter M (2005) No effect of MMR withdrawal on the incidence of autism: a total population study. *Journal of Child Psychology and Psychiatry* **46(6)**, 572–579.

9.   A list of articles, and other material relating to MMR, is given at: www.mmrthefacts.org.uk

10. ISD Scotland (2005) at: www.isdscotland.org

11. Cooke M K *et al* (2004) Influenza and other respiratory viruses surveillance in the United Kingdom: October 2003 to May 2004. *Communicable Diseases Review* (Supplement) Health Protection Agency at: www.hpa.org.uk/cdr

12. Chief Medical Officer (August 2000) Influenza immunisation. PL/CMO/2000/3. Department of Health at: www.dh.gov.uk

13. Chief Medical Officer (March 2005) *The pneumococcal immunisation programme for older people and risk groups*. PL/CMO/2005/1. Department of Health www.dh.gov.uk

14. Quinn M, Babb P, Brock A, Kirby L and Jones J (2001) *Cancer Trends in England and Wales 1950–1999*. Studies on Medical and Population Subjects no.66. Office for National Statistics: London. www.statistics.gov.uk

15. Quinn M and Allen E (on behalf of the United Kingdom Association of Cancer Registries) (1995) Changes in incidence of and mortality from breast cancer in England and Wales since the introduction of screening. *BMJ* **311**, 1391–1395.

16. Blanks R G, Moss S M, McGahan C E, Quinn M J and Babb P J (2000) Effect of NHS Breast screening programme on mortality from breast cancer in England and Wales, 1990-8: comparison of observed with predicted mortality. *BMJ* **321**, 665–669.

17. Sasieni P and Adams J (1999) Effect of screening on cervical cancer mortality in England and Wales: analysis of trends with an age period cohort model. *BMJ* **318**, 1244–1245.

18. Department of Health (2005) *Breast Screening Programme, England: 2003–04*. Statistical Bulletin 2005/06, at: www.dh.gov.uk

19. Department of Health (2000) *NHS Cancer Plan 2000* at: www.dh.gov.uk

20. Department of Health (2004) *Cervical Screening Programme, England: 2003–04*. Statistical Bulletin 2004/20 at: www.dh.gov.uk

21. World Health Organisation. Nutrition: Infant and young child - breastfeeding (review of evidence) at: www.who.int/child-adolescent-health/nut.htm

22. Department of Health (2003) *Infant Feeding Recommendation* at: www.dh.gov.uk

23. Hamlyn B *et al* (2002) *Infant Feeding 2000*, TSO: London. www.dh.gov.uk

24. Poswillo D (1998) *Report of the Scientific Committee On Tobacco and Health*, TSO: London. www.archive.official-documents.co.uk/document/doh/tobacco/report.htm

25. Report of the Swedish Presidency (2001) *A background report on relevant data on alcohol consumption, alcohol-related problems and relevant policies.*(Section 3.4, Pregnancy and drinking). European Commission at: http://europa.eu.int/comm/health

26. Twigg L, Moon G and Walker S (2004) *The smoking epidemic in England*. Health Development Agency at: www.publichealth.nice.org.uk

27. Office for National Statistics (2005) General Household Survey 2003, TSO: London. www.statistics.gov.uk

28. Department of Health (1998) *Smoking Kills: a White Paper on tobacco. Saving lives: Our Healthier Nation*, TSO: London. www.archive.official-documents.co.uk/document/cm41/4177/4177.htm

29. Department of Health (2004) Technical Note for the Spending Review 2004. Public Service Agreement at: www.dh.gov.uk

30. Health and Social Care Information Centre (2005) *Statistics on NHS Stop Smoking Services in England, April 2004 to March 2005*. Department of Health at: www.dh.gov.uk

31. Department of Health (2000) *Modernising NHS Dentistry – Implementing the NHS Plan*, at: www.dh.gov.uk

32. Department of Health (1994) *An Oral Health Strategy for England*. Central Print Unit, Department of Health.

33. Todd J E and Dodd T (1985) *Children's Dental Health in the United Kingdom* 1983, HMSO: London.

34. O'Brien M (1994) *Children's Dental Health in the United Kingdom 1993*, HMSO: London. www.statistics.gov.uk

35. Pitts N, Harker R *et al* (2005) *Children's Dental Health in the United Kingdom 2003* at: www.statistics.gov.uk/children/dentalhealth

36. Walker A and Cooper I (eds.) (2000) *Adult Dental Health Survey. Oral Health in the United Kingdom, 1998*, TSO: London. www.statistics.gov.uk/ssd/surveys/adult_dental_health_survey.asp

Use of services

Melissa Coulthard

chapter 11

Introduction

The National Health Service (NHS) was created in 1948 to provide universal healthcare based on medical need rather than the ability to pay. All taxpayers, employers and employees contribute to the cost. Most forms of treatment are provided free, but others such as prescription drugs, eye tests and dentistry may incur a charge. The NHS is made up of a wide range of health professionals, support workers and organisations. In England the NHS is managed by the Department of Health, which is responsible for developing and implementing policies and for the regulation and inspection of health services. The devolved administrations have similar responsibilities in other parts of the UK. *The official year book of the United Kingdom of Great Britain and Northern Ireland* provides a good summary of the structure of the NHS in each of the countries of the UK.[1]

Health care can be divided into primary and secondary care. Primary care is the first point of contact people have with health services, and includes the services provided by General Practitioner (GP) practices, dental practitioners, pharmacists and opticians. Most contacts with the NHS take place in primary care. Secondary health care services are hospital based and provide more specialist knowledge, skills and equipment than is provided by primary care.

Primary care

Primary care provides a range of health care services including diagnosis and management of acute and chronic conditions, family planning, preventive medicine and referrals to other services including secondary health care. Primary care is provided by a variety of people, including the GP, practice nurse, district or community nurse, midwife, health visitor and other attached staff such as counsellor or psychologist.

General Practitioners

The GP practice is one of the first contact points people have with health care services, and provides care throughout people's lives. GP surgeries offer a range of services including prevention, investigation, diagnosis and treatment. The GP can also refer patients to other health professionals for more specific diagnosis and treatment.

The General Household Survey (GHS) in Great Britain and the Continuous Household Survey (CHS) in Northern Ireland collect information on GP consultations. In the UK in 2003/04 there were on average four NHS GP consultations per person per year. Females had more consultations per year than males (five compared with three and a half) particularly among the 16–44 age group (Figure 11.1). The higher consultation rates by

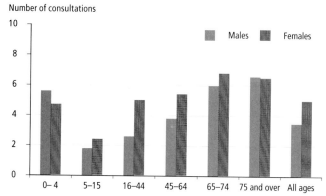

Figure 11.1

Average number of NHS GP consultations per person per year: by age and sex, 2003

United Kingdom

Source: General Household Survey, Office for National Statistics; Continuous Household Survey, Northern Ireland Statistics and Research Agency

females is evident in all age groups except preschool children and is distributed across a wide range of illnesses in addition to the obvious needs of women to consult for contraceptive and pregnancy care.

With the exception of children aged under five, GP consultation rates tended to increase with age. Children aged 5–15 had the lowest rate of consultations: two per year. The highest consultation rates (seven per year) were found among men aged 75 and over and women aged 65–74.

People aged 16 and over who were economically inactive were more likely to have consulted an NHS GP in the last two weeks than those who were working. This disparity was evident in each age group and was greater for men than women. Nineteen per cent of men living in the UK who were economically inactive had consulted their GP in the last fortnight, whereas among working men only 8 per cent had consulted their GP during this period. Economically inactive women were also more likely to consult a GP than those who were working (21 per cent compared with 14 per cent).

In Great Britain, the information collected by the GHS on the use of GPs shows that since 1972 the average number of consultations has remained relatively stable (either four or five). However the total number of GP consultations has risen over time as the population has increased, with a growing proportion of older people.[2]

In 1999 the Health Survey for England (HSfE) focused on the health of ethnic minority groups.[3] After age-standardisation, the average annual NHS GP contact rate was found to be higher for Black Caribbean men, and for Bangladeshi, Pakistani,

Indian men and women compared with men and women in the general population. The biggest difference was for Bangladeshi men, who had more than twice as many contacts per year with the GP than men in the general population.

Site of GP consultation

Over the past 30 years there has been a shift in the way that people access their GPs. In 2003/04 most GP consultations in Great Britain, 86 per cent, took place in surgeries or health centres, an increase of 13 percentage points since 1971 (Figure 11.2).

GP home visits in Great Britain decreased considerably over the same period, from 22 per cent of all consultations in 1971 to 4 per cent in 2003/04. Telephone consultations more than doubled from 4 per cent in 1971 to around 10 per cent from 1998/99 onwards. During this period phone ownership has increased and telephone consultations with GPs have been made more widely available.

A GP's decision on whether to visit a patient at home will depend upon a number of factors. These include the severity and urgency of the condition, as well as the patient's access to transport, distance from the practice and their ability to communicate over the phone.

People aged 75 and over are the most likely to receive a home visit. In the UK in 2003/04, 12 per cent of GP consultations for people in this age group were home visits (Figure 11.3). Older

Figure **11.2**

NHS GP consultations: percentage distribution by site of consultation,[1–3] 1971–2003

Great Britain

Percentages

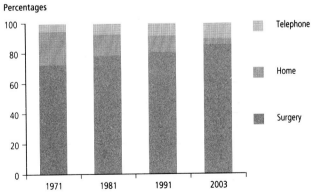

1 *Data prior to 1998 are unweighted.*
2 *NHS GP consultations in the 14 days before the interview.*
3 *'Surgery' includes consultations with a GP at a health centre and those who had answered 'elsewhere'.*

Source: General Household Survey, Office for National Statistics

Figure **11.3**

NHS GP consultations taking place at home: by age, 2003

United Kingdom

Percentages

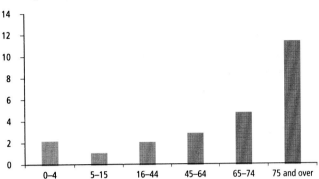

Source: General Household Survey, Office for National Statistics; Continuous Household Survey, Northern Ireland Statistics and Research Agency

people are more vulnerable to illness, are less likely to own a car, may be less willing or able to use a phone and are more likely to be housebound than younger age groups.

Practice nurses

A practice nurse is a nurse employed by a GP. The role of a practice nurse is wide ranging and includes giving injections, taking blood, participating in clinics and giving information and advice on topics such as contraception, pregnancy and health promotion.

The role of the practice nurse is changing. Practice nurses now take on more of the day-to-day work of general practice that was previously within the GPs workload. From March 2002 the range of medicines that nurses were able to prescribe was extended. In April 2004 the General Medical Services contract between general practices and Primary Care Trusts was implemented which allows nurses to extend their roles in areas such as chronic disease management, preventive services and first contact care. Nurses can specialise in providing particular services, such as sexual health or minor surgery, and can now provide out-of-hours services.

In 2003/04 5 per cent of people in the UK reported consulting a practice nurse during the fortnight before interview. This is less than the percentage of people who had consulted their GP (15 per cent), although the patterns of consultations by age and sex were similar. Older people were more likely to consult a practice nurse than younger people (Figure 11.4 – see overleaf). For example, people aged over 65 were twice as likely to have consulted a practice nurse than those aged 45–64. Among children, those under five years old were more likely to have

Figure **11.4**

Practice nurse consultations: by age, 2003

United Kingdom

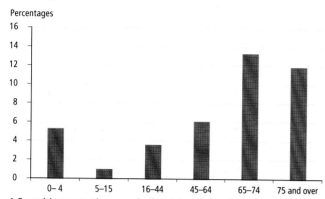

Percentages

1 Consulting a practice nurse in the 14 days before interview.

Source: General Household Survey, Office for National Statistics; Continuous Household Survey, Northern Ireland Statistics and Research Agency

visited a practice nurse (5 per cent) than those aged 5–15 (1 per cent). Females were more likely than males to have consulted a practice nurse (7 per cent compared with 4 per cent). The difference was greatest in the 16–44 age group, where women were over twice as likely as men to have consulted a practice nurse (5 per cent compared with 2 per cent). Consultations concerning family planning and pregnancy may account for some of this difference.

Consultations with a practice nurse tend to be longer than consultations with a GP. In 2003 the median consultation length in England was about seven minutes longer for a practice nurse than with a GP (20 minutes compared with 13 minutes).[4]

Prescriptions

Medicines are dispensed to patients in three main ways. First, they may be issued and dispensed by hospitals, both to inpatients and outpatients. Second, some GPs, known as dispensing doctors, can dispense medicines in their surgery. This occurs mainly in rural areas where patients may have to travel long distances to their nearest pharmacist. Third, prescriptions are written by GPs, and to a lesser extent by dentists, hospital doctors, nurses, pharmacists and chiropodists, and are dispensed by retail pharmacies (chemist and appliance contractors) who are contracted to the NHS. Appliance contractors provide items such as dressings, orthopaedic equipment and contraceptive devices. The majority of prescriptions are dispensed by community pharmacists and appliance contractors.

The prescription data in this section covers items dispensed by community pharmacists, appliance contractors and dispensing doctors including items personally administered and does not include prescriptions dispensed at hospitals. In 2003, the total number of prescription items dispensed were 701 million, 650 million in England and 51 million in Wales. This represents 13.3 prescription items per head of population England and Wales, with the number of prescription items per head one-third higher in Wales (17.5 items per head) than in England (13.1 items per head).[5, 6]

In terms of the number of prescription items dispensed, the six leading disease groups in England and Wales as categorised by British National Formulary chapters were: Cardiovascular System (195 million), Central Nervous System (128 million), Endocrine System (54 million), Respiratory System (54 million), Gastro-intestinal System (53 million) and Infections (45 million). Between them, these six chapters account for three-quarters of all prescription items (Figure 11.5).

The number of prescription items dispensed in England and Wales has been increasing year-on-year. Between 1996 and 2003, the items dispensed have increased by one-third (from 523 million to 701 million), increasing more rapidly since 2000 (Figure 11.6).[5, 6]

Figure **11.5**

Prescription items (millions):[1] by leading British National Formulary chapters,[2] 2003

England & Wales

Millions

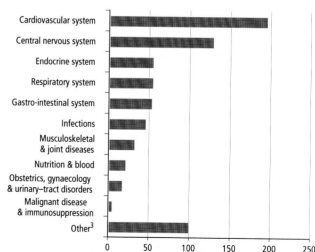

1. The data are from the Prescription Cost Analysis system and cover all prescription items dispensed by community pharmacists and appliance contractors, dispensing doctors, and personal administration.
2. Therapeutic classes are based on the British National Formulary (September 2002).
3. The 'Other' category covers drugs contained in BNF chapters 11–15 and pseudo British National Formulary chapters used by the Prescription Pricing Authority, eg homeopathic preparations.

Source: Health & Social Care Information Centre; National Assembly for Wales

Figure **11.6**

Number of prescription items dispensed, 1996–2003

England & Wales

Millions

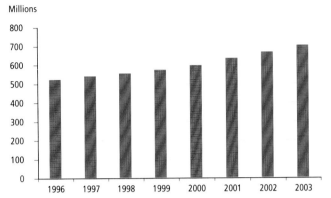

Source: Health & Social Care Information Centre; National Assembly for Wales

There are various reasons for the increase in the number of prescriptions dispensed, including: demographic changes, particularly the rising proportion of elderly people; new drugs or therapies becoming available (for example, the neuraminidase inhibitor anti-viral drugs for the treatment and prevention of influenza); wider use of existing drugs; changes to national policy (such as making nicotine replacement therapy available on prescription or the greater use of statins in the management of heart disease); increases in prescription for particular conditions, such as diabetes, following recommendations from the National Service Frameworks and the National Institute for Health and Clinical Effectiveness and the pressure from patients and the pharmaceutical industry.[7]

Information from the HSfE provides a more accurate picture of medication use than data collected by administrative sources as it describes the number and types of medication that people actually take, as opposed to information on items prescribed or dispensed.

As people get older they are more likely to use prescribed medicines. In 2000, the HSfE specifically focussed on the health of people aged 65 and over living in the community (private households) and in care institutions.[8] About four-fifths of older people living in private households took prescribed medicines (78 per cent of men and 80 per cent of women). However the proportion of people living in care homes who took prescribed medicines was much higher (93 per cent of men and 97 per cent of women). Although some of this difference was due to people living in care homes being older, the difference still remained after standardising for age. People living in care homes were far more likely to have health problems than those of a similar age in private households and, therefore, more likely to require medication.

Use of prescribed medication increased with age up to those in their mid-eighties: 84 per cent of men and 86 per cent of women aged 80 and over used prescribed medications compared with 76 per cent of men and 79 per cent of women aged 65–79. However, there was a decline in the percentage of people taking prescribed medications among those aged 90 and over.

Older people are also more likely to be taking a number of different drugs. Around a third of people aged 65 or over (31 per cent of men and 36 per cent of women) were on four or more prescribed medicines. The categories of prescribed medicine most frequently taken were those for the cardiovascular system, such as for high blood pressure or heart disease (55 per cent), followed by those for the central nervous system, including pain relief (31 per cent), gastrointestinal system (17 per cent), musculoskeletal disease (17 per cent), endocrine system (15 per cent) and respiratory system (13 per cent) (Figure 11.7).

The 1999 HSfE of ethnic minority people showed that, after taking age into account, South Asian men took a higher mean number of prescribed drugs per person than men in the general population. For example, after standardising for age, Bangladeshi men took twice as many prescribed drugs as men in the general population. Pakistani and Bangladeshi women used more prescribed medication, and Chinese women used less prescribed medication, relative to women in the general population.[3]

Figure **11.7**

Category of prescribed medicine taken by people aged 65 and over, 2000

England

Percentages

Source: Health Survey for England, 2000

Ophthalmic services

Until April 1989 free sight tests were offered by the NHS to the whole population, after which free tests were restricted to children under 16 years, full-time students aged under 19 years, people who need complex lenses, diagnosed diabetics and glaucoma sufferers, relatives (aged 40 and over) of glaucoma sufferers, people who are registered blind or partially-sighted and people receiving income support or family credit. From April 1999 free sight tests were reinstated for those aged 60 or over.

From 1993 (when the first Great Britain Sight Tests Volume and Workforce Survey was carried out) until 1998, about a half of sight tests in Great Britain were private (46–50 per cent). Since April 1999, when patients aged 60 or over became eligible for NHS sight tests, only a third of sight tests were paid for privately.[9] Similar results were found in Northern Ireland; in 2003 30 per cent of sight tests were private, compared with 44 per cent in 1998.[10]

In 1994/95 the GHS collected data on the percentage of people who had been for a sight test in the past year in Great Britain. Women were more likely than men to have had a sight test (34 per cent compared with 29 per cent) and to wear either glasses or contact lenses (69 per cent compared with 61 per cent). For both men and women, a higher proportion of adults in non-manual than manual occupations had gone for a sight test in the past year (Figure 11.8).[11]

Figure **11.8**

Sight tests in the year before interview: by own socio-economic group,[1] 1994

Great Britain

Percentages

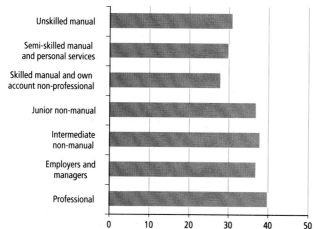

1 People aged 16 and over, classified into occupation-based Socio-Economic Group.

Source: General Houshold Survey, Office for National Statistics

In England and Wales in 2002 there were 10.3 million NHS sight tests paid for by Family Health Services Authorities or Health Authorities.[5]

Recent developments in primary care provision

One of the recent changes in primary care in England is the provision of services such as NHS Direct and NHS Walk-in Centres which offer more convenient access to health care and may result in more appropriate use of both primary and emergency services.[7]

NHS Direct was launched in England in March 1998. It is a 24-hour nurse-led telephone helpline, which provides quick and convenient access to health care information and advice. The nurse advises on the most appropriate course of action and for more serious problems whether and where the caller needs to seek further health advice, such as contacting their GP or visiting their local accident and emergency department (A&E). The number of calls handled by NHS Direct has increased dramatically since its launch, from around 100,000 calls in the financial year 1998/99 to 6.4 million in 2003/04 (Figure 11.9). Wales has a similar service, NHS Direct Wales, which offers advice in both English and Welsh. In Scotland, NHS 24 was launched in 2002. There is also an internet service called NHS Direct Online. This interactive site allows people to access information on health topics.

In England, NHS Walk-in Centres are nurse-led and offer health care advice as well as treatment for minor ailments and injuries without an appointment. They are open everyday, from early in the morning until late in the evening. They are intended to complement GP surgeries and help reduce pressure on GPs. In December 2000 there were 35 NHS Walk-in Centres that had

Figure **11.9**

Number of calls handled by NHS Direct, 1998/99–2003/04

England

Millions

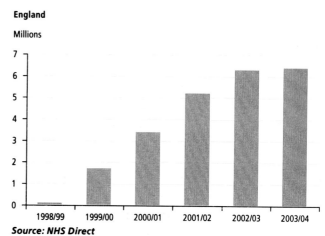

Source: NHS Direct

been open for at least six months and around 60,000 visits to these centres that month. By December 2004 this had increased to 52 Walk-in Centres and almost 165,000 visits.

Secondary care

Secondary health care services are hospital based and provide more specialised knowledge, skills and equipment than is provided by primary care. District general hospitals offer a broad spectrum of clinical specialities, supported by a range of other services such as anaesthetics, pathology and radiology. Almost all have facilities for the admission of emergency patients, either through accident and emergency departments or as direct referrals from GPs. Treatments are provided for inpatients, day cases, outpatients and patients who attend wards for treatment such as dialysis. Some hospitals also provide specialist services covering more than one region or district, for example for heart and liver transplants and rare eye and bone cancers.

There are two main data sources that inform the Government about the use of secondary health services: administrative and survey data. Administrative data are collected as a by-product of the service and are useful in giving an estimate of the number of people who use the health services. This information is then complemented by survey data which provides population-based data and is independent of whether or not someone makes contact with the health care system. Survey data is a good source of information on the demographics of those who use the health services. The GHS in Great Britain and the CHS in Northern Ireland provide data on how men and women of different ages use health services in the UK; the most recent data is for the financial year 2003/04. In 1999 the HSfE focused on the health of ethnic minority groups and is therefore the best source of survey data on use of health services by ethnic groups.[3] This section of the chapter draws on data from administrative sources and the surveys mentioned above. All information in this section relates to NHS secondary health care services.

Inpatients

In the UK, 7 per cent of people reported an inpatient stay in the 12 months prior to interview in 2003/04. At 14 per cent, people aged 75 and over were more likely to report an inpatient stay than any other age group. With the exception of children under the age of five, the percentage who reported an inpatient stay increased with age. In general, females were more likely to report an inpatient stay than males (8 per cent compared with 6 per cent). However, differences between males and females vary by age (Figure 11.10). For example, females in the 16–44 age group were significantly more likely

Figure **11.10**

Inpatient admissions in the 12 months before interview: by age and sex, 2003

United Kingdom

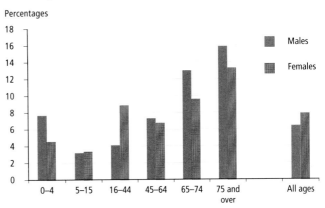

Source: General Household Survey, Office for National Statistics; Continuous Household Survey, Northern Ireland Statistics and Research Agency

than males to report an inpatient stay (9 per cent compared with 4 per cent). By contrast, males below the age of five and in the 65–74 age group were significantly more likely than females to report an inpatient stay. This is partly because stays related to maternity are included in inpatient stays.

Since the mid-1990s the number of inpatient admissions in NHS hospitals has been rising steadily year on year, except in 1996/97 and 2001/02. The data from Hospital Episodes Statistics for England shows that in 2003/04 there were a record number of 8.0 million patients discharged (excluding

Figure **11.11**

Hospital inpatient stay and day case admission rates[1] and mean length of stay, 1995/96–2003/04

England

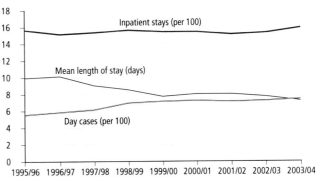

1 Due to continuous updating of the hospital inpatient databases estimates may vary slightly depending on timing of data extract.

Source: Hospital Episode Statistics, Health & Social Care Information Centre; Office for National Statistics day cases) from hospitals after treatment, representing an increase of 5.1 per cent over the 1995/96 figure of 7.6 million. This increase is well in excess of the population increase of 3 per cent for England over the same period. After allowing for population increase, this represents an increase of just over 2 per cent in the inpatient rate per 100 population over the nine-year period reported (Figure 11.11).

Among those treated as inpatients (i.e. excluding day cases) the length of stay in hospitals has been falling gradually: from an average of 10.1 days per stay in 1995/96 to 7.4 days per stay in 2003/04. The decline in the average length of inpatient stay during a period of increased inpatient activity may well be the result of a combination of factors such as technological

advances in medical diagnosis and treatment, reduction in the number of long-stay beds in hospitals and increased use of 'intermediate' care facilities.

Overall, the most common conditions treated as inpatient were 'Circulatory and Respiratory diseases'. In 2003/04, this diagnostic group accounted for 15.2 per cent of all finished consultant episodes, followed by 'Complications of pregnancy, etc and Perinatal conditions' (10.7 per cent) and 'Cancer' (10.5 per cent). Not surprisingly the leading diagnostic group accounting for the largest proportion of hospital inpatient activity varied with age. Among children aged 5–14 'Injury and poisoning' was the main diagnostic group for admission; among people aged 45–64 it was 'Cancer' closely followed by 'Circulatory and Respiratory diseases'; and among those aged 65 and over it was 'Circulatory and Respiratory diseases' (Table 11.12).

Table **11.12**

Finished consultant episodes:[1] by primary diagnostic group and age, 2003/04[2]

England

Percentages

ICD-10 Chapter	Main Diagnosis	Age								
		0–4	5–14	15–44	45–64	65–74	75–84	85–120	Age not known	All Ages
I	Infectious diseases A00–B99	4.6	2.7	0.9	0.7	0.6	0.8	1.1	3.8	1.2
II	Cancer C00–D48	1.6	5.7	4.8	17.0	18.2	13.1	7.5	2.4	10.5
III	Blood & blood-forming organs diseases D50–D89	0.6	2.2	1.2	1.5	1.8	2.1	1.9	0.5	1.5
IV	Endocrine & nutritional diseases E00–E90	0.4	2.6	1.1	1.6	1.4	1.3	1.4	0.6	1.3
V	Mental & behavioural disorders F00–F99	0.1	1.9	2.6	1.7	0.9	1.3	1.7	0.7	1.7
VI–VIII	Diseases of the nervous system, Eye and Ear G00–H95	3.0	9.5	2.9	5.8	7.7	10.6	8.9	0.6	6.0
IX–X	Circulatory and Respiratory diseases I00–J99	11.1	12.2	6.1	16.1	22.0	24.5	26.8	2.6	15.2
XI	Digestive diseases K00–K93	4.1	14.7	9.4	13.4	11.2	10.0	9.0	1.7	10.3
XII–XIII	Skin and Musculoskeletal diseases L00–M99	1.6	6.1	7.7	11.8	9.4	7.4	5.9	3.6	8.0
XIV	Genitourinary diseases N00–N99	1.6	4.9	7.1	8.3	6.2	5.7	5.8	17.0	6.4
XV–XVI	Complications of pregnancy etc and Perinatal conditions O00–P96	15.3	0.3	30.6	0.1	0.0	0.0	0.6	46.7	10.7
XVII	Congenital malformations, Q00–Q99	5.1	4.0	0.4	0.2	0.1	0.0	0.0	0.2	0.8
XX	Injury & poisoning S00–T98	3.7	15.6	7.5	4.7	3.8	5.7	9.8	1.5	6.2
	Other not mentioned above R00–R99, Z00–Z99	47.3	17.6	17.8	17.3	16.7	17.7	19.6	18.2	20.2
	All diagnosis A00–Z99	100.0	100.0	100.0	100.0	100.0	100.0	100.0	100.0	100.0
	Base (thousands)	1185	511	3981	2884	1914	1954	860	31	13320

1 Due to continuous updating of the hospital episode statistics database, data extracted at different time points may differ slightly.
2 Year for hospital activity runs from 1st April to 31st March.

Source: Hospital Episode Statistics, Health & Social Care Information Centre

There is considerable variation in hospital inpatient activity by ethnic group. According to the Health Survey for England 1999, after standardising for age and excluding admissions relating to maternity, Pakistani men were more likely, and Chinese men and women were less likely to have been admitted as inpatients compared to the general population.[3]

Day cases

Day cases are patients who receive planned investigation, treatment or operation that does not require an overnight stay in a hospital. In 2003/04, the number of day cases as recorded in HES for England was 3.8 million. The number of day cases have been increasing at a much faster pace than inpatient admissions. Between 1995/96 and 2003/04, the increase in the rates of day cases (34 per cent) was 17 times the increase in the rates of patients staying overnight (2 per cent) (Figure 11.11).

The data from GHS and CHS shows that in 2003/04, 7 per cent of people in the UK reported treatment as day cases in the past year. Patterns were similar for men and women. Like many other health services, the likelihood of having day case treatment is related to age (Figure 11.13). With the exception of children aged under five, the percentage who had day case treatment increased with age. Children aged 5–15 were least likely to have had day case treatment (4 per cent) and people aged over 75 were most likely (11 per cent).

There were no significant differences in hospital admission rates for day cases by ethnic minority group in England.[3]

Figure **11.13**

Day case admission in the 12 months before interview: by age, 2003

United Kingdom

Percentages

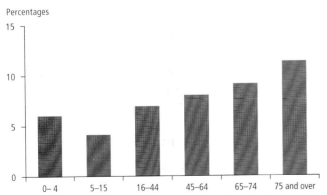

Source: *General Household Survey, Office for National Statistics; Continuous Household Survey, Northern Ireland Statistics and Research Agency*

Outpatient and casualty

An outpatient is a person who is seen by a consultant for treatment or advice. The total number of outpatient attendances has been rising steadily year-on-year, from 43.4 million in 1996/97 to 47.4 million in 2002/03.[5, 6] After allowing for population increase, this represents an increase of 7 per cent in the rate of outpatient attendances over the same period (Figure 11.14). In comparison, the total number of casualty or A&E attendances has remained relatively stable, fluctuating between 15.0 million and 15.7 million between 1997/98 and 2002/03.[5, 6]

Figure **11.14**

Outpatient attendance rates, 1996/97–2002/03

England & Wales

Rate per 100 population

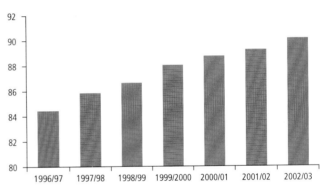

Source: *Department of Health; National Assembly for Wales*

Fourteen per cent of people in the UK reported visiting an outpatient or casualty (A&E) department at least once in the three-month period before interview. With the exception of the youngest age group, the percentage of people attending an outpatient or casualty department increased with age. For example, 9 per cent of 5- to 15-year-olds had attended an outpatient or casualty department in the three months before interview compared with 22 per cent of people aged 75 and over. Women aged 16–64 were more likely than men to attend an outpatient or casualty department, resulting in a higher overall attendance rate among females than males (15 per cent compared with 13 per cent) (Figure 11.15 – see overleaf).

In 1999 the HSfE found that overall, the levels of age-standardised ratios of outpatient or casualty attendance among most ethnic minority groups were similar to the general population. The exceptions were Chinese people, Bangladeshi men and Pakistani women all of whom had lower age-standardised ratios relative to the general population.[3]

Figure **11.15**

Outpatient or casualty department attendance in the three months before interview: by age and sex, 2002

United Kingdom

Percentages

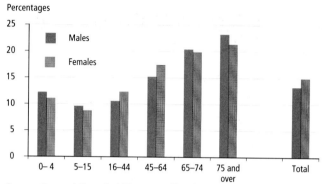

Source: General Household Survey, Office for National Statistics; Continuous Household Survey, Northern Ireland Statistics and Research Agency

Among those aged 16–34 levels of outpatient or casualty attendance for men and women in most ethnic minority groups were significantly lower than that of the general population in that age group (Figure 11.16). The exceptions were Irish men and women, and Black Caribbean women who had similar rates to that of the general population at about 30 per cent. Chinese and Bangladeshi people had the lowest rates in the same age group, with rates around half the general population level (14 per cent of Bangladeshi men, 15 per cent of Bangladeshi women, 16 per cent of Chinese men and 13 per cent of Chinese women). However, among those aged over 55

Figure **11.16**

Outpatient or casualty department attendance in the past year (excluding maternity) for adults aged 16–34: by sex and ethnic group, 1999

England

Percentages

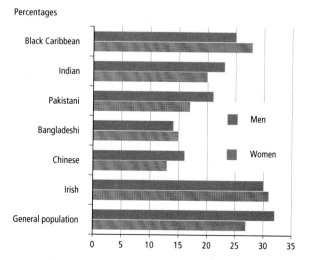

Source: Health Survey for England, Department of Health

all ethnic minority groups (with the exception of Chinese people) had similar or higher levels than those in the general population.[3]

Access to services

According to a World Health Organisation report, along with the primary goal of better health, health systems should also have the goal of fairness. "Fairness means that it responds equally well to everyone, without discrimination or differences in how people are treated."[12] The NHS was founded on a principle of equity, where provision and access to services should be based on medical need, rather than status or ability to pay.

In some areas of health care, especially primary health services, there is evidence that access to services is based on medical need, rather than any other factor.[13, 14] For example acute and chronic illness were found to be better predictors of children's use of primary health service rather than socio-economic status or ethnicity.[15, 16]

However, there is also evidence that access to, and utilisation of, health services do not always reflect health needs. Inequalities in accessing health services may relate to various factors, including social class, age, sex, ethnicity and geography. The Department of Health's report *Addressing Inequalities – Reaching the Hard-to-Reach Groups*, noted that marginalised groups, including homeless people, travellers, asylum seekers, refugees, people with disabilities, those living in deprivation and prisoners, can face difficulties in accessing health care services.[17]

The *NHS Plan* states that "The inverse care law, where communities in greatest need are least likely to receive the health services that they require still applies in too many parts of the country... Many deprived communities are less likely than affluent ones to receive heart surgery, hip replacements and many other services including screening."[18] For example, a study using data for England and Wales from 1994 to 1998 found that the prevalence of treated coronary heart disease was approximately 40 per cent higher in deprived areas than in affluent areas. In contrast, coronary heart disease was approximately 25 per cent less likely to be treated with a statin (a drug that can reduce cholesterol levels) in the most deprived areas than in the affluent areas.[19] The Audit Commission report, *A Focus on General Practice in England*, found evidence that areas with greater health needs had fewer GPs.[7]

There are many reasons why some individuals or groups have less access to health services than others in the population. The *Independent Inquiry into Inequalities in Health* stated that access to services, such as primary care, is influenced by 'supply' and 'demand' factors. 'Supply' factors include the range of facilities in an area, the ability to recruit staff, timing and organisation of services and the availability of affordable and safe transport. 'Demand' factors include knowledge of what facilities are available, as well as socio-economic influences, such as financial insecurity and social mobility.[20]

The Department of Health's cross cutting review, *Tackling Health Inequalities*,[21] suggested that unequal access to public services was often due to a lack of responsiveness to the needs of users, including:

- "Inadequate provision or poor affordability of services in disadvantaged areas.

- Low quality of services in disadvantaged areas.

- Poor transport to services, particularly for those without use of a car or with special needs, such as the elderly or disabled people.

- Locational disadvantage, including dispersed populations and poor public transport, low access to shops providing affordable food for a healthy diet, fear of crime.

- Discrimination, for example on grounds of race, gender, age, sexual identity, disability and long-term illness etc.

- Lack of cultural sensitivity: services which do not meet the cultural, language or religious needs of all parts of the population served.

- Gender bias: gender differences in accessing services, in some cases related to the way the service is delivered.

- Poor knowledge and access to information: lack of recognition or knowledge about the importance of symptoms and their meaning, or about the availability of services.

- Complex problems: services are often unable to respond to the complex and multiple needs of some parts of the population, eg a person with a combination of physical heath needs, substance misuse problems, housing problems and mental health problems."

The ONS Omnibus Survey, carried out in 2000 and 2001 in Great Britain, examined how poor transport affects use of health services. It found that one in five people (20 per cent) reported difficulties in travelling to hospital. People without access to a car were more likely to report difficulty travelling to hospital, their GP or to the chemist than those living in a household with access to a car (Figure 11.17).[22] Lack of access to transport is experienced disproportionately by older people.[20]

Figure **11.17**

Difficulty in getting to services:[1] by household car ownership, 2000–2001

Great Britain

Percentages

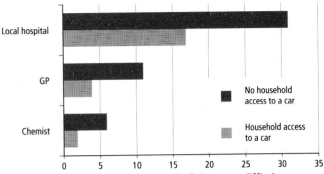

1 Adults aged 16 and over finding service farly or very difficult to access.

Source: ONS Omnibus Survey, January and March, 2000–01

Public perception

The British Social Attitudes Survey showed that people in Britain consistently rated satisfaction with their GP higher than hospital services, and that satisfaction in individual services is greater than satisfaction with the NHS overall.[23] In 2003, the majority of people said they were satisfied with the way GP services are run (72 per cent). Over half of people were satisfied with the way inpatient and outpatient services are run (52 and 54 per cent, respectively) and just under half were satisfied with the way accident and emergency departments were run (45 per cent) (Figure 11.18 – see overleaf).[24] Generally, recent users were more satisfied than those without such experience and older people were more satisfied than younger people.[23]

In 1998, the first national survey of NHS patients was carried out in England looking at people's experiences of their GP service and was repeated four years later in 2002.[25, 26] On the whole people viewed their GP and practice nurse positively, the large majority of people (around nine out of 10) had positive views of their GP's skills, knowledge, attitude and ability to communicate as well as the amount of time the GP spent with them. For example, 95 per cent of patients felt their GP treated them as they would wish all or most of the time.

In the four-year period between the two surveys, patients' views have become more critical of certain aspects of GP services.[26] These mainly relate to waiting times – waiting for an appointment with their GP, waiting to see a hospital doctor and waiting for an out of hours visit. Nearly three-quarters (72 per cent) reported waiting two or more days for an appointment with the preferred GP, an increase from 63 per cent in 1998. Likewise, a considerably higher proportion

Figure **11.18**

Satisfaction with selected NHS services:[1] by sex, 2003

Great Britain

Percentages

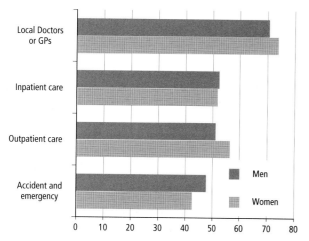

1 Adults aged 18 and over who said they were 'very satisfied' or 'quite satisfied' when asked 'From your own experience, or from what you have heard, please say how satisfied or dissatisfied you are with the way in which each of these parts of the National Health Service runs nowdays'.

Source: British Social Attitudes, National Centre for Social Research

reported waiting more than a month to see a hospital doctor in 2002 (58 per cent) than in 1998 (53 per cent). More significantly, patients contacting out of hours service were less likely to receive a home visit from a GP in 2002 (33 per cent) than in 1998 (47 per cent). Those receiving home visits were also more likely to wait an hour or more for a doctor to arrive in 2002 than in 1998 (55 per cent in 2002 compared with 47 per cent in 1998).

There was also some indication that making contact with the surgery has become more difficult. Overall, there were very few regional differences in opinions of GP services. The main difference was between London and other regions. For example, waiting times were longer in London: in 2002, 77 per cent had to wait two or more days for a GP appointment, compared with the overall figure for the rest of the country of 67 per cent.[26]

A survey of acute inpatients in England in 2001/02 found that overall, patients had a positive view of their experience. The majority of patients rated the care they received as excellent or very good (74 per cent), felt they had always been treated with respect and dignity throughout their stay (79 per cent) and felt that the ward was very or fairly clean (93 per cent).[27]

A survey of cancer patients in England found that the majority of patients (86 per cent) had confidence and trust in all doctors responsible for their treatment, however 11 per cent of patients would like to have been more involved in decisions about their care.[28]

A general finding across all these surveys is that women, younger people and ethnic minority groups were more sceptical about the quality of care received than men, older people, or people who reported their background as White. Ethnic minority respondents, particularly the Pakistani and Bangladeshi group, tended to take a less favourable view of their GP service than the White population. For example, the Pakistani and Bangladeshi group were less likely to report getting an appointment on the day they wanted, felt the doctor did not answer their questions and were more likely to have been put off going to see the GP because of inconvenient surgery hours.[26]

Conclusion

The demand for NHS services, whether provided in the primary care setting or in the secondary care setting (hospitals), is on the increase. There is a complex interplay of factors such as population ageing and the availability of a wider range of treatments leading to an increase in demand for health care services. All the indicators reported in this chapter – number of GP consultations, volume of prescriptions dispensed, and hospital inpatient, day case and outpatient admissions – confirm this general trend.

Certain sections of the population are more likely to use NHS services than others. Not surprisingly, GP consultation rates and hospital inpatient admission rates for elderly people were the highest. Among ethnic minority groups, GP consultation rates were higher for South Asian men and women, Black Caribbean men and Irish women than the general population.

Over the years there have been important changes to the way primary care services are accessed and delivered. While the average number of GP consultations per head of the population has remained fairly stable since the early 1970s, there has been a shift in the site of consultations with more than four in five consultations taking place in the surgery and fewer home visits. Practice nurses have an expanded role in patient care in areas such as chronic disease management and preventive services. In addition, NHS Direct and NHS Walk-in Centres, set up to compliment GP services, are gaining in popularity. NHS Direct has seen a year-on-year increase in the number of calls received since its introduction in 1998. Likewise, visits to NHS Walk-in Centres have increased almost three-fold in the four years since being set up in 2000.

In general, satisfaction with health services remains high, with higher levels of satisfaction with primary care services than secondary care services. There is some evidence to suggest that the move away from GP home visits may not be popular with the general public. In the four year period between the first (1998) and second (2002) NHS surveys of patients, people had become more critical of 'out of hours services'. GPs were reported to be far less likely to visit people in their homes than in 1998, and when they did, spent less time with them than before.

Despite the efforts to reduce geographical variations in service provision, certain aspects of the 'inverse care law' still apply. It was found that some areas with greater health needs had fewer GPs and patients living in the most deprived areas although more likely to have coronary heart diseases were less likely to receive preventive care such as statin prescription.

References

1. ONS (2003) Chapter 13, in *UK 2004. The official year book of the United Kingdom of Great Britain and Northern Ireland*, TSO: London.
   www.statistics.gov.uk

2. Atkinson T (2004) *Atkinson Review: Interim Report*, TSO: London, p70.
   www.statistics.gov.uk

3. Erens B, Primatesta P and Prior G (2000) *Health Survey for England: the Health of Minority Ethnic Groups 1999*, TSO: London.
   www.archive.official-documents.co.uk/document/doh

4. Audit Commission (2004) *Transforming Primary Care: the Role of PCTs in Shaping and Supporting General Practice*, Audit Commission: London, p.33.
   www.audit-commission.gov.uk/reports

5. Department of Health Bulletin (2004) *Prescriptions Dispensed in the Community Statistics for 1993 to 2003: England*.

6. National Assembly for Wales (2004) *Prescriptions Dispensed in the Community in Wales, 2002 to 2003*.
   www.wales.gov.uk/keypublicationsforwales

7. Audit Commission (2002) *A Focus On General Practice in England, July 2002*, Audit Commission: London.
   www.healthcarecommission.org.uk

8. Falaschetti E, Malbut K and Primatesta P (2002) *Health Survey for England 2000: The general health of older people and their use of health services*, TSO: London.
   www.official-documents.co.uk/document/deps/doh

9. Department of Health (2004) *Sight tests volume and workforce survey 2003-04 optometrists & ophthalmic medical practitioners* at: www.gnn.gov.uk/imagelibrary

10. Department of Health, Social Services and Public Safety (2003) *Northern Ireland Sight Test Survey 2003*, Department of Health, Social Services and Public Safety: Belfast at www.dhsspsni.gov.uk/publications and Department of Health, Social Services and Public Safety (2001) *Northern Ireland Sight Test Survey 2000*, Department of Health, Social Services and Public Safety: Belfast.

11. Bennett N, Jarvis L, Rowlands O, Singleton N and Haselden L (1996) *Living in Britain 1994*, HSMO: London.

12. *World Health Organisation (2000) World Health Report 2000: Health systems: improving performance*, World Health Organisation: Geneva, p26. www.who.int/whr

13. Goddard M and Smith P (2001) Equity and access to health care services: theory and evidence from the UK. *Social Science and Medicine*, **Vol. 53**, 1149–1162.

14. Baker D, Mead N and Campbell S (2002) Inequalities in morbidity and consulting behaviour for socially vulnerable groups. *British Journal of General Practice*, **Vol. 52**, 124–130.

15. Sonia Saxena, Joseph Eliahoo and Azeem Majeed (2002) Socioeconomic and ethnic group differences in self reported health status and use of health services by children and young people in England: cross sectional study. *BMJ* **325**, 520.

16. Cooper H, Smaje C and Arber S (1999) Equity in Health service use by children: examining the ethnic paradox. *Jnl Soc Pol* **28, 3**, 457–478.

17. Department of Health (2002) *Addressing inequalities – reaching the hard-to-reach groups. National Service Frameworks. A practical aid to implementation in primary care*, Department of Health: London, p.1.
   www.dh.gov.uk/PublicationsAndStatistics/Publications/PublicationsPolicyAndGuidance

18. Department of Health (2000) *The NHS Plan: A Plan for Investment, A Plan for Reform*, Department of Health: London. p.107.
   www.dh.gov.uk/PublicationsAndStatistics/Publications/PublicationsPolicyAndGuidance

19. Ryan R and Majeed A (2001) Prevalence of ischaemic heart disease and its management with statins and aspirins in general practice in England and Wales, 1994 and 1998. *Health Statistics Quarterly* **12**, 34–39.

20. Acheson D (1998) *Independent Inquiry into Inequalities in Health*, TSO: London.

21. Department of Health (2002) Paragraph C70, in *Tackling health inequalities: Cross cutting review*, TSO: London.

22. Ruston D (2002) *Difficulty in Accessing Key Services*, ONS: London. p.7.
   www.statistics.gov.uk/StatBase

23. Appleby P and Alvarez Rosete A (2003) The NHS: keeping up with public expectations? In Park A *et al* (eds.) *British Social Attitudes. 20th Report*, SAGE: London.

24. Office for National Statistics (2005) *Social Trends 35,* Palgrave Macmillan: Basingstoke.

25. Airey C and Erens B (eds.) (1999) *National survey of NHS patients. General Practice* 1998, Department of Health: London. www.dh.gov.uk/PublicationsAndStatistics/PublishedSurvey

26. Boreham R et al (eds.) (2003) *National survey of NHS patients. General Practice 2002*, Department of Health: London. www.dh.gov.uk/PublicationsAndStatistics/PublishedSurvey

27. Bullen N and Reeves R (2003) *National surveys of NHS patients – Acute inpatient survey: 2001/02* at: www.dh.gov.uk

28. Department of Health (2002) *National surveys of NHS patients – Cancer patients, 1999/2000* at: www.dh.gov.uk/PublicationsAndStatistics/PublishedSurvey

Caring and carers

Levin Wheller

chapter 12

Background

Caring, whether provided informally by individuals, or formally through services to support people living in their own homes or care homes, is provided to those in need of support and assistance in living their daily lives. Carers are defined as people who look after and support family members, friends or neighbours in need of help because of long-term physical or mental illness or disability or problems related to old age. In 2001, the Census asked a question on caring (see below) for the first time which sought not only to identify the number of informal carers in the UK, but also (in three broad bands) the number of hours of care they provided each week.

Do you look after, or give any help or support to family members, friends, neighbours or others because of;

- **long-term physical or mental ill-health or disability, or**
- **problems related to old age?**

- ◆ Do not count anything you do as part of your paid employment;
- ◆ ✓ time spent in typical week
  - ☐ No
  - ☐ Yes, 1 - 19 hours a week
  - ☐ Yes, 20 - 49 hours a week
  - ☐ Yes, 50+ hours a week

Carers are a diverse group; people from all social backgrounds and situations are likely to provide care at some point in their life. With the number of people aged 75 and over projected to rise from 4.4 million in 2001 to 6.9 million in 2031 (from 8 to 11 per cent of the UK population),[1] the care of the sick and elderly is an increasingly important social policy concern. The demographic shift towards an older population distribution raises important questions of who will care for whom in the future.

This chapter first looks at the provision of informal, or unpaid care, along with the social, economic, and health characteristics of carers in the UK. In later sections, the chapter examines the provision of formal care, through care in the community provided by local authorities, and through institutions such as nursing and residential care homes. The chapter uses age-standardised rates where indicated.

Informal care

Prevalence of caring

According to the Census, around six million people in the UK (11 per cent of the population aged five years and over) were providing unpaid care for a friend or relative in 2001. The majority (approximately four million people, and 67 per cent of carers) were providing between one and 19 hours of care per week. A further 11 per cent spent 20–49 hours (700,000 people), whereas 21 per cent of carers (1.3 million people) spent 50 or more hours per week providing informal care. These 1.3 million people represent around 2 per cent of the UK population aged five years and over.

Sociodemographic profile of carers

Age and sex

While the vast majority of carers (65 per cent) were aged between 35 and 64, a number of the very young and very old were also carers. There were 114,000 children aged 5–15 years providing care, with 9,000 (8 per cent) of these caring for 50 or more hours a week. Among the oldest old, around 44,000 people aged 85 and over provided care, with around half of these (51 per cent) spending 50 or more hours a week.

More females than males were carers. In 2001, 12 per cent of females (3.4 million) and 9 per cent of males (2.5 million) were providing informal care. Females make up 58 per cent of all informal carers (3.4 million people) in the UK. The majority of carers in all age groups were females, except in the oldest age groups. Males represented 51 per cent of carers aged 75–84, and 54 per cent of all carers aged over 85 in 2001. As the amount of care provided (in hours) increases, the proportion of female carers also rises. Females made up 57 per cent of people caring for 1–19 hours, 60 per cent of those caring for 20–49 hours, and 61 per cent of people caring for 50 hours or more.

The proportion of people providing informal care varies by age group. In 2001, around one per cent of both females and males aged 5–15 were providing care (Figure 12.1). This increases to 10 per cent of males and 15 per cent of females aged 35–44, rising to a peak of 17 per cent for men aged 55–64 and 23 per cent of females aged 45–54. The proportion of people providing care decreases in older age groups. Fourteen per cent of both males and females aged 65–74 provide informal care. Higher proportions of females than males provide care in all age groups up to 74 years. Among those aged 75–84, 12 per cent of males and 8 per cent of females provide care, whereas among those aged 85 and over, 9 per cent of males and only 3 per cent of females provide care.

Figure **12.1**

Percentage of population providing unpaid care: by age and sex, 2001

United Kingdom
Percentages

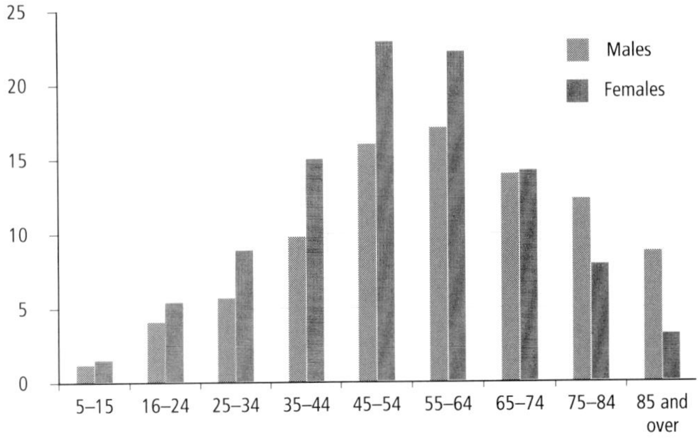

The number of hours of care giving is also related to age, with a higher percentage of older carers providing more intensive levels of care. The proportion of carers providing more intensive levels of care rises sharply from age 65. A third (33 per cent) of carers aged 65–74 provide 50 or more hours of care per week, rising to 44 per cent for carers aged 75– 84, and 51 per cent for carers in the oldest (85 and over) age group (Figure 12.2).

Figure **12.2**

Percentage distribution of care provision (in hours): by age of carer, 2001

United Kingdom
Percentages

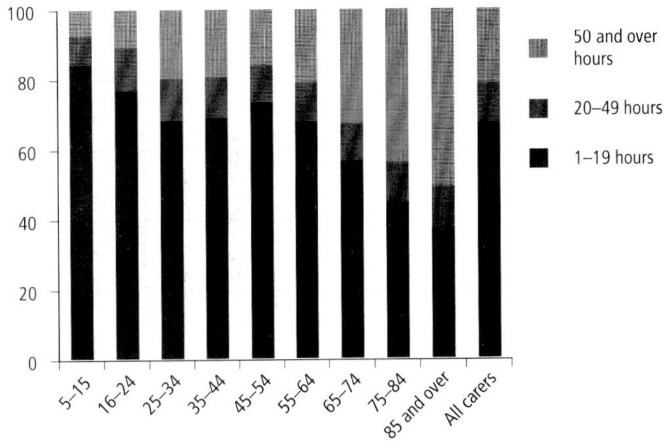

Overall, while 14 per cent of all carers providing 1–19 hours of care per week were aged 65 and over, 31 per cent of carers providing 50 hours or more of care were found in this age group. This suggests that on the whole, older people, though less likely to provide care in the first place, tend to provide more hours of care if they are carers. This is possibly because older people are predominantly looking after their partners, who they are more likely to live with, and who, by virtue of their age, are more likely to have long-term health problems.

Although more women than men were care givers, the levels of care provided were similar for male and female carers. About two-thirds of carers provided 1–19 hours of care (males 69 per cent, females 66 per cent), a tenth 20–49 hours a week (males 11 per cent, females 12 per cent), and a fifth 50 or more hours per week (males 20 per cent, females 22 per cent).

After age-standardisation, the same proportion of males and females aged 5 and over provided care as in the age-specific rates discussed earlier (12 per cent of females and 9 per cent of males). As with non-standardised data, the intensity of care provided for males and females was very similar.

Marital status

In 2001, over two-thirds of all carers aged 16 and over were married (68 per cent) whereas 17 per cent were single, 8 per cent divorced, 4 per cent widowed and 2 per cent separated. Compared with the general population (aged 16 and over) carers were more likely to be married (51 versus 68 per cent).

After age-standardisation, around one in six (15 per cent) married people provided unpaid care in 2001, a higher proportion than for all other marital status groups (Figure 12.3 – see overleaf). In all other marital status groups, around one in ten people provided care, with slightly higher proportion of people who were widowed (12 per cent) providing care than those who were divorced, single (both 11 per cent) or separated (10 per cent). In all marital status groups, a higher percentage of females than males provided care.

Married people were also more likely to provide a higher intensity of care than individuals in other groups. One in four married carers (24 per cent) spent 50 or more hours per week caring compared with a slightly lower proportion of widowed (23 per cent) and divorced carers (22 per cent). Around one in five separated (20 per cent) and single (19 per cent) people provided 50 or more hours of care per week (Figure 12.4 – see overleaf).

Figure **12.3**

Percentage of adults¹ providing unpaid care (age-standardised): by marital status and sex, 2001

United Kingdom
Percentages

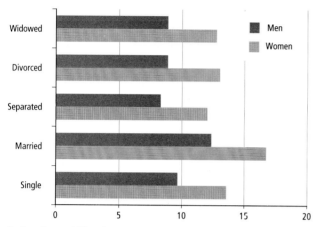

1 People aged 16 and over.

Source: Census 2001, Office for National Statistics; Census 2001, General Register Office for Scotland; Census 2001, Northern Ireland Statistics and Research Agency

Figure **12.4**

Percentage distribution of care provision (in hours): by marital status (age-standardised), 2001

United Kingdom
Percentages

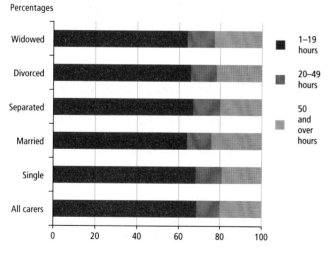

1 People 16 and over.

Source: Census 2001, Office for National Statistics; Census 2001, General Register Office for Scotland; Census 2001, Northern Ireland Statistics and Research Agency

Ethnicity

After age-standardisation, White and Asian populations had the highest proportion of people aged 16 and over providing care (13 per cent) in 2001. The Mixed and Black ethnic groups had rates of 11 and 9 per cent respectively, whereas 7 per cent of those in Chinese and other ethnic groups were care

Figure **12.5**

Percentage of adults¹ providing unpaid care (age-standardised): by ethnic group and sex, 2001

United Kingdom
Percentages

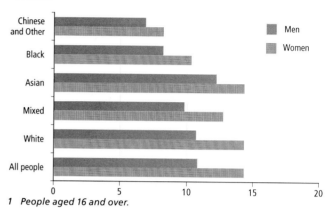

1 People aged 16 and over.

Source: Census 2001, Office for National Statistics; Census 2001, General Register Office for Scotland; Census 2001, Northern Ireland Statistics and Research Agency

providers. A higher percentage of females than males were providing care in all ethnic groups (Figure 12.5).

Overall about one in five carers in all ethnic groups provided the highest intensity of care (50 and over hours per week). However, there are interesting gender differences in intensive care provision between ethnic groups. Over a quarter of Asian female carers (29 per cent) provided 50 or more hours of care compared with less than a fifth (18 per cent) of Asian male carers, a difference of 11 percentage points (Figure 12.6). The difference between the sexes in Chinese and other ethnic

Figure **12.6**

Percentage of adult¹ carers providing 50 or more hours of unpaid care per week (age-standardised): by ethnic group and sex, 2001

United Kingdom
Percentages

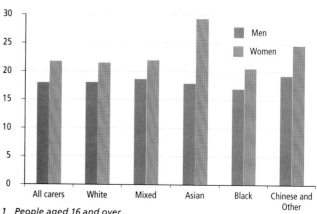

1 People aged 16 and over.

Source: Census 2001, Office for National Statistics; Census 2001, General Register Office for Scotland; Census 2001, Northern Ireland Statistics and Research Agency groups was six percentage points (males 18, females 24 per cent), while there was a difference of three percentage points between the sexes in the white (males 18 per cent, females 21 per cent), black (males 17 per cent, females 20 per cent) and mixed (males 19 per cent, females 22 per cent) ethnic groups.

Socio-economic status

The percentage of people aged 16–64 providing unpaid care does not vary greatly by social position. As Figure 12.7 illustrates, a higher percentage of females than males were providing care in all socio-economic groups. However, for both males and females there is a difference of only two percentage points between those groups with the lowest and the highest proportion of people providing unpaid care.

Among females, the higher managerial and professional group had the lowest percentage of carers at 14 per cent, the group with the highest proportion providing care were small employers and own account workers (16 per cent). For males, people in routine occupations were least likely to provide care (9 per cent), while the intermediate occupations group had the highest proportion of carers (11 per cent). For all people, the highest proportion providing care were found in intermediate

occupations (13 per cent) and the lowest proportion in higher managerial and professional groups (11 per cent).

Despite overall similarities in the likelihood of providing any amount of care, there are interesting differences between the socio-economic groups when we look at the intensity of care provision. Here there is a clear gradient, with lower social groups providing a greater number of hours of care. Around a fifth (22 per cent) of carers in routine occupations and two-fifths (37 per cent) of carers who had never worked or were long-term unemployed provided 50 or more hours of care per week (Figure 12.8). This compares to only 8 per cent of carers in the higher managerial and professional group.

This pattern is equally apparent among both males and females, with the proportions of male and female carers providing 50 or more hours of care a week very similar in most socio-economic groups. However, a noticeably higher percentage of female carers who had never worked or were long-term unemployed provided 50 or more hours of care per week. Over a quarter (28 per cent) of male carers in this group provided the most intense levels of care compared with two-fifths (41 per cent) of female carers.

Figure **12.7**

Percentage of adults¹ providing unpaid care (age-standardised): by NS-SEC and sex, 2001

United Kingdom
Percentages

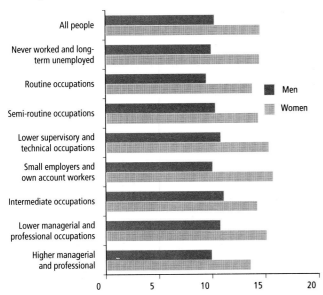

1 People aged 16–64.

Source: Census 2001, Office for National Statistics; Census 2001, General Register Office for Scotland; Census 2001, Northern Ireland Statistics and Research Agency

Figure **12.8**

Percentage distribution of care provision (in hours): by NS-SEC of carer (age-standardised), 2001

United Kingdom
Percentages

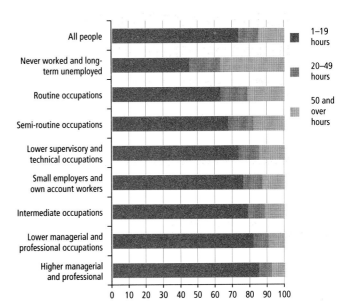

Source: Census 2001, Office for National Statistics; Census 2001, General Register Office for Scotland; Census 2001, Northern Ireland Statistics and Research Agency

Household tenure

A similar percentage of people resident in owned and social housing provided care in 2001. After age-standardisation, around one in 10 males (9 per cent) and females (12 per cent) in owned accommodation provided unpaid care, compared with only very slightly higher proportions of males (10 per cent) and of females (13 per cent) resident in social housing (Figure 12.9). Only 7 per cent of males and 10 per cent of females living in privately rented accommodation provided unpaid care. Greater proportions of residents in social housing were providing a higher intensity of care when compared with residents of owned accommodation. Twice the proportion of carers living in social housing (31 per cent) provided the highest intensity of care (50 or more hours per week) compared with carers resident in owned accommodation (15 per cent). Around a fifth (22 per cent) of carers resident in private rented accommodation cared for 50 or more hours per week.

Figure **12.9**

Percentage distribution of care provision (in hours): by housing tenure (age-standardised), 2001

United Kingdom
Percentages

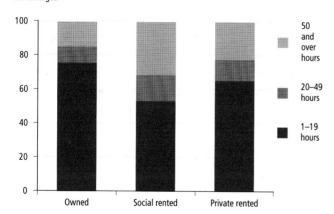

Source: Census 2001, Office for National Statistics; Census 2001, General Register Office for Scotland; Census 2001, Northern Ireland Statistics and Research Agency

Caring commitments

Relationship to person cared for

The Census tells us a great deal about individuals who provide unpaid care. However, it offers no information about the actual recipients of care. The General Household Survey (GHS) asks a specific module on caring every five years, with the last Carers survey completed in 2000. Respondents to the GHS are asked if they look after or give special help to anyone, such as a sick or disabled (or elderly) relative/ friend/ partner.[2] In 2000, the

GHS reported that 16 per cent of people aged 16 and over were carers.

According to the 2000 GHS, over half of all carers (52 per cent) were caring for a parent (38 per cent) or parent-in-law (14 per cent), whereas around one in five (18 per cent) looked after their spouse (Figure 12.10). One-fifth of carers provided care to other relatives (21 per cent), with the same proportion (21 per cent) helping friends or relatives. Smaller percentages provided care for children: 3 per cent of carers for children under 16, and 5 per cent for children 16 and over.[2]

Two-thirds of carers (67 per cent) were caring for people living in another private household, with one-third (33 per cent) caring for people living in the same household. As we might expect, carers looking after people in the same household were more likely to be caring for members of their immediate family. Over half of all carers (55 per cent) looking after someone in the same household provide care for their spouse, whereas another 9 per cent care for children under 16, and a further 11 per cent for children aged 16 and over.

Almost two-thirds (65 per cent) of carers looking after people in another household were caring for a parent (46 per cent) or parent-in-law (19 per cent). Other relatives (27 per cent) and friends or neighbours (29 per cent) were both cared for by more than one in four carers who supported people in other private households, but only very few carers caring for people in the same household (9 and 4 per cent respectively).[2]

Figure **12.10**

Relationship of carer to person cared for:[1] by residence of care recipient, 2000

Great Britain
Percentages

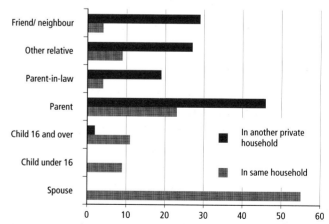

1 *Totals may add to more than 100 per cent as people may care for more than one individual.*

Source: GHS Carers 2000, Office for National Statistics

Health of person being cared for

The GHS gives us details about the health problems of people receiving care. In 2000, over ten times as many carers were looking after someone with a physical disability only (62 per cent) than with a mental disability only (6 per cent) (Figure 12.11). A further 18 per cent of carers were looking after people with both physical and mental disabilities. Old age, rather than a type of disability, was given as a reason for providing care in 14 per cent of cases.

Carers looking after someone in the same household were more likely to be looking after someone with a mental or both mental and physical disability than carers looking after people in a different household (30 per cent compared with 21 per cent). Carers providing care for people simply because of old age made up a greater proportion of people caring for those in another household (18 per cent) than in the same household (4 per cent).

Figure **12.11**

Disability of main person cared for, 2000

Great Britain
Percentages

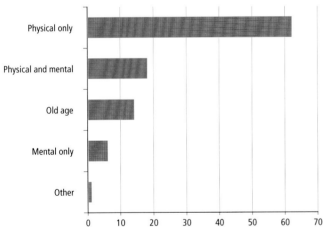

Source: GHS Carers 2000, Office for National Statistics

Type of care provided

Over two-thirds (71 per cent) of carers provided practical help such as preparing meals, shopping and doing laundry, 60 per cent kept an eye on the person cared for, and 55 per cent provided company (Figure 12.12). Smaller proportions of carers provided more intimate or personal forms of help. Around a quarter of carers gave assistance with personal care (26 per cent), whereas one in five (22 per cent) helped administer medicines. Over a third of carers (35 per cent) provided physical help, for example with walking.

Figure **12.12**

Type of unpaid care provided to person cared for: by residence of care recipient,[1] 2000

Great Britain
Percentages

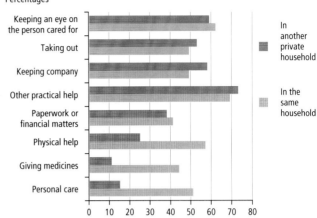

1   Totals may add to more than 100 per cent as people may provide more than one type of care.

Source: GHS Carers 2000, Office for National Statistics

The nature of the tasks carers provided help with differed between carers looking after someone in the same household and those caring for someone in another household. The former were more likely than the latter to undertake personal care tasks (51 compared with 15 per cent) and physical tasks (57 compared with 25 per cent). Carers looking after someone in the same household were less likely to say they provided practical assistance or company (69 per cent compared with 73 per cent and 49 per cent compared with 58 per cent). However, carers looking after someone they lived with may not have considered the provision of company or help with practical tasks as an extra responsibility.

Impacts of caring

Economic status

The 2001 Census asked all respondents aged 16–74 about their economic activity. There was a marked difference in the distribution of carers and non-carers by economic activity status. A higher percentage of non-carers were working full-time. Full-time employees and the full-time self-employed made up 39 per cent of all carers compared with 48 per cent of all non-carers. Conversely, 18 per cent of all carers were part-time employees or part-time self-employed compared with only 13 per cent of all non-carers. People who were retired (18 per cent) or looking after the home or family (12 per cent) made up a greater proportion of carers than non-carers (13 and 6 per cent respectively). The unemployed made up 3 per cent of all carers and 4 per cent of non-carers.

Prevalence of caring varied by working status (full and part-time workers, for example) and whether people were economically active or inactive (such as the retired). Economically inactive individuals were more likely to provide care than their economically active counterparts. In 2001, 10 per cent of economically active males and 14 per cent of economically active females provided care. Rates among economically inactive males and females were higher, at 14 and 16 per cent respectively.

Economically active individuals were less likely to provide more intensive levels of care. Around one in three economically inactive carers (34 per cent of males and females) spent 50 or more hours per week providing care compared with only one in 10 (11 per cent of males and females) economically active carers.

A higher percentage of people who worked part-time provided care compared with people working full-time. Among full-time employees, 10 per cent of males and 12 per cent of females provided unpaid care. This compares to 13 and 17 per cent of male and female part-time employees. This pattern is repeated amongs the self-employed.

Males and females looking after the home or family were most likely to provide unpaid care. Half of all males (50 per cent) and one in five females (22 per cent) in this group were carers. Economically inactive students were least likely to provide care. Only 4 per cent of males and 5 per cent of females in this group provided care.

Health status of carers

In 2001, 1.5 million carers (25 per cent of carers) had a limiting long-term illness (LLTI), while 700,000 carers (12 per cent of carers) reported having 'not good health'. Since rates of poor health tend to be higher in older age groups, the figures presented below on general health and LLTI are age-standardised to control for the different age-structures of caring and non-caring population.

Overall, a lower proportion of carers reported 'good health' than non-carers. Whereas 63 per cent of carers rated their general health as 'good', 70 per cent of non-carers reported good health after age-standardisation. Carers appear to be more likely than non-carers to describe their health as 'fairly good' than 'not good'. Over a quarter (28 per cent) of carers reported 'fairly good health' compared with around a fifth of non-carers (21 per cent). The rate of 'not good health' among both carers and non-carers was 9 per cent.

Rates of 'not good' general health increased as hours of care provided rose (Figure 12.13). While only 7 per cent of people providing care for 1–19 hours a week reported 'not good

Figure **12.13**

General health (age-standardised): by hours of care provided per week,[1] 2001

United Kingdom
Percentages

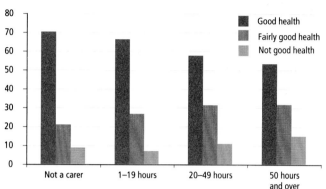

1 All people aged 5 and over.

Source: Census 2001, Office for National Statistics; Census 2001, General Register Office for Scotland; Census 2001, Northern Ireland Statistics and Research Agency

health', this rose to 11 per cent of people caring for 20–49 hours per week and 15 per cent of those caring for 50 hours or more. People providing the most intensive levels of care were more likely to be in poor health than those providing no care at all (15 compared to 9 per cent). Low intensity carers (1–19 hours per week) actually had lower levels of 'not good health' than those who did not provide care (7 compared with 9 per cent), but a rate of 'good health' four percentage points lower (66 compared with 70 per cent).

Carers also had higher rates of LLTI than non-carers did. Overall, 19 per cent of carers had an LLTI compared with 17 per cent of non-carers. Rates of LLTI were higher among those providing more intensive levels of care (Figure 12.14). Whereas 17 per cent of carers providing 1–19 hours of care per week had an LLTI, this rose to 22 per cent of those providing 20–49 hours and 27 per cent of those providing 50 or more hours of care. Carers providing the most intensive level of assistance therefore had a rate of LLTI 10 percentage points higher than those who did not provide care at all. Males providing care had higher rates of LLTI than females, with greater differences found in those groups providing more intensive care. For all carers, 20 per cent of males compared with 19 per cent of females had an LLTI, whereas for those providing 50 or more hours of care per week, 29 per cent of males had an LLTI compared to 25 per cent of females.

The 2000 GHS also asks carers how their health is affected by being a carer. The questions deal with more specific health issues than those covered by the Census questions on general health and LLTI. The percentage of carers saying that their health was not affected by being a carer decreased as the hours of care they provided went up. Of those carers providing under 20 hours of care per week, 72 per cent said their health had not been affected, compared with 39 per cent of people providing 20–49 hours, and 28 per cent of carers providing 50 or more hours of care per week.

Figure **12.14**

Percentage of population[1] with limiting long-term illness (age-standardised): by hours per week of care provided and sex, 2001

United Kingdom
Percentages

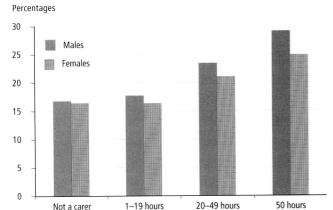

1 All people aged 5 and over.

Source: Census 2001, Office for National Statistics; Census 2001, General Register Office for Scotland; Census 2001, Northern Ireland Statistics and Research Agency

Over half of carers (52 per cent) providing 50 or more hours of care a week reported feeling tired, and around one in five (17 per cent) had had to see their own GP as a result of the time they dedicated to caring. Overall, 39 per cent of carers reported that their physical or mental health had been affected as a result of caring (Figure 12.15). A fifth of carers (20 per cent) reported feeling tired, the same proportion that reported they had a general feeling of strain. Carers also reported being short-tempered (17 per cent), feeling depressed (14 per cent) and having disturbed sleep (14 per cent).

Geographical variations

Overall, after age-standardisation, 13 per cent of adults (persons aged 16 and over) in the UK provide unpaid care. There are, however, regional variations in care provision. The proportion of people providing care in both Scotland (10 per cent) and England (11 per cent) were lower than the overall UK rate. The proportion of people providing unpaid care in Wales was 13 per cent, whereas the UK country with the highest proportion providing care was Northern Ireland (15 per cent).

Variations are also found between the various English Government Office Regions (GORs). The lowest proportions were found in the South East, London, the East and the South

Figure **12.15**

Effect of caring on health of carer, 2000

Great Britain
Percentages

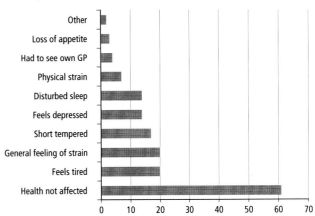

Source: GHS Carers 2000, Office for National Statistics

West where one in 10 people (10 per cent) provided care. Slightly higher proportions of people provided care in the East Midlands and Yorkshire and the Humber (11 per cent), while the highest proportion of carers were found in the West Midlands, the North West and the North East (12 per cent). The proportion of people providing care in all English GORs was lower than for both Wales and Northern Ireland. (Table 12.16 – see over).

These regional differences may be explained in part by the fact that those areas with a higher percentage of people providing care have on the whole higher rates of both 'not good' general health and of LLTI. The four regions with the highest rates of not good health and LLTI (Wales, Northern Ireland, North West, North East) were also the four areas with the highest proportions of people providing unpaid care in 2001. (Table 12.16 – see over).

Geographical variations at local authority (LA) level, shown in Map 12.17 (see overleaf), are even more pronounced than at regional level. At regional level, there is a difference of only five percentage points between the highest (Northern Ireland, 15 per cent) and lowest (South East, 10 per cent) rates of care provision. However, at LA level there is a difference of eight percentage points between Kensington and Chelsea in London, where only 8 per cent of people provide unpaid care, and Castlereagh in Northern Ireland, where 16 per cent of adults provide care.

Six of the 10 LAs with the lowest proportion of adults providing care were found in London. Outside of London, Bracknell Forest, Wokingham and Hart in the South East; and Forest Heath in the East were among the 10 LAs with the

Table **12.16**

Percentage of people (age-standardised): (a) providing unpaid care (b) with a limiting long-term illness (c) with not good general health, by Region,[1] 2001

United Kingdom

Percentages

	Providing care (aged 16 and over)	With an LLTI (all ages)	With 'not good health' (all ages)	LLTI rank	Caring rank	'Not good health' rank
Northern Ireland	14.56	19.48	10.49	1	1	2
Wales	12.56	19.41	10.55	2	2	1
North East	11.84	19.36	10.36	3	3	3
North West	11.77	17.83	9.58	4	4	4
West Midlands	11.56	16.04	8.42	7	5	7
Yorkshire and the Humber	11.39	16.55	8.91	6	6	5
East Midlands	11.17	15.42	7.79	8	7	9
Scotland	10.46	17.31	8.88	5	8	6
South West	10.34	13.96	6.76	10	9	10
East	10.23	13.27	6.37	11	10	11
London	9.79	15.14	8.19	9	11	8
South East	9.76	12.55	5.93	12	12	12
England	10.75	15.21	7.82	-	-	-
United Kingdom	12.51	15.73	8.12	-	-	-

1 Regions have been ranked by percentage providing care.

Source: Census 2001, Office for National Statistics; Census 2001, General Register Office for Scotland; Census 2001, Northern Ireland Statistics and Research Agency

lowest percentage of people providing care. Of the 10 LAs with the highest rates of informal care provision, nine were in Northern Ireland, the region with the highest overall rate of care provision after age-standardisation. Neath Port Talbot in Wales also featured among those LAs with the highest proportion of unpaid carers.

Trends in caring

Since questions about care have only been asked in the most recent Census, trends in the overall percentage of people providing care are taken from the GHS. For both males and females, the highest percentage of adults providing care was found in 2000 (males 14 per cent, females 18 per cent) and the lowest in 1995 (males 11 per cent, females 14 per cent). However, since the GHS began recording data on carers in 1985, the percentage of people in Great Britain who were carers has been fairly constant.

In 1985, 14 per cent of all people aged 16 and over were carers compared with 15 per cent in 1990, 13 per cent in 1995, and 16 per cent in 2000. The percentage of people providing care has therefore remained stable, with around 15 per cent of people providing care in all surveyed years. The proportion of people providing 20 or more hours of care per week has also

remained stable at around 4 per cent.[2] In all years a higher percentage of females than males were providing care.

Formal care

While family and friends may provide care informally, a number of people receive formal or paid care services either in institutions or their own homes. LAs and central government, as well as both private and charitable organisations have a role in providing formal care. In one week of September 2004, Councils with Social Service Responsibilities (CSSRs) in England provided 3.4 million contact hours of care to 368,400 clients in 355,600 households:[3] an average of 9.5 hours per household per week. As well as the home care provided by CSSRs, other individuals receive formal care in medical establishments and institutions.

Care in the community[3]

The purpose of Community Care Reforms of 1993 (the National Health Service and Community Care Act 1990 fully enacted 1993)[4] was to enable more people in need of personal care and assistance to live in their homes as independently as possible. Home care is provided by CSSRs and is defined as 'services that assist the client to function as independently as

Map **12.17**

Proportion of adults[1] providing unpaid care (age-standardised): by local authority,[2] 2001

United Kingdom

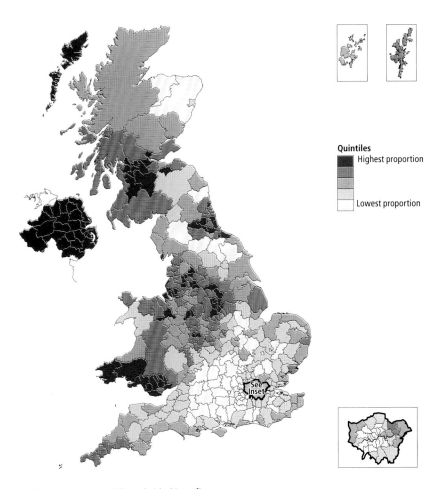

Quintiles
- Highest proportion
- Lowest proportion

See Inset

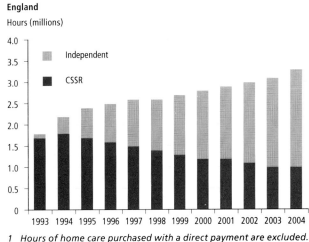

1 People aged 16 and over.
2 Local authorities ranked from highest to lowest and then divided into five groups.

Source: Office for National Statistics
© *crown copyright. All rights reserved (ONS.GD272183.2005).*

possible and/or continue to live in their own home'. Services provided by CSSRs may involve routine household tasks inside or outside the home, personal care of the client, or respite care in support of the regular (informal) carers.

The Department of Health has provided information on home care services purchased or provided by CSSRs across England since 1993. Services such as day care, meals, transport and equipment are not included in the DH returns on home care. People receiving direct payments and arranging their own care, independent of providers used by the CSSR they live in, are also excluded.[5]

Community care

CSSRs provided or purchased an estimated 3.4 million contact hours of home help or home care during the survey week in September 2004. This represents an increase of 90 per cent

Figure **12.18**

Number of hours of home care[1] and home help provided: by sector, 1993–2004

England
Hours (millions)

Independent

CSSR

1993 1994 1995 1996 1997 1998 1999 2000 2001 2002 2003 2004

1 *Hours of home care purchased with a direct payment are excluded.*

Source: Department of Health

since 1993 when 1.8 million contact hours of care per week were provided (Figure 12.18).

In 1993, CSSRs directly provided 95 per cent of all home care contact hours, whereas 5 per cent were provided by the independent sector. The percentage of care provided directly by CSSRs has fallen rapidly since 1993, and by 1999, provision of home care was divided equally between CSSRs and the independent sector (49 compared with 51 per cent). In 2004, more than two-thirds (69 per cent) of all home care was provided by the independent sector with less than one-third (31 per cent) directly provided by CSSRs.

Number of households visited

Overall, the number of hours of home care being provided is on the increase, with an increasing proportion of care being purchased from the independent sector. However, contrary to the increasing number of hours of care CSSRs are purchasing or providing, the actual number of households receiving home care is decreasing. Between 2000 and 2004, the number of households receiving home care fell by 11 per cent from 398,100 to 355,600. Similarly, the number of clients receiving home care is decreasing, with CSSRs having 11 per cent fewer clients in 2004 (368,400) than in 2000 (414,700).

Intensity of home care provision

The rise in total hours of care being purchased or provided, along with the decreasing number of households receiving care means that the average number of hours of care provided to each household per week has been increasing. In 2000, CSSRs were providing an average of 5.5 hours per household per week, while the independent sector was on average providing 8.2 hours per household per week. By 2004, CSSRs were providing on average 7.7 hours of care per household (up 2.2 hours), whereas the independent sector was providing 9.9 hours of home care per household (up 1.7 hours).

Along with the overall increase in the average number of hours of care provided to each household, there has also been an increase in the number of households receiving intensive home care packages since 2000. Intensive home care is defined as more than ten contact hours and six or more home visits in one week. About a quarter (26 per cent) of households receiving assistance were being provided with intensive home care in 2004 compared with 18 per cent in 2000. This represents an increase of 28 per cent in households in England receiving intensive home care between 2000 and 2004 (from 72,300 to 92,300 households) (Figure 12.19).

Figure **12.19**

Proportion of households¹ receiving high and low intensity of home care, 1993–2004

England
Percentages

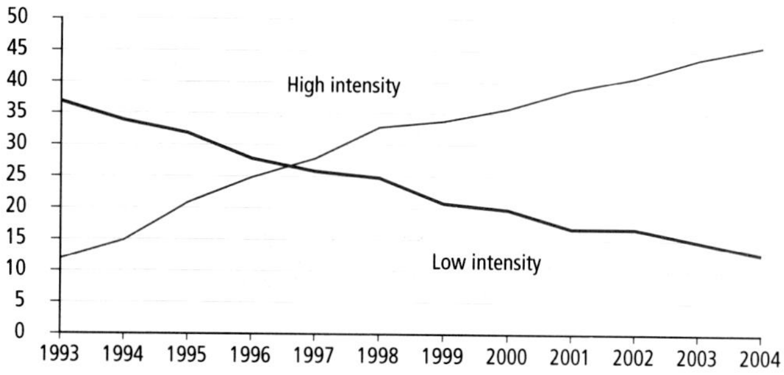

1 Households receiving income for home care purchased with a direct payment are excluded.

Source: Department of Health

Medical and care establishments

As well as commissioning the provision of home care services, LAs, along with the National Health Service (and private and charitable organisations) – also provide institutional care for people unable to continue living independently in their own homes. In 2001, the Census identified around 510,000 people in the UK living in medical and care establishments, with 91 per cent of these people reporting an LLTI.

Females made up 69 per cent of those living in medical and care establishments, outnumbering males (30 per cent) by more than two to one. Two-fifths (43 per cent) of people living in medical and care establishments were aged 85 and over, contributing to the total of 78 per cent of all people living in establishments who were aged 65 and over. Children under 16 made up one per cent of those living in medical and care establishments.

Most people in medical and care establishments were living in nursing homes (35 per cent) and residential care homes (52 per cent) (Figure 12.20). The remaining 13 per cent of people lived in other medical and care establishments, such as psychiatric hospitals or children's homes. Rates of LLTI were highest in nursing homes (97 per cent), residential care homes (92 per cent) and psychiatric hospitals (91 per cent). Rates in general hospitals (29 per cent) and children's homes (17 per cent) were relatively lower by comparison.

Figure **12.20**

Distribution of persons living in medical and care establishments by establishment type, 2001

United Kingdom
Percentages

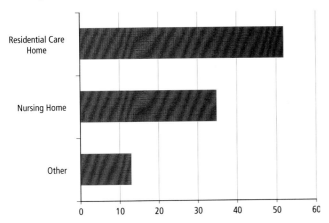

Source: Census 2001, Office for National Statistics; Census 2001, General Register Office for Scotland; Census 2001, Northern Ireland Statistics and Research Agency

Conclusion

Informal care was provided by around 6 million people in the UK in 2001, representing over one in ten people (11 per cent) over 5 years of age. One-fifth of carers (around 1.3 million people) spent 50 or more hours a week providing care. The majority of carers were aged between 35 and 64 years (65 per cent), female (58 per cent) and married (68 per cent of carers aged 16 and over).

In 2000, over half of all carers were looking after a parent (38 per cent) or parent in law (14 per cent), with a fifth (18 per cent) caring for their spouse. Two-thirds of carers (67 per cent) were looking after people living in another household, rather than their own (33 per cent). Most carers were looking after someone with a physical disability only (62 per cent) and provided practical help with tasks like preparing meals, shopping and doing laundry (71 per cent).

Though the overall proportion of people providing care does not vary greatly by social position or household tenure, a higher proportion of carers in lower socio-economic groups and in social housing provided the most intensive levels of care. Carers were less likely to be economically active or to work full-time than non-carers, and were more likely to say their health was 'not good', or to have a limiting illness or disability than those who did not provide care. In 2000, 28 per cent of carers said their health had been affected by their caring commitments, with 14 per cent of carers reporting that they felt depressed as a result of their responsibilities.

Typically, the areas with the highest levels of 'not good health' and limiting long-term illness rates also had the highest proportions of people providing care. Higher proportions of people were carers in Northern Ireland, Wales, the North West and the North East compared to the UK average. The South East had the lowest proportion of carers in the UK.

In 2003, CSSRs provided formal home care to around 375,000 individuals in England. The number of contact hours funded by CSSRs has increased by 75 per cent since 1993, with an increasing percentage of care being provided by the independent sector (but still funded by CSSRs). The proportion of households receiving intensive home care is also rising. Around 510,000 people in England and Wales live in medical and care establishments. Ninety per cent of people living in these institutions in 2001 were disabled or had a chronic illness.

Overall, what is most apparent is that all sections of society are affected by the need to provide care to family and friends who are elderly or in poor health. The amount of formal care provided by CSSRs in England increased dramatically between 1993 and 2003. With the UK population in older age groups set to increase, the burden on available care services, whether formal or informal is set to increase as well.

References

1. Population projections from the Government Actuary's Depatment (GAD) for the UK available at: www.gad.gov.uk/population/2001/uk/wuk015y.xls

2. Maher J and Green H (2002) *Carers 2000*, TSO: London. www.statistics.gov.uk/statbase/Product.asp?vlnk=5756

3. Department of Health (2004) *Community Care Statistics 2004: Home Care Services for Adults* at: www.publications.doh.gov.uk/public/Hh2004.htm

4. National Health Service and Community Care Act 1990 (c. 19) at: www.opsi.gov.uk/acts/acts1990/Ukpga_19900019_en_1.htm

5. Direct payments at: www.dh.gov.uk/PolicyAndGuidance/OrganisationPolicy/FinanceAndPlanning/DirectPayments/fs/en

Mortality

Anita Brock and Clare Griffiths

Chapter 13

Introduction

There is a long history of mortality analysis in the UK. Before the introduction of civil registration, the main sources of information available on deaths were the Bills of Mortality. These were published for various large cities by local companies – in London, for example, they were published weekly when plague threatened the city in 1592 and 1603. With the introduction of civil registration in 1837 for England and Wales, 1855 for Scotland, and 1864 for Northern Ireland, statisticians and physicians were able to analyse more reliable mortality data countrywide. Examples of the use of mortality data include John Snow's identification of contaminated water supply as the chief source of cholera epidemics in 1854,[1] the study of the effects of London fog which brought about the Clean Air Act of 1956,[2] and the effect that temperature and weather had on mortality rates.[3,4] More recently, mortality data are used extensively to assess trends in the population's health, and, for example, to set and monitor Government health targets to improve health outcomes such as those to reduce ischaemic heart disease, stroke and cancer death rates[5] and for the suicide prevention strategy.[6]

This chapter examines trends in mortality between 1979 and 2003. Over this period the age distribution of the population of the UK has changed: the elderly population (aged 85 and over) has almost doubled, whereas the fertility rate has declined.[7] As the population structure changes the major causes of death also change. This chapter therefore analyses the most common causes of death by age group starting with infants, moving onto children aged under 15, young adults aged 15–44, older adults aged 45–64 and 65–84, and finally the elderly.

Data sources and methods

Mortality data

The UK is composed of England, Wales, Scotland and Northern Ireland. Mortality data, which are collated from death certification and registration, are collected and processed by the Office for National Statistics (ONS) for England and Wales, the General Register Office for Scotland (GROS), and the General Register Office for Northern Ireland (GRONI), which is part of the Northern Ireland Statistics and Research Agency (NISRA). In this chapter the data from these countries have been aggregated to produce results for the UK on the numbers of death in each calendar year from 1979 to 2003. Data are for registrations of death in each calendar year for Scotland and Northern Ireland and for the years 1979 to 1992 for England and Wales. From 1993 onwards, occurrences of death in each calendar year have been used for England and Wales.

Approximately 88 per cent of deaths in the UK are registered in England and Wales, 10 per cent in Scotland, and 2 per cent in Northern Ireland each year.

Population data

The population figures used to calculate death rates are the annual mid-year estimates re-based every ten years on Censuses of Population for the UK and refer to the resident population. The mid-year estimates back to 1982 have been revised in light of the 2001 Census. These analyses use the most recent revised mid-year population estimates which were published in March 2003 for the years 1982–91; in October 2004 for the years 1992–2000; and in September 2004 for the years 2001–03.

Mortality rates

This chapter mainly examines age-standardised mortality rates, which have been standardised to a fixed reference or standard population. Using the direct method of standardisation, the age-standardised rate for a particular condition is that which would have occurred if the observed age-specific rates for the condition applied in a given standard population. The standard population used in this chapter is the European standard population and is the same for both males and females, so that rates may be compared over time, across sex, and across different countries or areas. Age-standardised rates have been calculated separately for males and females for age groups under 85. For the elderly (aged 85 and over), age-specific rates have been analysed.

The infant mortality rate is defined as the number of deaths at ages under one year per 1,000 live births in the same period.

Coding causes of death

William Farr, eminent medical statistician and the first appointed 'compiler of abstracts' at the General Register Office, initiated a uniform framework for disease classification, which culminated in an internationally agreed classification of diseases, injuries and causes of death in 1855. Since 1921, in England and Wales, the underlying cause of death has been coded to the International Classification of Diseases (ICD).[8] The World Health Organisation (WHO) was formed as an office of the United Nations in 1948 and has been responsible for publishing the ICD from 1950. As 'new' diseases (such as HIV/AIDS) are discovered and medical knowledge of the aetiology, pathology and natural history of diseases change, WHO produce revisions of the ICD. Currently, ONS, GROS and GRONI use the Tenth Revision of the ICD.[9]

The ICD is used to code the underlying cause of death in the UK. WHO define the underlying cause of death as:

a) the disease which initiated the train of events directly leading to death; or

b) the circumstances of the accident or violence which produced the fatal injury.

There have been two revisions of the ICD in use during the period covered by this chapter. The Ninth Revision (ICD-9) was used in all of the countries of the United Kingdom from 1979. The Tenth Revision (ICD-10) was introduced in Scotland in 2000 and in England and Wales and Northern Ireland in 2001.

There are some significant differences between ICD-9 and ICD-10 and how the accompanying rules are used to code the underlying cause of death. A list of the ICD codes used in this analysis can be found in Appendix Table 13A at the end of this chapter. Comparability ratios have been produced by GROS, GRONI and ONS, using bridgecoded data, so that comparable figures can be analysed between ICD-9 and ICD-10. These ratios adjust ICD-9-coded deaths to be comparable with ICD-10. Figure 13.1 shows the adjusted and unadjusted age-standardised mortality rates for persons where the ICD-9 coded underlying cause of death was from respiratory diseases.

Figure **13.1**

Respiratory disease mortality rates (age-standardised), 1979–2003

United Kingdom

Rate per 100,000 population

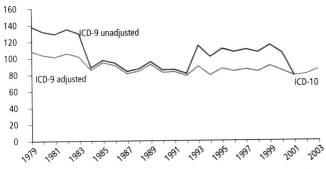

Source: Office for National Statistics; General Records Office Scotland; Northern Ireland Statistics and Research Agency

Between 1984 and 1992, ONS used a different interpretation of the ICD-9 selection rule 3 to code underlying cause of death in England and Wales to that used internationally. This interpretation was more in line with the selection rules used for ICD-10. ONS reverted back to the original interpretation of this rule from 1993 to coincide with the installation of an automated coding system.[10] This makes mortality data for England and Wales not directly comparable with mortality data for Scotland and Northern Ireland between 1984 and 1992.

Figure 13.1 shows the ICD-9 coded data where it has been adjusted to be comparable with ICD-10 and where it has been left unadjusted. The unadjusted rates are roughly 27 per cent higher than rates for years where ICD-10 has been used to code the underlying cause of death. In this chapter all rates and numbers have been adjusted so that they are comparable with ICD-10.

More information on bridgecoding and the differences between ICD-9 and ICD-10 can be found on the ONS,[11] GROS[12] and GRONI[13] websites as well as comparability ratios by age, sex and underlying cause of death. Various articles have also been published which analyse in more depth the effect of the introduction of ICD-10 on trends in major causes of death.[14–18]

This chapter mainly examines broad cause of death groups (Chapters of the ICD) but individual causes within these groups have also been analysed. Comparability ratios have been used so that data can be compared across ICD-9 and ICD-10. All neoplasms (Chapter II of ICD-9 and ICD-10) has been defined as cancer even though it includes benign neoplasms as well as malignant neoplasms. Where suicide deaths have been analysed, figures include deaths from injury of undetermined intent, otherwise known as open verdicts. It is thought that most open verdicts are cases where the harm was self-inflicted but there was insufficient evidence to prove that the deceased deliberately intended to kill themselves.[19]

Results

All cause mortality

Life expectancy at birth in 1980–82 was 71 years for males and 77 years for females. In 2001–03 life expectancy had increased to 76 and 81 years, respectively.[20] This is as a result of declining infant mortality (deaths in the first year of life) and falling mortality rates at most ages, which means that more people survive to older ages before eventually dying. Table 13.2 (see overleaf) shows the percentage of all deaths by age group and sex for the years 1981, 1991 and 2001. The proportion of all deaths occurring in the younger age groups fell whilst an increasing number were occurring in the oldest age group (aged 85 and over) in both sexes. Almost a third (31 per cent) of all deaths in the UK in 2001 occurred among those aged 85 and over compared with 17 per cent two decades earlier. This reflects the increase in life expectancy over this period.

Between 1979 and 2003, the overall age-standardised mortality rate for all causes of death fell for both males and females in the UK (Figure 13.3 – see overleaf). Between 1979 and 2003, death rates decreased by 38 per cent in males (from 1,311 to 814 per 100,000) and 29 per cent in females (from

Table **13.2**

Deaths: by sex and age, 1981, 1991 and 2001

United Kingdom

	Percentages						Number of deaths
	Under 1	1–14	15–44	45–64	65–84	85 and over	
Males							
1981	1.4	0.6	4.3	22.3	61.6	9.7	329,145
1991	1.1	0.5	4.7	17.7	62.2	13.9	314,427
2001	0.7	0.3	4.9	16.6	57.2	20.4	286,757
Females							
1981	1.0	0.4	2.4	14.0	57.9	24.1	328,829
1991	0.7	0.3	2.3	10.4	54.0	32.2	331,754
2001	0.5	0.2	2.3	9.8	46.9	40.4	315,510
Persons							
1981	1.2	0.5	3.4	17.8	59.7	17.4	657,974
1991	0.9	0.4	3.5	14.0	58.0	23.3	646,181
2001	0.6	0.3	3.5	13.0	51.8	30.8	602,267

Source: Office for National Statistics; General Records Office Scotland; Northern Ireland Statistics and Research Agency

798 to 567 per 100,000). Females had lower mortality than males throughout the period after allowing for differences in the age structure of the population (age-standardisation).

Figures 13.4 and 13.5 shows the all cause age-standardised mortality rate by age group and sex in the United Kingdom from 1979 to 2003. Figure 13.4 shows the age-standardised rates for ages under 65 – the rates in most of the age groups have shown a steady decline across the study period except for rates among young adult men aged 15–44. The all cause mortality rates for this group increased from 1987 to 1990 by 4

per cent, from 116 to 121 per 100,000. Another slight increase was seen in 1995 but rates have since declined. Figure 13.5 shows the age-standardised rates for ages over 64. A steady decrease in all cause mortality rates was seen in both men and women aged 65–84 across the study period. Among men and women aged 85 and over there was a declining trend up until 2000 since when rates stabilised and began to increase.

Figure **13.4**

All cause mortality rates (age-standardised): by sex and age for people under 65, 1979–2003

United Kingdom

Rate per 100,000 population

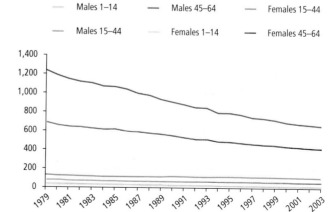

Figure **13.3**

All cause mortality rates (age-standardised): by sex, 1979–2003

United Kingdom

Rate per 100,000 population

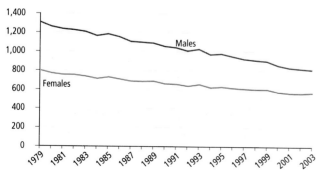

Source: Office for National Statistics; General Records Office Scotland; Northern Ireland Statistics and Research Agency

Source: Office for National Statistics; General Records Office Scotland; Northern Ireland Statistics and Research Agency

Figure **13.5**

All cause mortality rates (age-standardised): by sex and age for people over 64, 1979–2003

United Kingdom

Rate per 100,000 population

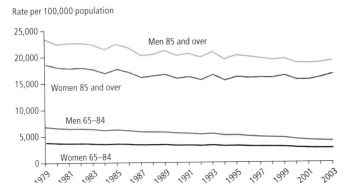

Source: Office for National Statistics; General Records Office Scotland; Northern Ireland Statistics and Research Agency

Infant mortality (aged under 1 year)

Infant mortality is defined as all deaths at ages less than one year after live birth. They can be subdivided into neonatal deaths at ages under 28 days and postneonatal deaths at ages 28 days and over but under one year. Infant mortality data as a whole are not available by underlying cause of death from 1986 onwards due to the introduction of a new certificate for registering neonatal deaths in England and Wales from this date.

Infant mortality decreased by nearly 60 per cent from 12.9 deaths per 1,000 live births in 1979 to 5.3 in 2003 (Figure 13.6). A rise in infant mortality rates in 1986 has been associated with exceptionally cold weather in February of that year[21] which was mainly seen in postneonates. Neonatal death

Figure **13.6**

Infant mortality rate, 1979–2003

United Kingdom

Rate per 1,000 live births

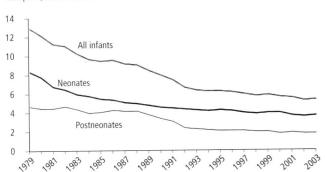

Source: Office for National Statistics; General Records Office Scotland; Northern Ireland Statistics and Research Agency

rates were higher than postneonatal death rates across the study period, and rates for both neonates and postneonates fell by over half between 1979 and 2003.

Infant mortality varies by social and biological factors. Regular analysis published annually by ONS has long shown that risk of infant death is higher for babies with low birthweight (less than 2,500 grams), for babies of mothers aged under 20 and 40 and over and for babies registered solely by the mother. Where the birth was registered jointly with the father, babies of fathers in semi-routine occupations have a higher risk of mortality than babies of fathers in professional occupations.[22] A multivariate analysis including all of these risk factors for neonatal mortality showed that birthweight is the strongest and most important risk factor.[23]

Major causes of infant death are events occurring in pregnancy (congenital anomalies, antepartum infections and immaturity-related conditions).[22]

Childhood mortality (aged 1–14 years)

Children aged between one and 14 formed just under a fifth of the population of the UK between 1979 and 2003. Deaths in children accounted for less than half a per cent of all deaths registered in the UK between 1979 and 2003. More boys than girls died each year, with 1.3 deaths among boys for every one death among girls in 2001–03. Mortality rates in children fell by 57 per cent in boys and halved in girls between 1979 and 2003 (from 39 to 17 per 100,000, and from 29 to 15 per 100,000, respectively), although the rate had stabilised from 2000.

Appendix Table 13B at the end of this chapter, shows the proportion of all deaths by age, sex, and chapter of the ICD for the years 1979 and 2003. The table shows the percentage of all deaths by chapter, the rank for each year, and the total number of deaths in each sex and age group. The data for 1979, which was originally coded in ICD-9, has been adjusted using comparability ratios to be comparable with 2003, which was coded in ICD-10.

Although the numbers of deaths in children halved over the study period, the greatest proportion of deaths for both 1979 and 2003 were due to injury and poisoning, and cancer. Although the proportion of deaths attributed to cancer stayed the same in both 1979 and 2003 (roughly 20 per cent), the proportion attributed to injury and poisoning almost halved from 40 per cent in 1979 to 24 per cent in 2003. The proportion of childhood deaths from congenital anomalies increased from 2 per cent in 1979 to 11 per cent in 2003, although there were under 200 deaths from these causes in 2003.

Figure 13.7 shows the age-standardised mortality rates for children from injury and poisoning, and cancer from 1979 to 2003. Across the period, a quarter of all deaths in girls and a third of all deaths in boys were from injury and poisoning. In both boys and girls the majority (almost 90 per cent) of these deaths were from accidents, with over half of these occurring from land transport accidents. Child death rates from injury and poisoning decreased and in 2003 stood at roughly a third of the rate seen in 1979 for both boys and girls (from 15 to four per 100,000, and from eight to three per 100,000, respectively).

Although cancer is rare in childhood compared to older age groups, with around one in 200 cancers occurring in children,[24] it accounted for just under a fifth of all childhood deaths across the period. Roughly one-third of all childhood cancers are leukaemias, and around a fifth brain and spinal tumours. Other common cancers in children are embryonal tumours (which include neuroblastoma and Wilm's tumour) and lymphomas.[25] Between 1979 and 2003, childhood mortality from cancer fell at a slower rate than deaths from injury and poisoning, and in 2003 roughly the same number of boys and girls died from cancer as from injury and poisoning.

Young adult mortality (aged 15–44 years)

Young adults, or those aged between 15 and 44 years of age, formed just over 40 per cent of the population of the UK between 1979 and 2003. Deaths in young adults accounted for 5 per cent of all male deaths and 2 per cent of all female deaths across this period. There were roughly two deaths in young men for each death in young women. For young men, death rates stopped falling in the mid-1980s and increased to a peak of 121 deaths per 100,000 in 1990 and a smaller peak of

119 per 100,000 in 1995. The decline in death rates for young women slowed from the mid-1980s but continued to fall.

Appendix Table 13B shows that for young adults the chapters with the highest proportion of deaths in both 1979 and 2003 were injury and poisoning, cancer and circulatory diseases. The proportion of injury and poisoning deaths stayed roughly the same (a third of all deaths), whereas the proportion of circulatory disease and cancer deaths decreased. In 2003, there were increased proportions of deaths from infectious diseases (from 1 per cent in 1979 to 2 per cent in 2003), mental disorders (from 1 to 5 per cent) and diseases of the digestive system (from 3 to 8 per cent).

Figure 13.8 shows the age-standardised mortality rate by ICD chapter and sex for the three main causes of death in young adults between 1979 and 2003 – injury and poisoning, cancer and circulatory diseases. However, the order in which these cause chapters rank are different for young adult men and women. They are therefore discussed separately.

Young adult men

Among young men, deaths from injury and poisoning were the most common cause of death accounting for 43 per cent of all young male deaths across the study period. The age-standardised death rate for this cause stopped declining and began to rise from the mid-1980s to peaks in 1990, 1995 and 1998, since when it has fallen. Previous research[26] has shown that although the 1990 peak was owing to increases in both land transport accidents and suicide, the peak in 1998 was

Figure **13.7**

Mortality rates (age-standardised): by cause and sex for children aged 1–14, 1979–2003

United Kingdom

Rate per 10,000 population

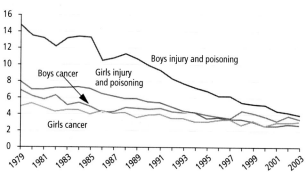

Source: Office for National Statistics; General Records Office Scotland; Northern Ireland Statistics and Research Agency

Figure **13.8**

Mortality rates (age-standardised): by cause and sex for people aged 15–44, 1979–2003

United Kingdom

Rate per 100,000 population

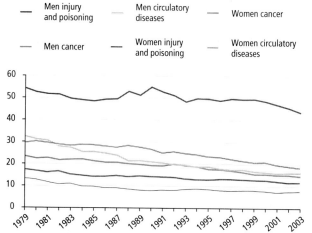

Source: Office for National Statistics; General Records Office Scotland; Northern Ireland Statistics and Research Agency

almost entirely due to an increase in suicide in young men, although deaths from accidental drug poisoning also increased rapidly. In the early 1980s, just under half of all injury and poisoning deaths were due to land transport accidents, and just over a quarter were from suicide. By the late 1990s, these figures were transposed with almost half of these deaths due to suicide and a quarter from land transport accidents. Deaths from land transport accidents decreased over the last 25 years but the number of deaths from suicide had seen an increase up until 2000.[27] The age-standardised death rate from land transport accidents almost halved between 1979 and 1994 (from 25 to 13 per 100,000) but has since stabilised. The rate for suicide, however, increased by almost 50 per cent between 1979 and the highest peak in 1998 (from 15 to 23 per 100,000) but has since declined. The age-standardised rate for accidental poisoning saw a four-fold increase between 1979 and a peak in 1999 (from one to four per 100,000).

The second most common cause of death at chapter level in young men was circulatory diseases. In the late 1970s these diseases accounted for almost a quarter of all deaths in young men, but by 2003 this had fallen to 15 per cent. The age-standardised death rate over this period halved from 32 per 100,000 in 1979 to 16 per 100,000 in 2003. Ischaemic heart disease was the most common cause of death in the circulatory disease chapter in young men. Over half of all circulatory disease deaths were due to ischaemic heart disease, and just under a fifth were from stroke across the study period. Between 1979 and 2003 the age-standardised death rate for ischaemic heart disease fell by almost two-thirds and that for stroke almost halved, from 22 to eight per 100,000 and from five to three per 100,000, respectively.

The third most common cause of death at chapter level was cancer. During the early 1980s cancer accounted for 17 per cent of all deaths in young men. By 2003 this had decreased slightly to 14 per cent. The age-standardised death rate fell by just over a third from 23 per 100,000 in 1979 to 15 in 2003. The most common cancers in young men were cancers of the brain (15 per cent of all cancer deaths in 2003), the lung (8 per cent), colon and rectum (7 per cent), leukaemia (9 per cent) and non-Hodgkin's lymphoma (6 per cent). These cancers combined accounted for almost half of all cancer deaths in young men over the period covered.

Young adult women

Among young women aged 15–44, cancer was the most common cause of death and accounted for just over a third of all deaths in this age group across the study period. The death rate from cancer in young women decreased gradually during the 1980s, but fell more rapidly during the 1990s. In 1988 the age-standardised death rate was 28 per 100,000 but by 2003

this had fallen to 18 per 100,000. Almost a third of these deaths were due to breast cancer in each year. Other common cancers in young women include cancer of the cervix (7 per cent of all cancer deaths in 2003), brain (7 per cent), lung (6 per cent), colon and rectum, and ovaries (5 per cent each), as well as leukaemia (5 per cent) and non-Hodgkin's lymphoma (4 per cent). These cancers accounted for 74 per cent of all cancer deaths in young women between 1979 and 2003.

The second most common cause of death at chapter level was injury and poisoning, accounting for a fifth of all deaths in young women in 2003. Unlike the trend seen in young men, deaths from this cause fell among young women over the study period. The death rate fell by a third between 1979 and 2003, from 17 to 12 per 100,000, respectively. During the early 1980s, half of the deaths in this chapter were due to accidents (mostly land transport accidents) and 39 per cent were as a result of suicide. By 2003, the proportion due to accidents and suicide were roughly the same (43 and 45 per cent, respectively). As seen in young men, the age-standardised death rate from land transport accidents decreased over the period, from five to three per 100,000, but unlike young men the suicide rate in young women also fell, from seven to five per 100,000, but not as rapidly as for land transport accidents. As also seen in men, the age-standardised death rate from accidental drug poisoning increased up to a peak in 1999 of 1.1 per 100,000; a doubling of the rate from a low seen in the mid-1980s of 0.5 per 100,000.

The third most common cause of death at chapter level was circulatory diseases. In the late 1970s these diseases accounted for 16 per cent of all deaths in young women, but by 2003 this had decreased slightly to 14 per cent. The age-standardised death rate over this period fell from 13 per 100,000 in 1979 to eight per 100,000 in 2003. Unlike men, stroke rather than ischaemic heart disease, was the most common cause of death in the circulatory disease chapter in young women. Across the study period, 40 per cent of all circulatory disease deaths were due to stroke, and just over a quarter were due to ischaemic heart disease. Between 1979 and 2003 the age-standardised death rates for ischaemic heart disease and stroke halved, from 3.8 to 1.8 per 100,000 and from 5.1 to 2.5 per 100,000, respectively.

Older adult mortality – aged 45–64 and 65–84

Older adults have been separated into two groups in this chapter – those aged 45–64 who were of working age, and those aged 65–84 who were of pensionable age. As the proportion of the population living to 85 or older has been steadily increasing over the study period, this age group has been analysed separately.

Older adults aged 45–64

People in this age group formed just under a quarter of the population of the UK across the period covered. There has been a decreasing number of deaths and an increasing proportion of the population in this age group. This has affected the age-standardised death rates which have fallen by over 40 per cent in both sexes across the period covered by this analysis. In the early 1980s, deaths in this age group accounted for 22 per cent of all male deaths and 13 per cent of all female deaths. By 2003, this had decreased to 16 and 10 per cent respectively. There were approximately 1.6 male deaths for each female death in this age group.

Appendix 13B shows that the chapters with the highest proportion of deaths for persons aged 45–64 in both 1979 and 2003 were circulatory diseases, cancer, respiratory diseases and deaths from injury and poisoning. Although the proportion for circulatory diseases decreased (from 46 per cent in 1979 to 29 per cent in 2003), that for cancer and respiratory diseases increased, although the number of deaths from these diseases fell by a quarter. A major increase was also seen in the proportion of deaths from diseases of the digestive system – from 3 to 8 per cent – due to the number of deaths due to these causes increasing by nearly two-thirds. By 2003, digestive diseases (which include chronic liver disease and ulcers) formed a greater proportion of deaths in this age group than deaths from respiratory diseases or injury and poisoning.

Figure 13.9 shows the age-standardised mortality rates for the five most common causes of deaths between 1979 to 2003 for men and women aged 45–64 separately. Up to 2000, the most common cause of death for men at chapter level was circulatory diseases (Figure 13.9). Due to a sustained decrease

in deaths from circulatory diseases in men – the death rate fell by two-thirds between 1979 and 2003 – cancer became the most common cause from 2001 onwards. The death rate for cancer also declined over this period – by 34 per cent – but not as rapidly as for circulatory diseases. Across the period, deaths from ischaemic heart disease accounted for 75 per cent of all circulatory disease deaths seen in men in this age group and stroke for 12 per cent. Between 1979 and 2003 the age-standardised death rates for ischaemic heart disease and stroke each fell by two-thirds, from 494 to 155 per 100,000 and from 83 to 31 per 100,000, respectively. In men aged 45–64, the most common cancer sites were lung (26 per cent of all cancer deaths in 2003), colon and rectum (10 per cent), oesophagus (8 per cent) and pancreas (5 per cent). Together these sites accounted for half of all cancer deaths in 45- to 64-year-old men in 2003. Between 1979 and 2003, the age-standardised death rate for lung cancer fell by 60 per cent from 151 to 61 per 100,000 but remained the most common cancer site in 2003.

Among women aged 45–64, cancer accounted for almost half of all deaths and circulatory diseases for almost a third (Figure 13.9). The death rate for cancer in women was roughly the same as that for men but the rate for circulatory diseases was much lower. However, decreases in death rates in women were of a similar magnitude to those in men – 65 per cent fall in circulatory diseases between 1979 and 2003, and 29 per cent for cancers. Ischaemic heart disease accounted for over half of the circulatory disease deaths across the period and stroke for roughly a quarter. Between 1979 and 2003 the age-standardised death rates for ischaemic heart disease and stroke each fell by two-thirds, from 127 to 40 per 100,000 and from 63 to 23 per 100,000, respectively. In women aged 45–64, the

Figure 13.9

Mortality rates (age-standardised): by cause and sex for ages 45–64, 1979–2003

United Kingdom

Rate per 100,000 population

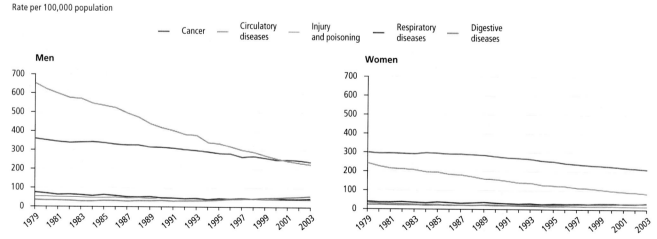

Source: Office for National Statistics; General Records Office Scotland; Northern Ireland Statistics and Research Agency

most common cancer sites were breast (24 per cent of all cancer deaths in 2003), lung (18 per cent), ovaries (9 per cent), colon and rectum (8 per cent), and pancreas (4 per cent). Together these sites accounted for almost two thirds of all cancer deaths in women aged 45–64 in 2003. The age-standardised death rate for breast cancer was static during the early 1980s but started to fall in 1987, since when it had decreased by just over a third, from 80 per 100,000 in 1987 to 51 per 100,000 in 2003.

Up until the late 1990s, the third most common cause of death at chapter level in both men and women was diseases of the respiratory system, although deaths from injury and poisoning had only marginally lower rates. Indeed, in 1990, 1992 and 1994 the death rate for men was slightly higher for injury and poisoning than for respiratory diseases. Between 1979 and 1994, the age-standardised death rates from respiratory disease almost halved for men and fell by over a third for women. From 1995 onwards, however, these rates stabilised. The death rates for injury and poisoning also fell up to the mid-1990s but then levelled off for both men and women. This is in contrast to age-standardised death rates from digestive diseases, which increased by 68 per cent in men and 38 per cent in women between 1994 and 2003. Indeed, from 1998 onwards the death rate for men in this age group was higher for digestive diseases than respiratory diseases and became the third most common cause of death at chapter level.

The most common cause of death in the respiratory disease chapter was chronic lower respiratory diseases, which accounted for two-thirds of these deaths in both sexes across the period. This group of diseases includes bronchitis, emphysema and other chronic obstructive pulmonary diseases. Between 1979 and 2002 the age-standardised death rates in men for chronic lower respiratory diseases fell by 62 per cent, from 54 to 21 per 100,000, and the rate in women fell by almost a third, from 25 to 18 per 100,000. However, the rates for both sexes rose by 10 per cent in 2003. Pneumonia accounted for almost a quarter of all respiratory disease deaths in both men and women in this age group across the study period. There was a downward trend in the age-standardised death rate for both sexes between 1979 and 1993, but between 1994 and 2003 the rates for both men and women increased, by 46 per cent in men and by 28 per cent in women (from nine to 14 per 100,000 and from six to eight per 100,000, respectively).

The distribution of deaths from injury and poisoning by intent altered by sex over the period covered. In 1979, the age-standardised rate in men due to accidents was 33 per 100,000 and the suicide rate was 20 per 100,000. By 2003, the male

age-standardised rate from accidents had decreased by 43 per cent whilst that for suicide had only fallen by 15 per cent, although the rate for accidents was still higher. In women in 1979, the age-standardised rate from suicide and accidental causes was 17 and 15 per 100,000, respectively. During the 1980s the rates in women fell by over a third for accidents and almost halved for suicide, from 15 to nine per 100,000 and from 17 to nine per 100,000, respectively. Since the early 1990s the female rates for both of these causes had stabilised and from 1990 onwards the rate was higher for accidents than for suicide.

Alcoholic liver disease was the most common cause of digestive disease death across the period. The proportion of these deaths increased annually in both sexes until 2003 when this cause accounted for half of all digestive disease deaths in men and 40 per cent in women. Between 1979 and 2003, the age-standardised rate increased almost six-fold in men, from five to 29 per 100,000, and four-fold in women, from three to 13 per 100,000.

Adults aged 65–84

People in this age group formed 14 per cent of the population of the UK across the period. There has been a decreasing number of deaths and an increasing proportion of men of this age in the population. In women, however, although the numbers of deaths were also decreasing, the proportion of the population has remained relatively stable. Between 1979 and 2003, age-standardised death rates fell by 41 per cent in men (from 6,794 to 3,997 per 100,000) and almost a third in women (from 3,832 to 2,620 per 100,000). In the early 1980s men in this age group accounted for 61 per cent of all male deaths, and women 58 per cent of all female deaths. By 2003, these proportions had decreased to 57 and 47 per cent respectively, although the largest proportion of deaths in the UK still occurred at these ages. There were approximately 1.1 male deaths for each female death in this age group.

Appendix 13B shows that the chapters with the highest proportion of deaths in this age group in both 1979 and 2003 were circulatory diseases, cancer, and respiratory diseases. As with those aged 45–64, the proportion of deaths due to circulatory diseases decreased (from 55 per cent in 1979 to 40 per cent in 2003) in those aged 65–84, whilst the proportions for cancer and respiratory diseases increased. An increase was also seen in the proportion of deaths due to diseases of the digestive system, although this was not as great as was seen in those aged 45–64.

Figure 13.10 shows the age-standardised mortality rates for the three most common causes of death, by sex, from 1979 to 2003. For men aged 65–84, as with the previous age group, the most common cause of death was circulatory diseases. But for women, unlike the previous age group, circulatory diseases had exceeded cancer as the most common cause of death. Age-standardised death rates from circulatory diseases fell by 55 per cent in both men and women between 1979 and 2003, from 3,603 to 1,619 per 100,000, and from 2,182 to 971 per 100,000, respectively. Ischaemic heart disease was the most common cause within this disease chapter accounting for over 60 per cent of male deaths and half of female deaths across the study period, followed by stroke which accounted for almost a quarter of all circulatory disease deaths in men and almost a third in women. Between 1979 and 2003, the age-standardised death rate for ischaemic heart disease halved and that for stroke fell by 59 per cent, in both men and women aged 65–84.

Cancer was the second most common cause of death in both men and women in this age group. In men, a peak in death rates from cancer was seen in the mid-1980s, since when rates declined steadily. In contrast, age-standardised death rates for women increased by 12 per cent between 1979 and 1992. The rates have since fallen but are still higher than those seen in the early 1980s. The most common cancer sites in men were lung (26 per cent of all cancer deaths in 2003), prostate (13 per cent), colon and rectum (11 per cent), stomach and oesophagus (5 per cent each). Together these sites accounted

Figure **13.10**

Mortality rates (age-standardised): by cause and sex for people aged 65–84, 1979–2003

United Kingdom

Rate per 100,000 population

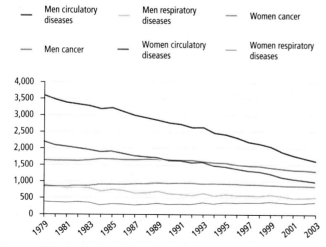

Source: Office for National Statistics; General Records Office Scotland; Northern Ireland Statistics and Research Agency

for 60 per cent of all cancer deaths in men aged 65–84 in 2003. Between 1979 and 2003, the age-standardised rate for lung cancer in men fell by 46 per cent, from 632 to 343 per 100,000, respectively. Up until 1987, the death rate was higher for colorectal cancer than prostate cancer. From 1987, however, the death rate was higher from prostate cancer. This was due to a fall in colorectal cancer deaths and an increase in deaths attributable to prostate cancer during the late 1980s. In women, the most common cancer sites were lung (21 per cent of all cancer deaths in 2003), breast (13 per cent), colon and rectum (10 per cent), ovaries (6 per cent), and pancreas (5 per cent). Combined these sites accounted for just over half of all cancer deaths in women in this age group in 2003. During the early 1980s, the age-standardised rate for lung cancer was lower than that for breast or colon and rectum cancer. Between 1979 and 1996, however, the rate for lung cancer increased by 65 per cent (from 113 to 186 per 100,000, respectively). Since then the rate for lung cancer had stabilised, but in 2003 was still higher than that seen during the 1980s. The age-standardised rate for breast cancer increased between 1979 and 1987 by 11 per cent but had since fallen by a quarter.

The third most common cause of death at chapter level in both sexes was respiratory diseases. In men, the age-standardised death rate for these diseases fell – by 41 per cent between 1979 and 2003 (from 888 to 521 per 100,000, respectively). For women, the rates fell between 1979 and the mid-1980s, but then increased, so that in 2003 the rate was only 1 per cent lower than that seen in 1979. In men, the most common causes of respiratory disease death were chronic lower respiratory diseases, which accounted for 60 per cent of all respiratory deaths across the period, and pneumonia, which was responsible for just under a third. The age-standardised rate almost halved for chronic lower respiratory diseases and pneumonia between 1979 and 2003, from 532 to 271 per 100,000 and 297 to 156 per 100,000, respectively. For women, both of these causes were also the most common but the proportions changed over time. Between 1979 and 2003, the age-standardised rate for pneumonia in women aged 65–84 fell by over a third (from 188 to 117 per 100,000). The rate for chronic lower respiratory diseases, however, increased by 77 per cent between 1979 and a peak in 1999 (from 108 to 190 per 100,000). Since 1999, the rate has fluctuated and in 2003 was not much lower than the rate seen for pneumonia in 1979 at 183 per 100,000.

Mortality in the elderly – aged 85 and over

In 2003, people in this age group formed 2 per cent of the population of the UK. The number of people aged 85 years and over has almost doubled since 1979. Deaths in this age group accounted for almost a third of all deaths in 2003 with a higher proportion in women than in men. There were just over 2.4 female deaths for each male death in the elderly. From 1979 to 2001, the death rate fell by 20 per cent in men and 16 per cent in women but has since shown a slight increase.

Appendix 13B shows that the chapters with the highest proportion of deaths in the elderly in both 1979 and 2003 were circulatory diseases, respiratory diseases, and cancer. As seen with the previous two age groups, although the proportion for circulatory diseases decreased, the proportions for respiratory diseases and cancer increased. There was a general increase in the proportions for all other chapters in 2003 compared to 1979. In particular, increases were seen in mental disorders (from 1 per cent in 1979 to 5 per cent in 2003) and symptoms, signs and ill-defined conditions (from 1 to 6 per cent).

Figure 13.11 shows the age-specific rates for the three most common causes of death by sex from 1979 to 2003. The most common cause of death at chapter level in the elderly was circulatory diseases. Death rates in both elderly men and women fell by over a third between 1979 and 1999 (from 12,999 to 8,346 per 100,000 and 11,451 to 7,335 per 100,000, respectively) but have since increased slightly. In men, 46 per cent of all circulatory disease deaths resulted from ischaemic heart disease and almost a third resulted from stroke across the period. The male age-specific rate for ischaemic heart disease increased slightly up until 1985 but then fell by almost a third between 1985 and 2003 (from 5,287 to 3,674 per 100,000, respectively). The male rate for stroke fell by 38 per cent across the study period (from 3,840 per 100,000 in

Figure **13.11**

Mortality rates: by cause and sex for people aged 85 and over, 1979–2003

United Kingdom

Rate per 100,000 population

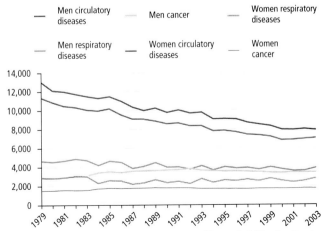

Source: Office for National Statistics; General Records Office Scotland; Northern Ireland Statistics and Research Agency

1979, to 2,393 per 100,000 in 2003) although the rate had stabilised from 2000 onwards. In women, ischaemic heart disease and stroke each composed almost 40 per cent of all circulatory disease deaths. Up until 1981, the female age-specific rate for stroke was higher than the rate for ischaemic heart disease. From 1982 onwards, however, the rate for ischaemic heart disease was slightly higher. As seen in elderly men, the rate for ischaemic heart disease increased slightly during the early 1980s and then fell, from a peak in 1985, by almost a third up to 2003 (from 3,906 to 2,702 per 100,000, respectively). The rate for stroke fell by 31 per cent across the study period (from 3,836 per 100,000 in 1979, to 2,656 per 100,000 in 2003) although, as also seen in elderly men, the rate stabilised and stopped declining from 2000 onwards.

The second most common cause of death in the elderly was respiratory diseases. In men, the age-specific death rate from all respiratory diseases fell by 16 per cent between 1979 and 2003 (from 4,642 to 3,897 per 100,000), but in women the rate was fairly stable. Pneumonia was responsible for over half of these deaths in men and chronic lower respiratory diseases for a third across the period. After a slight increase to peaks of 2,590 and 1,706 per 100,000, respectively, in 1985, the age-specific male rates for both pneumonia and chronic lower respiratory diseases began to fall. This downward trend continued for chronic lower respiratory diseases and rates fell by two-thirds between 1985 and 2003. Pneumonia rates in elderly men, however, increased between the mid-1990s and 2003 by 21 per cent.

In women, the majority (68 per cent) of deaths were due to pneumonia and 14 per cent from chronic lower respiratory diseases. Age-specific female rates for pneumonia fluctuated up until the late 1980s then began to fall. Pneumonia rates fell by a quarter between 1989 and 1994, from 2,054 to 1,559 per 100,000, but then started to rise. The age-specific rate in 2003, 1,938 per 100,000, was just below that seen in the late 1980s. Chronic lower respiratory disease rates had shown an upward trend throughout the study period. Rates increased by 32 per cent between 1979 and 2003, from 352 to 464 per 100,000, respectively.

The third most common cause of death in the elderly was cancer, which accounted for 17 per cent of all elderly male and 11 per cent of all elderly female deaths across the period. The death rate for cancer in elderly men increased by a third between 1979 and a peak in the early 1990s, from 2,871 to 3,827 per 100,000 in 1992. Since then it has fallen, but in 2003 was still a fifth higher than in 1979. The most common cancer sites in men were prostate (25 per cent of all cancer deaths in 2003), lung (16 per cent), colon and rectum (10 per cent), bladder (6 per cent), and stomach (4 per cent). These sites combined accounted for 62 per cent of all cancer deaths in elderly men in 2003. During the 1980s the age-specific rate for lung cancer in elderly men was higher than that for prostate cancer. As prostate cancer rates increased (by 71 per cent between 1979 and 2003; from 502 to 858 per 100,000), lung cancer rates began to decline from the mid-1980s onwards.

In elderly women, the death rate from cancer increased by 21 per cent from 1979 up to the late 1980s, from 1,598 to 1,936 in 1989, but then stabilised. The most common cancer sites were breast (17 per cent of all cancer deaths in 2003), colon and rectum (13 per cent), lung (10 per cent), pancreas (5 per cent), stomach and bladder (4 per cent each). These sites together accounted for over half of all cancer deaths in elderly women in 2003. Up until 1988, the age-specific rate for colon and rectum cancer in elderly women was higher than that for breast cancer. As breast cancer rates increased (by 35 per cent between 1979 and 1991; from 265 to 358 per 100,000), colon and rectum cancer rates began to decline from the mid-1980s. Breast cancer rates fell between 1991 and 1995 but have since stabilised at around 300 per 100,000 annually.

Conclusion

Over the last 25 years mortality rates at younger ages have fallen in both men and women in the UK resulting in more people living longer and an increasing proportion of deaths occurring in the elderly. When trends were examined by age and sex, the only group that saw a rise in death rates during the period 1979 to 2003 was young men aged 15–44.

The most common underlying cause of death changed by age group examined. Infant mortality rates fell by 60 per cent from 1979 to 2003, alongside awareness campaigns such as 'Reduce the risk.'[28] In children, the most common causes of death across the period were from land transport accidents and leukaemia. The mortality rates had fallen for both of these causes alongside Government road safety campaigns[29, 30] and major improvements in treatment, and consequent large gains in survival, for childhood leukaemia.[24]

In young adults there was a divergence by sex in the pattern of causes of death. In young men, although there was a fall in death rates from most diseases, this was offset by a rise in death rates from injury and poisoning – almost half of all deaths across the period were from these causes which are thought of as 'avoidable.'[26] In the 1980s, most injury and poisoning deaths in young men were from land transport accidents, but by the 1990s suicide was the main cause. This was partly due to a fall in the death rate from land transport accidents, but also owing to an increase in the death rate due to self-harm. Suicide also accounted for almost half of all injury

and poisoning deaths in young women although the mortality rates were much lower than those seen in men. The decrease seen in land transport accidents may in part be due to Government legislation, including the compulsory wearing of seatbelts for back-seat passengers in 1991, and drink-drive campaigns[31] but the reasons for the increase in suicide are less obvious. It has been suggested that there is a relationship between suicide and access to methods to commit suicide.[32] In 2002, the Government produced a 'National Suicide Prevention Strategy'[6] to identify ways of reducing the number of deaths in England from this cause and to monitor trends in suicide.

In young adult women, cancer was the most common cause of death across the period. The age-standardised rate was stable until the mid-1980s and then began to decline. The most common cancer site in young adult women was breast cancer, which accounted for a third of all cancer deaths each year.

In older adults aged 45–64 and 65–84, the two most common causes of death were circulatory diseases and cancer. Nearly all of the circulatory disease deaths were due to ischaemic heart disease and stroke and the main cancer sites were lung in men, and lung and breast in women. In men and women aged 45–64, age-standardised mortality rates for ischaemic heart disease and stroke fell by two-thirds, and in men and women aged 65–84 rates halved for both of these causes, between 1979 and 2003. Among men, lung cancer rates also saw a dramatic fall for both age groups. Lung cancer rates gradually fell in women aged 45–64, but increased up until the 1990s in women aged 65–84. Breast cancer rates fell from the late-1980s among women aged 45–64 and from the early-1990s in women aged 65–84.

One major risk factor that circulatory diseases and lung cancer share is cigarette smoking.[33, 34] Other risk factors for ischaemic heart disease and stroke include obesity and high saturated fat diets, high blood pressure, diabetes and family history of the disease. Most of the known risk factors for breast cancer relate to a women's reproductive history.[35] In the early 1980s breast cancer was the most common form of cancer in women in the 65–84 year age group, but during the 1990s lung cancer became the most common cancer site. Secular changes in mortality risk may result from a combination of factors such as improvements in health care – for example the NHS breast screening programme in 1988,[36] and better treatment – and lagged effects of risky behaviour – for example the increase in smoking among women over the course of the 20th century.

Circulatory diseases were also the main cause of death in the elderly (aged 85 and over) but respiratory diseases were the second most common. Pneumonia was responsible for half of these deaths in men and over two-thirds in women. It has been suggested that the increased risk of death resulting from pneumonia among the elderly may be the manifestation of a cohort effect[37] and that people born after the middle of the 20th century will show a decreasing mortality rate from this disease.

The increase in deaths from digestive diseases was noted through all of the adult age groups examined – including young adults aged 15–44. Most of the increase in these deaths were due to alcoholic liver disease. Previous research[38] has suggested that this rise is not only caused by increased alcohol consumption, but may be linked to changing consumption patterns, such as binge drinking, to changes in the types of alcohol consumed, and changing drinking habits in the young.

This chapter has presented mortality by year of death (registration or occurrence). However, many diseases have strong cohort as well as period patterns, for example lung cancer which is strongly affected by the timing of smoking take-up and cessation by different population groups. A recent analysis[39] by the Government Actuary's Department (GAD) showed that cohorts of men and women born between 1925 and 1945 appeared to have the greatest rates of mortality improvement compared to cohorts born before or after.

The analysis of trends at national level can mask differences between population subgroups across the country. Examples of this include differences in mortality by socio-economic status and by area. Geographical variations in mortality have been analysed in Decennial Supplements since the 1800s, the most recent publication being *Geographic Variations in Health*, which showed that inequalities in mortality by area have persisted over time. Mortality from the major causes of death is generally higher in Scotland, Wales and Northern Ireland than in England, and within England the north-south divide in mortality persists. Variations at local level within regions are generally greater than variations between regions.[40] However, variations in mortality at area level are partially explained by individual circumstances, most often characterised by Social Class, based on occupation. There is a gradient of increasing mortality from major causes of death, such as ischaemic heart disease, stroke and lung cancer, between professionals and unskilled manual workers nationally and within countries and regions. However, there is little geographic variation in mortality within the professional group.[41] Recent work using the Longitudinal Study has shown that inequalities in overall male mortality between professionals, managers and technical workers and partly-skilled and unskilled workers increased 3.6 per cent between 1986 and 1999. This was due to a greater decline in mortality among professional, managers and technical workers compared with partly-skilled and unskilled workers. Diseases contributing most to this widening are major

causes of death – ischaemic heart disease, cerebrovascular disease, respiratory diseases and lung cancer. Among females, there was a narrowing of this inequality over the same time period.[42]

References

1. Nissel M (1987) *People Count: a history of the General Register Office*, HMSO: London.

2. McFarlane A (1976) Daily deaths in Greater London. *Population Trends* **05**, 20–25.

3. Curwen M (1997) Chapter 13: Excess winter mortality in England and Wales with special reference to the effects of temperature and influenza, in *The Health of Adult Britain, 1841–1994*, volume 1, TSO: London.

4. Johnson H, Kovats S, McGregor G, Stedman J, Gibbs M, Walton H, Cook L and Black E (2005) The impact of the 2003 heat wave on mortality and hospital admissions in England. *Health Statistics Quarterly* **25**, 6–11.

5. Department of Health (1999) White Paper, *Saving Lives: Our Healthier Nation*, TSO: London.

6. Department of Health (2002) *National Suicide Prevention Strategy for England*, Department for Health Publications: London.

7. Office for National Statistics (2005) Table 2.2: Key demographic and health indicators. *Health Statistics Quarterly* **25**, 42.

8. General Register Office (1912) *Manual of the international list of causes of death, as adapted for use in England and Wales, based on the second decennial revision by the International Commission, Paris, 1909*, HMSO: London.

9. World Health Organisation (1994). *Manual of the International Statistical Classification of Diseases and Related Health Problems*, Tenth Revision, Volume 1, WHO: Geneva.

10. Rooney C and Devis T (1996) Mortality trends by cause of death in England and Wales 1980-94: the impact of introducing automated cause coding and related changes in 1993. *Population Trends* **86**, 29–35.

11. www.statistics.gov.uk/about/classifications/ICD10/default.asp

12. www.gro-scotland.gov.uk/statistics/library/annrep/00annrep/00app2.html

13. www.nisra.gov.uk/statistics/financeandpersonnel/DMB/2002RG_Report/appendix7.pdf

14. Rooney C, Griffiths C and Cook L (2002) The implementation of ICD-10 for cause of death coding – some preliminary results from the bridge coding study. *Health Statistics Quarterly* **13**, 31–41.

15. Office for National Statistics (2002) Report: Results of the ICD-10 bridge coding study, England and Wales 1999. *Health Statistics Quarterly* **14**, 75–83.

16. Griffiths C and Rooney C (2003) The effect of the introduction of ICD-10 on trends in mortality from injury and poisoning in England and Wales. *Health Statistics Quarterly* **19,** 10–21.

17. Griffiths C, Brock A and Rooney C (2004) The impact of introducing ICD-10 on trends in mortality from the circulatory diseases in England and Wales. *Health Statistics Quarterly* **22**, 14–20.

18. Brock A, Griffiths C and Rooney C (2004) The effect of the introduction of ICD-10 on cancer mortality trends in England and Wales. *Health Statistics Quarterly* **23**, 7–17.

19. Adelstein A and Mardon C (1975) Suicides 1961–74. *Population Trends* **02**, 13–18.

20. Office for National Statistics (2005) Table 5.1: Expectation of life at birth and selected ages. *Health Statistics Quarterly* **25**, 47.

21. MacFarlane A and Mugford M (2000) Chapter 3: Variations in births and deaths, *Birth Counts: statistics of pregnancy and childbirth. Second edition.* TSO: London.

22. Office for National Statistics (2004) Report: Infant and perinatal mortality by social and biological factors, 2003. *Health Statistics Quarterly* **24**, 66–70.

23. Dattani N, Cooper N, Rooney C, Rodrigues L and Campbell C (2000) Analysis of risk factors for neonatal mortality in England and Wales, 1993–97: based on singleton babies weighing 2,500–5,499 grams. *Health Statistics Quarterly* **08**, 29–35.

24. Stiller C, Quinn M and Rowan S (2004) Chapter 13: Childhood cancer. *The health of children and young people*, ONS: London.

25. Quinn M, Babb P, Brock A, Kirby L and Jones J (2001) Chapter 23: in Childhood cancers, *Cancer Trends in England and Wales, 1950–1999*, TSO: London.

26. Brock A and Griffiths C (2003) Trends in the mortality of young adults aged 15–44 in England and Wales, 1961 to 2001. *Health Statistics Quarterly* **19**, 22–31.

27. Brock A and Griffiths C (2003) Trends in suicide by method in England and Wales, 1979 to 2001. *Health Statistics Quarterly* **20**, 7–18.

28. www.sids.org.uk/fsid/rtrabr.htm

29. www.thinkroadsafety.gov.uk/campaigns/introduction.htm

30. www.srsc.org.uk/

31. www.thinkroadsafety.gov.uk

32. Kelly S and Bunting J (1998) Trends in suicide in England and Wales, 1982–96. *Population Trends* **92**, 29–41.

33. Charlton J and Murphy M (1997) Chapter 18: Cardiovascular diseases, in *The Health of Adult Britain 1841–1994*. Volume 2, TSO: London.

34. Quinn M, Babb P, Brock A, Kirby L and Jones J (2001) Chapter 12: Lung in *Cancer Trends in England and Wales, 1950–1999*, TSO: London.

35. Quinn M, Babb P, Brock A, Kirby L and Jones J (2001) Chapter 5: Breast in *Cancer Trends in England and Wales, 1950–1999*. TSO: London.

36. www.cancerscreening.nhs.uk/breastscreen/

37. Marks G and Burney P (1997) Chapter 20: Diseases of the respiratory system in *The Health of Adult Britain 1841–1994*. Volume 2. TSO: London.

38. Baker A and Rooney C (2003) Recent trends in alcohol-related mortality, and the impact of ICD-10 on the monitoring of these deaths in England and Wales. *Health Statistics Quarterly* **17**, 5–14.

39. Government Actuary's Department (2002) *National Population Projections: Review of Methodology for Projecting Mortality.* National Statistics Quarterly Review Series Report No. 8, Government Actuary's Department: London.

40. Fitzpatrick J, Griffiths C, Kelleher M and McEvoy S (2001) Descriptive analysis of geographic variations in adult mortality by cause of death, in Griffiths C and Fitzpatrick J (eds.) *Geographic Variations in Health*, TSO: London.

41. Uren Z, Fitzpatrick J, Reid A and Goldblatt P (2001) Geographic variation in mortality by Social Class and alternative social classifications, in Griffiths C and Fitzpatrick J (eds.) *Geographic Variations in Health*, TSO: London.

42. Coulthard M, Chow Y H, Dattani N, White C, Baker A and Johnson B (2004) Health, in Babb P, Martin J and Haezewindt P (eds.) *Focus on Social Inequalities*, TSO: London.

Appendix Table **13A**

ICD codes used to examine trends by cause of death

Cause of death	ICD-10 code	ICD-9 code
Infectious diseases	**A00–B99**	**001–139**
Cancer	**C00–D48**	**140–239**
Oesophageal caner	C15	150
Stomach cancer	C16	151
Colon and rectum cancer	C18–C21	153–154
Pancreatic cancer	C25	157
Lung cancer	C33–C34	162
Breast cancer	C50	174–175
Cervical cancer	C53	180
Ovarian cancer	C56	183
Prostate cancer	C61	185
Bladder cancer	C67	188
Brain cancer	C71	191
Non–Hodgkin's lymphoma	C82–C85	200, 202
Leukaemia	C91–C95	204–208
Blood & blood–forming organs diseases	**D50–D89**	**280–289**
Endocrine & nutritional diseases	**E00–E90**	**240–279**
Mental & behavioural disorders	**F00–F99**	**290–319**
Diseases of the nervous system	**G00–G99**	**320–359**
Diseases of the eye	**H00–H59**	**360–379**
Diseases of the ear	**H60–H95**	**380–389**
Circulatory diseases	**I00–I99**	**390–459**
Ischaemic heart diseases	I20–I25	410–414
Stroke	I60–I69	430–438
Respiratory diseases	**J00–J99**	**460–519**
Pneumonia	J12–J18	480–486
Chronic lower respiratory diseases	J40–J47	490–494, 496
Digestive diseases	**K00–K93**	**520–579**
Alcoholic liver disease	K70	571.0–571.3
Skin diseases	**L00–L99**	**680–709**
Musculoskeletal diseases	**M00–M99**	**710–739**
Genitourinary diseases	**N00–N99**	**580–629**
Complications of pregnancy, etc	**O00–O99**	**630–676**
Perinatal conditions	**P00–P96**	**760–779**
Congenital malformations	**Q00–Q99**	**740–759**
Symptoms & ill–defined conditions	**R00–R99**	**780–799**
Injury & poisoning	**V01–Y89**	**E800–E999**
Accidents	V01–X59	E800–E928, excluding E870–E879
Land transport accidents	V01–V89	E800–E829
Accidental poisoning by drugs and medicaments	X40–X44	E850–E858
Suicide	X60–X84, Y10–Y34*	E950–E959, E980–E989†

Note
* *Excludes pending verdicts coded to Y33.9 for England and Wales.*
† *Excludes code E988.8 for England and Wales.*

Appendix Table 13B

Percentage of deaths by age and ICD chapter, 1979 and 2003

United Kingdom

ICD-9 chapter	ICD-10 chapter	Chapter text	All ages 1979 %	All ages 1979 Rank	All ages 2003 %	All ages 2003 Rank	1–14 1979 %	1–14 1979 Rank	1–14 2003 %	1–14 2003 Rank	15–44 1979 %	15–44 1979 Rank	15–44 2003 %	15–44 2003 Rank	45–64 1979 %	45–64 1979 Rank	45–64 2003 %	45–64 2003 Rank	65–84 1979 %	65–84 1979 Rank	65–84 2003 %	65–84 2003 Rank	85 plus 1979 %	85 plus 1979 Rank	85 plus 2003 %	85 plus 2003 Rank
I	I	Infectious diseases	0.4	12	1	11	4	6	6	6	1	9	2	8	1	9	1	8	0	11	1	10	0	12	1	12
II	II	Cancer	22.7	2	26	2	20	2	21	2	24	2	20	2	34	2	42	1	23	2	30	2	10	3	13	3
IV	III	Blood & blood-forming organs	1.2	8	0	15	1	11	2	11	0	13	0	14	0	12	0	14	0	12	0	14	0	13	0	14
III	IV	Endocrine & nutritional	0.2	13	2	10	5	5	5	5	2	7	2	9	1	7	1	7	1	8	2	8	1	11	1	10
V	V	Mental & behavioural disorders	0.7	10	3	6	0	14	0	15	1	8	5	6	0	11	1	9	1	10	2	6	1	7	5	5
VI (part)	VI	Nervous system diseases	1.6	6	3	7	10	3	14	3	5	4	5	5	2	6	3	6	1	7	3	5	1	8	3	7
VI (part)	VII	Diseases of eye	0.0	19	0	18	0	17	-	17	0	18	0	19	-	-	0	16	0	17	0	17	0	16	0	16
VI (part)	VIII	Diseases of ear	0.0	18	0	19	0	15	-	18	0	17	0	17	0	16	0	17	0	16	0	16	0	15	0	17
VII	IX	Circulatory diseases	53.1	1	38	1	4	7	6	7	20	3	15	3	46	1	29	2	55	1	40	1	60	1	43	1
VIII	X	Respiratory diseases	11.2	3	14	3	9	4	8	5	4	5	3	7	6	3	7	4	11	3	14	3	17	2	18	2
IX	XI	Digestive diseases	2.9	5	5	4	2	8	3	9	3	6	9	3	3	5	8	3	3	4	4	4	3	4	4	6
XII	XII	Skin diseases	1.3	7	0	13	0	16	0	16	0	16	0	16	0	14	0	15	0	14	0	13	0	14	0	13
XIII	XIII	Musculoskeletal diseases	0.0	17	1	12	0	13	1	13	1	11	1	13	1	10	1	12	1	9	1	11	1	9	1	11
X	XIV	Genitourinary diseases	0.1	16	2	9	1	12	1	14	1	10	1	12	1	8	1	10	1	6	2	7	2	6	3	8
XI	XV	Complications of pregnancy, etc	0.7	9	0	17	-	-	-	-	0	12	0	15	-	-	-	-	-	-	-	-	-	-	-	-
XV	XVI	Perinatal conditions	0.1	14	0	16	-	-	1	12	-	-	0	18	-	-	-	-	-	-	-	-	-	-	-	-
XIV	XVII	Congenital malformations	0.1	15	0	14	2	9	11	4	0	15	2	10	0	15	0	13	0	15	0	15	0	17	0	15
XVI	XVIII	Symptoms & ill-defined conditions	0.4	11	2	8	1	10	2	10	0	14	1	11	0	13	1	11	0	13	1	12	1	10	6	4
E	XX	Injury & poisoning	3.9	4	3	5	39	1	21	1	37	1	33	1	5	4	5	5	1	5	1	9	2	5	2	9
		Total number of deaths	675,576		608,924		3,670		1,563		23,118		20,914		125,713		78,306		400,666		315,029		112,936		191,687	

Glossary

Glossary

Acute illness

An acute condition typically has a rapid onset, relatively short duration and usually ends with recovery or death. See also **Morbidity**.

Age-specific rate

The number of cases (of a disease, deaths) in a particular age-group divided by the total number of persons in that age group.

Age-standardisation

Disease incidence, mortality and survival rates are usually strongly related to the age composition of the population. It is therefore misleading to use overall rates (crude rates) when comparing two different populations unless they have the same age structure. Age-standardised rates, calculated by making adjustments for different population structures, allow for comparisons to be made between geographical areas, over time and between the sexes. There are two methods of age standardisation: direct age-standardisation and indirect age-standardisation. Direct age standardisation is used throughout in this volume. In direct age-standardisation, age-specific rates for the study population are multiplied by the standard or reference population in that age group. These are then summed and divided by the total standard population for these age groups to give the overall age-standardised rate. See also **European Standard Population**.

Alcohol-related mortality

Alcohol-related mortality reported in this volume uses the ONS definition, which includes those causes regarded as being most directly due to alcohol consumption. The definition includes deaths from chronic liver disease and cirrhosis (even when alcohol is not specifically mentioned on the death certificate) and deaths due to accidental poisoning with alcohol. It does not include diseases where alcohol has been shown to have some causal relationship, such as pancreatitis or cancers of the mouth, pharynx, larynx, oesophagus and liver. The definition also excludes external causes of death, such as road traffic deaths and other accidents, and alcohol-related suicides and homicides. The ICD-9 and ICD-10 codes used to define alcohol related deaths are:

ICD-9 Code	Description
291	Alcoholic psychoses
303	Alcohol dependence syndrome
305.0	Non-dependent abuse of alcohol
425.5	Alcoholic cardiomyopathy
571	Chronic liver disease and cirrhosis
E860	Accidental poisoning by alcohol

ICD-10 code	Description
F10	Mental and behavioural disorders due to use of alcohol
I42.6	Alcoholic cardiomyopathy
K70	Alcoholic liver disease
K73	Chronic hepatitis, not elsewhere classified
K74	Fibrosis and cirrhosis of liver
X45	Accidental poisoning and exposure to alcohol

Alcohol Use Disorders Identification Test (AUDIT) score

AUDIT score is used to assess the prevalence of alcohol misuse. An AUDIT score of eight or above indicates hazardous alcohol use or a pattern of drinking carrying with it a high risk of damage to health in the future. For calculation of AUDIT score from survey questions refer to *Tobacco, Alcohol and Drug Use and Mental Health* at www.statistics.gov.uk/statbase

Antipsychotic medication

Drugs used in the treatment of psychoses and related conditions, also known as 'neuroleptics'. In the short term they are used to quieten disturbed patients whatever the underlying psychopathology. Also included in this group are antimanic drugs, which are used to control acute attacks of mania and prevent their recurrence. Treatment can also be administered via depot injections. See also **Depot Injections**.

Area definitions

Depending upon the nature and availability of data varying geographies have been used in this volume. The 2001 Census data are mostly reported at the UK level, at country level (England, Wales, Scotland and Northern Ireland), at government office region (GOR) level and sometimes at the local authority level.

Local authority definitions:

> England – district council/ unitary authority/ borough council
> Wales – unitary authority
> Scotland - council areas
> Northern Ireland – government districts (also known as District Councils)

For boundaries and more detailed definition refer to *Beginners' Guide to UK Geography.*
www.statistics.gov.uk/geography/beginners_guide.asp

Body mass index (BMI)

BMI is calculated as weight in kilogrammes divided by the square of height in metres. In adults, if the resulting value is more than 25 but no greater than 30, the condition is defined as 'overweight'. If it exceeds 30, the condition is defined as 'obese'. If it exceeds 40, the condition is defined as 'morbid obesity'.

Bridge coding

Bridge coding establishes correspondence between two coding schemas, for example between ICD-9 and ICD-10. In order to compare cause-specific mortality rates between the two schemas, a sample of death certificates is coded independently according to both classifications, and the resulting underlying causes of death compared. The first step in this process is to identify equivalent codes or code groups in the two revisions which represent the same causes. The results can then be presented as comparability ratios of the numbers of deaths assigned to a given disease or group of diseases in the two revisions. Bridge coding is useful when comparing rates over time when it is not feasible to calculate rates using a single coding scheme. See also **Chapter 13, Appendix Table 13A**.

British National Formulary (BNF)

The BNF is a publication by the Royal Pharmaceutical Society and the British Medical Association which summarises information on the prescribing, dispensing and administration of prescription drugs in the UK. It classifies all prescription drugs into 15 chapters with additional categories for items such as dressings and appliances and is revised twice a year.

Burden of disease

The term 'burden of disease' refers to the overall impact of diseases and injuries at the societal level, or to the economic costs of diseases. Diseases present two different forms of burdens on society. The first is the loss of duration and quality of life due to the effects of diseases and disorders. The second is the cost of health, social care and other services concerned with the prevention and treatment of disease and assisting people with diseases and disorders.

Chronic disease, illness or condition

A chronic disease, illness or condition is one that increases the risk of long-term disability, handicap, or death and is unlikely to remit, although the occurrence and/or severity of its manifestations may vary over time. The distinction between a chronic illness and a non-chronic illness is generally made according to the likelihood of its lasting for 12 months or more and resulting in functional limitations and/or need for ongoing medical care. See also **Morbidity**.

Chronic Obstructive Pulmonary Disease (COPD)

COPD is a chronic, progressive disease, especially prevalent among those aged 45 and over, most commonly resulting from a history of smoking or inhalation of airborne pollution. COPD is characterised by breathing difficulty, wheezing and a chronic cough. It is diagnosed when the forced expiratory volume (FEV1) is less than 60 per cent of the predicted value for the patient's age and height and the patient does not respond to steroid drugs or bronchodilators.

Clinical Interview Schedule – revised version (CIS-R)

The CIS-R is a survey instrument designed to measure neurotic symptoms and disorders, such as anxiety and depression. It is based on 14 sections each covering a particular type of neurotic symptom. Scores are obtained for each symptom based on frequency, duration and severity in the past week. Individual symptom scores can be summed to provide an overall score for the level of neurotic symptoms. A score of 12 or more indicates the presence of significant levels of neurotic symptoms while a score of 18 or more indicates symptoms of a level likely to require treatment. If required, diagnoses of six specific neurotic disorders can be obtained by looking at answers to the various sections of the CIS-R and applying algorithms based on the ICD-10 diagnostic criteria for research. For further details see Lewis G and Pelosi A J (1990) *Manual of the revised clinical interview schedule (CIS–R)*, Institute of Psychiatry; London.

Cognitive behaviour therapy (CBT)

CBT is a psychological treatment for people suffering from mental health problems. CBT is based on the assumption that most unwanted thinking patterns and emotional and behavioural reactions are learned over a long period of time. The aim is to identify the thinking that is causing unwanted feelings and behaviours and to learn to replace this thinking with more positive thoughts. It is a combination of cognitive therapy, which helps to modify or eliminate unwanted thoughts and beliefs, and behavioural therapy, which helps to modify behaviour in response to those thoughts. The treatment usually takes between 8 and 20 sessions.

Cohort

A cohort is a group of people who have an event, attribute or experience in common. For example, a birth-cohort would include all those born within a specified time period (e.g. a year). Other examples would include all those who joined an organisation on the same day.

Cohort effect

The cohort effect is the variation in outcomes between people of the same age, but living in different periods. It is therefore a measure of the age-specific difference between one birth cohort, compared with a preceding or successive birth cohort of the same age. Each cohort is exposed to a different environment which coincides with its life span. Cohort effects are also termed generation effects. See also **Period effect**.

Communal establishment

In the 2001 Census a communal establishment was defined as an establishment providing managed residential accommodation. Managed means full-time or part-time supervision of the accommodation.

The definition has changed since the 1991 Census, where a communal establishment was defined as an establishment in which some form of communal catering was provided. In 2001, establishments with self-catering facilities (e.g. nurses homes, student hostels, etc) were enumerated as communal establishments only if there was someone in charge to take responsibility for issuing the Census forms. Otherwise, each person or group of people sharing meals or accommodation was treated as a separate household.

Comorbidity

The term is used to describe the presence of multiple diseases in an individual.

Correlation coefficient

A correlation coefficient is a number between -1 and 1 which measures the degree to which two variables are linearly related. The correlation between two variables is said to be positive if 'large' values of the two occur together, and is said to be negative if 'large' values of one variable tend to occur with 'small' values of another variable. A correlation of zero means that there is no linear relationship between the two variables.

Day case

A day case is a patient admitted electively (as a planned admission) who does not require the use of a hospital bed overnight, and who returns home as scheduled on the same day.

Depot injections

When antipsychotic medication is given by injections on a monthly basis, these are sometimes termed depot injections.

Determinants of health

Determinants of health include the wide variety of interacting proximate (more immediate e.g. health behaviours) and distal (wider effects e.g. education) influences on the health of individuals and populations, including but not limited to policies, social and physical environments, health systems and services, as well as genetic, biological and historico-cultural characteristics.

Dietary reference values

Dietary reference values (DRVs) comprise a series of estimates of the amount of energy and nutrients needed per day by different groups of healthy people in the UK population. DRVs are benchmark intakes of energy and nutrients, averaged over several days, given as guidance but are not exact recommendations.

Drink driving limit

The legal limit for the alcohol level for driving is 80 milligrammes of alcohol in 100 millilitres of blood. There is, however, no failsafe guide as to how much alcohol can be consumed to remain under the limit, as the absorption of alcohol in the bloodstream depends upon a variety of factors including the type of alcoholic drink, a person's weight, sex, age, food intake and metabolism.

Drinking guidelines

In 1992, the Government introduced the **weekly guideline** that men should drink less than 21 units of alcohol per week and women under 14 units of alcohol per week. In 1995, the weekly guidelines were changed to the **daily guideline** advising that men should drink no more than 4 units per day and women no more than 3 units per day. A unit of alcohol is defined as 8 grammes of alcohol which is equivalent to half a pint of ordinary strength beer, a small (125ml) glass of wine (at 9 per cent strength) or one measure of spirits.

Drug-related deaths

The ICD-9 and ICD-10 codes used to define drug-related deaths were:

ICD-9 code	ICD-10 code	Cause
292, 304, 305.2–305.9	F11–F16, F18–F19	Mental and behavioural disorders due to drug use (excluding alcohol and tobacco)
E850–E858	X40–X44	Accidental poisoning by drugs, medicaments and biological substances
E950.0–E950.5	X60–X64	Intentional self-poisoning by drugs, medicaments and biological substances
E980.0–E980.5	Y10–Y14	Poisoning by drugs, medicaments and biological substances, undetermined intent
E962.0	X85	Assault by drugs, medicaments and biological substances

Drugs (illicit)

Under the Misuse of Drugs Act 1971, drugs have been classified into three categories, A, B and C depending upon their harmfulness: drugs in class A being most harmful followed by Class B and Class C. The classification of certain drugs depends on the method of delivery used. For example, amphetamines are a Class B drug if taken orally and a Class A drug if injected. Cannabis was reclassified from Class B to C in January 2004.

Drug	Mode of use	Classification
Speed and other amphetamines	Inject	A
Ecstasy	Oral	A
Cocaine	Sniff or inject	A
Crack	Inject or smoke	A
Heroin	Smoke, sniff or inject	A
LSD	Oral	A
Magic Mushrooms	Oral	A
Methadone	Oral	A
Speed and other amphetamines	Sniff or oral	B
Tranquillisers	Oral or inject	B/C (depends on drug)
Anabolic steroids	Oral or inject	C
Cannabis	Smoke or oral	C
Poppers	Sniff	It is an offence to supply these substances if it is likely that the product is intended for abuse
Glue	Sniff	
Gas	Sniff	

Economic activity

Economic activity relates to whether a person is economically active or economically inactive. In the 2001 Census, the economic activity questions were only asked of people aged 16–74. This definition of economic activity is compatible with the International Labour Organisation (ILO) definition.

Economically active – All people who were working in the week before the Census were described as economically active. The category also includes people who were not working but were looking for work (unemployed) and were available to start work within 2 weeks. It also includes full-time students who are economically active. These are identified separately in the classification.

Economically inactive – Specific categories of economic inactivity were: Retired, Student (excludes those students who were working or in some other way were economically active), Looking after family/home, Permanently sick/ disabled and Other. A person who is looking for work but is not available to start work within 2 weeks is counted as economically inactive.

Ethnic group

The 2001 Census included a question on (self-defined) ethnic origin. Although the format of questions differed somewhat between the different parts of the UK, the same detailed codes were used across the UK to code the write-in responses. In the 2001 Census standard output tables the most detailed classification used was 16 groups (England and Wales), 14 groups (Scotland) and 12 groups (Northern Ireland) and these groups were not identical. To produce the 2001 Census data for the UK, the level 1 ethnic group classification (5 categories, listed overleaf) derived from the more detailed categories of individual countries was used.

UK	England and Wales	Scotland	Northern Ireland
White	British, Irish, Other White	White Scottish, Other White British, White Irish, Other White	White
Mixed	White and Black Caribbean, White and Black African, White and Asian, Other Mixed	Any Mixed Background	Mixed
Asian	Indian, Pakistani, Bangladeshi, Other Asian	Indian, Pakistani, Bangladeshi, Other South Asian	Asian
Black	Black Caribbean Black African Other Black	Caribbean, African, Black Scottish or Other Black	Black
Chinese or other ethnic group	Chinese Other Ethnic Group	Chinese Other Ethnic Group	Chinese or other ethnic group

European Standard Population

Age-standardised rates reported in this volume were calculated using the direct age-standardisation method employing the European Standard Population (ESP). The ESP is used as it is closest to the demographic profile of the United Kingdom. The same population was used for both males and females. See also **Age-standardisation.**

Age group	European Standard Population
0	1,600
1–4	6,400
5–9	7,000
10–14	7,000
15–19	7,000
20–24	7,000
25–29	7,000
30–34	7,000
35–39	7,000
40–44	7,000
45–49	7,000
50–54	7,000
55–59	6,000
60–64	5,000
65–69	4,000
70–74	3,000
75–79	2,000
80–84	1,000
85 and over	1,000
Total	100,000

Family status

A family comprises a group of people consisting of a married or cohabiting couple with or without child(ren), or a lone parent with child(ren). It also includes a married or cohabiting couple with their grandchild(ren) or a lone grandparent with his or her grandchild(ren) where there are no children in the intervening generation in the household. Cohabiting couples include same sex couples. Children in couple families include dependent or non-dependent children of one or both members of the couple. The categories used in this volume to describe the family circumstances of a person are:

Not in a family – of pensionable age
Not in a family – other

In a couple family – member of couple
In a couple family – dependent child of one or both members of the couple
In a couple family – non dependent child of one or both members of the couple

In lone parent family – parent
In lone parent family – dependent child of parent
In lone parent family – non dependent child of parent

Finished consultant episode (FCE)

In hospital episode statistics data, an FCE is defined as an episode of care under one consultant within one healthcare provider. FCEs do not represent the number of patients admitted to hospital, as a person may have more than one episode of care within a spell of treatment (e.g. if they are transferred from one consultant to another) or within a year.

General population

In this report, the general population refers to the population resident in households (i.e. excluding residents of communal establishments such as boarding schools, prisons, care homes, hotels etc).

Government Office Regions

The Government Office Regions (GORs), established in England in 1994 and revised in 1998, divide England into 9 regions comprising the North East, North West, Yorkshire and the Humber, East Midlands, West Midlands, East of England, South East, South West and London. Scotland, Wales and Northern Ireland are not subdivided into GORs but are listed separately as regions in UK-wide statistical comparisons.

GP consultation rate

The consultation rate is the number of consultations with a general practitioner (GP) or family doctor within a reference period divided by the study population. In the General Household Survey, the reference period is the previous two weeks.

Household

A household is a person living alone or a group of people who have the address as their only or main residence and who either share one meal a day or share the living accommodation.

Household reference person

The harmonised definition of the household reference person used in Government Social Surveys is as follows:

a) In households with a sole householder that person is the household reference person.

b) In households with joint householders the person with the highest income is taken as the household reference person.

c) If both householders have exactly the same income, the older is taken as household reference person.

For more details, see the ONS website: www.statistics.gov.uk/harmonisation

Household tenure

The categories of household tenure used in this volume are defined as follows:

Owned – Accommodation either owned outright, owned with a mortgage or loan, or shared ownership (paying part rent and part mortgage).

Private Rented – Accommodation rented from a private landlord or letting agency, employer of a household member, relative or friend of a household member, or other.

Social Rented – Accommodation that is rented from a council (local authority, Scottish Homes, Northern Ireland Housing Executive) or a housing association, housing co-operative, charitable trust, non-profit housing company or registered social landlord.

Housing deprivation

In the 2001 Census, a household was defined as deprived in the housing dimension if it was either overcrowded (actual number of rooms minus rooms required is less than or equal to -1); or was a shared dwelling; or did not have sole use of a bath/ shower or toilet; or did not have central heating.

To calculate overcrowding, the room requirement for a household was calculated as follows:

1) A one-person household is assumed to require three rooms (two common rooms and a bedroom).

2) Where there are two or more residents it is assumed that they require a minimum of two common rooms plus one bedroom for:

   i.   each couple (as determined by the relationship question)

   ii.   each lone parent

   iii. any other person aged 16 or over

   iv.   each pair aged 10–15 of the same sex

   v.   each pair formed from a remaining person aged 10–15 with a child aged under 10 of the same sex

   vi.   each pair of children aged under 10 remaining

   vii. each remaining person (either aged 10–15 or under 10).

Hyperkinetic disorder

Hyperkinetic disorder is a mental disorder, usually of children, characterised by a grossly excessive level of activity and a marked impairment of the ability to pay attention. Learning is impaired as a result and behaviour is disruptive and may be defiant or aggressive.

Incidence

Incidence is a measure of the rate at which new cases occur in the population, i.e the number of new cases of a disease in a specified period, divided by the population at risk of getting the disease during the specified period (usually a calendar year).

Infant mortality rate

Infant mortality rate is the number of deaths of children aged less than one year during a given time period, divided by the number of live births reported during the same period. It is usually expressed as rate per 1,000 live births.

Informal care (unpaid care)

Alternatively known as 'unpaid care'. Within the Census 2001, the term 'unpaid care' covers any help provided looking after or supporting family members, friends, neighbours or others because of long-term physical or mental ill-health or disability or problems related to old age.

Inpatients

In hospital statistics data, inpatients include all admissions to hospital resulting in an overnight stay. Infants born in a maternity department, healthy persons accompanying inpatients and sick staff treated in their own quarters are not included.

International Classification of Diseases

International Classification of Diseases (ICD) is a coding scheme for classifying diseases and causes of death. The tenth revision of the ICD (ICD-10) was introduced for coding the underlying cause of death in Scotland from 2000 and in the rest of the UK from 2001. The ICD-10 replaces the ninth revision of the ICD (ICD-9).

Inverse care law

In 1971, a UK general practitioner, Julian Tudor Hart, coined the term 'inverse care law' which stated that 'the availability of good medical care tends to vary inversely with the need for it in the population served'.

Kilocalorie

Kilocalorie is a measure of energy-producing potential in food. It is defined as a unit of heat equal to the amount of heat required to raise the temperature of one kilogramme of water by one degree at one atmosphere pressure.

Life expectancy

Life expectancy is the average number of years a person would live if they experienced current mortality rates for the remainder of their life. Life expectancy is usually computed on the basis of a life table showing the probability of dying at each age for a given population according to the age-specific death rates prevailing at a given period.

Mean length of stay

In hospital episodes statistics data the mean length of stay in hospital is calculated as the sum of the duration of all spells in hospitals divided by the number of spells. A spell comprises a patient's entire continuous stay in a hospital. If a patient dies or is discharged from hospital or is transferred to another hospital, the spell ends. The duration of a spell is calculated as the difference in days between the admission date and the discharge date, where both are given. Day cases and other cases where the admission and discharge dates are the same, are excluded from this calculation.

Mental health

Mental health refers to the successful performance of mental function, resulting in productive activities, fulfilling relationships with other people, and the ability to adapt to change and cope with adversity. Good mental health is contrasted with mental disorders, which are health conditions characterised by alterations in thinking, mood or behaviour associated with distress and/or impaired functioning.

Morbidity

Morbidity is a broad term used to describe the presence of a health condition (any departure from a state of physiological or psychological health and well-being) in an individual, whether disease, injury or an impairment. Specifically, it covers both acute and chronic conditions.

Mortality rate

Mortality rate is a measure of the frequency of occurrence of deaths in a defined population during a specified time interval. In its simplest form, the crude mortality rate is defined as the total number of deaths in a given year divided by the total population. The value of crude rates is limited, particularly when comparing between two populations (e.g. population groups, geographical areas, or over time), with different age structures. In these circumstances, it is usual to age-standardise or to compare age-specific rates.

National Service Frameworks

National Service Frameworks are a set of policy documents setting out national standards for the best ways of providing health and social care services for particular diseases (e.g. cancer) or population groups (e.g. older people).

National Statistics Socio-Economic Classification

From April 2001, the National Statistics Socio-Economic Classification (NS-SEC) was introduced for all official statistics and surveys, replacing social class and socio-economic groups (SEG) based on occupation. The classification includes 17 categories, of which the last four (L14–L17) include people who are excluded when the classification is collapsed into its analytical classes (e.g. long-term unemployed, full-time students). Most of the statistical outputs only use the first eight classes, defined in column 1 below, known as analytical classes or a collapsed version of these as defined in column 3. Full details can be found in *The National Statistics Socio-Economic Classification User Manual 2002.*

Neurotic disorders

Neurotic disorders are mental disorders without any demonstrable organic basis in which there is no serious disturbance in the perception or understanding of external reality. Behaviour may be greatly affected although usually remaining within socially acceptable limits, but personality is not disorganised. The principal manifestations include excessive anxiety, hysterical symptoms, phobias, obsessional and compulsive symptoms, and depression.

Notifications of infectious diseases

The Infectious Disease (Notification) Act 1889 was introduced to identify and prevent the spread of infectious diseases in England and Wales. A doctor who makes a diagnosis (confirmed or suspected) of a notifiable infectious disease is required by statute to notify the 'Proper Officer' of their local authority (a person defined under the Public Health (Control of Disease) Act 1984). The list of notifiable diseases now covers 29 infections.

NS-SEC category Description	NS-SEC Category	Combined NS-SEC category Description
Large employers and higher managerial occupations	L1, L2	Managerial and professional occupations
Higher professional occupations	L3	
Lower managerial and professional occupations	L4, L5, L6	
Intermediate occupations	L7	Intermediate occupations
Small employers and own account workers	L8, L9	
Lower supervisory and technical occupations	L10, L11	Routine and manual occupations
Semi-routine occupations	L12	
Routine occupations	L13	
Never worked and long-term unemployed	L14	Excluded when the classification is collapsed into its analytical classes.
Full time students	L15	
Occupation not stated or inadequately described	L16	
Not classifiable for other reasons	L17	

Oral health

A standard of health of the oral (mouth) and related tissues which enables an individual to eat, speak and socialise without active disease, discomfort or embarrassment and which contributes to general well-being. Dental health is included.

Outpatient

An outpatient is defined as a person visiting hospital for treatment or to see a consultant for treatment or advice without being admitted.

Outpatient attendance rate

There are two types of sources used to calculate outpatient attendance rates in this volume:

- Rates based on NHS administrative data were calculated by dividing the total number of outpatient attendances by the mid-year population estimate for the year (expressed per 100 population). Outpatient attendances include both NHS and private patients seen for their first appointments as well as for subsequent or follow up appointments. Persons attending more than one department in the same visit (for unrelated conditions) are counted in each department separately. Patients attending Accident & Emergency (or Casualty) are not included.

- Rates based on survey data (i.e. General Household Survey and Health Survey for England) were based on the reported number of 'casualty or outpatient' attendances in the past year, divided by the number of respondents in the survey.

Pensionable age

In this volume pensionable age is defined as age 60 for women and 65 for men.

Period effect

A period effect is the impact of an event or conditions occurring at a particular point in time which affects people of all ages or different generations. Examples would include famines, epidemics, food rationing, etc. It would also include changes in disease classification, or coding, introduction of screening, efficacy of treatment. See also **Cohort effect**.

Personality disorder

A condition in which the sufferer fails to learn from experience or to adapt to changes. The outcome is impaired social functioning and personal distress.

Prevalence

Prevalence is a measure of the number of people with a disease in a defined population at a specified time. It includes all cases of the disease existing at a point in time (point prevalence), or over a period of time (period prevalence), in a defined population. Other than in epidemiology, it is often used as a measure of the commonality of an activity (such as smoking) or an attribute (such as obesity). See also **Incidence**.

Preventive healthcare

Preventive healthcare can be variously defined but here it focuses on measures aimed at promoting health and preventing disease in individuals and defined populations. It forms part of public health comprising activities such as screening, immunisation, health education and promotion. Other aspects of public health such as housing, water supplies, sanitation and food hygiene are not included.

Primary care

Primary care includes those health services which provide the first (or primary) point of contact for patients. In the UK, these include family health services provided by general practitioners (GPs), community nurses, dentists, pharmacists, optometrists and ophthalmic medical practitioners.

Primary diagnostic groups

In hospital episodes statistics data, the main health condition for which the patient is admitted to hospital is entered as the primary diagnosis. The diagnosis is coded into groups according to the International Classification of Diseases, tenth revision (ICD-10).

Psychiatric morbidity

The prevalence of mental health problems such as anxiety, depression, schizophrenia and personality disorders.

Psychoses

Psychoses are mental disorders that produce disturbances in thinking and perception that are severe enough to distort the person's perception of the world and the relationship of events within it. Psychoses are normally divided into two groups: organic psychoses, such as dementia and Alzheimer's disease, and functional psychoses, which mainly cover schizophrenia and manic depression. See also **Neurotic disorders**.

Qualifications

To assess educational attainment, the 2001 Census asked what qualifications respondents had in some detail, although there were some differences between the types of qualifications covered in the question between the UK countries. (In addition, in England and Wales there was a separate question which recorded teaching, nursing, medical and dental professional qualifications.)

In this report, respondents have been grouped into two broad categories based on their highest qualification attained: 'Lower level qualifications' (from one or more O levels/CSEs/ GCSEs to two or more A levels, or four or more AS levels, in England and Wales and equivalents in the other UK countries); and 'Higher level qualifications' covering first degree or higher NVQ levels 1 to 5, and other qualifications.

Quintile, Quartile

Quintiles divide an ordered set of data values (say from highest to lowest) into five equal groups. Likewise, quartiles partition an ordered data set into four equal groups. Commonly, references to quartiles relate to just the outer two: the upper and lower quartiles. The lower quartile defines the cut-point below which lie the lowest 25 per cent of the data values; and the upper quartile is the cut-point above which lies the highest 25 per cent of the data values.

Relative survival

Relative survival is the ratio of the observed survival rate in the group being studied (e.g. with a specific cancer) to the expected survival rate had they been subject only to the mortality rates of the general population. The relative survival rate is an estimate of the chance of surviving the effects of disease after taking into account general mortality rates.

Risk factor

A risk factor is an aspect of personal behaviour or lifestyle, an environmental exposure, or a hereditary characteristic that is associated with an increase in the likelihood of a particular disease, chronic condition, or injury occurring.

Screening

Screening is the routine examination of apparently healthy people in the population in order to detect a particular disease at an early stage, before symptoms develop.

Secondary care

Secondary or specialist care is, typically, provided in a hospital setting following referral from a primary or community health professional.

Sexually transmitted infections

Sexually transmitted infections (STIs) are infections that can be passed on through sexual contact, whether intimate physical

contact or sexual intercourse including sexual foreplay, anal and oral sex. The most well-known STIs are chlamydia, gonorrhoea, genital warts and syphilis.

Social class

Social class, or more specifically known as Registrar General's Social Class, has been in use in the UK official statistics since its first appearance in the Registrar General's Annual Report of 1911. Social class is derived from the individual's current or last occupation and employment status (such as employee, manager, or self-employed). The size of the organisation is also used when that information is available, such as in the Census. There are six categories in the Registrar General's Social Class defined as follows

Descriptive Definition	Social Class
Professional	I
Intermediate occupations	II
Skilled occupations – non-manual	III NM
Skilled occupation – manual	III M
Partly-skilled	IV
Unskilled occupations	V

Sometimes, the six-category social class is summarised into two groups: non-manual (Social Class I, II, IIINM) and manual (Social Class IIIM, IV, V).

Socio-economic grouping

The Registrar General's socio-economic grouping (SEG) was the occupational classification used in UK Censuses and surveys until 2001 when it was replaced by NS-SEC. For persons aged 16 or over, including full-time students with employment experience, socio-economic group corresponds to their own present job, or, for those not currently working, to their last job. Persons whose occupation was inadequately described, the Armed Forces and full-time students are excluded. Most statistical outputs use an 8-categories abridged version of SEG.

Descriptive definition	SEG number
Professional	3,4
Employers and managers	1,2,13
Intermediate non-manual	5
Junior non-manual	6
Skilled manual (including foremen and supervisors and own account non-professional)	8,9,12,14
Semi-skilled manual and personal service	7,10,15
Unskilled manual	11

These categories can be further collapsed into two categories Non-Manual (SEGs 1–6,13) Manual (SEGs 7–12,14–15).

Standardised patient consultation rate (SPCR)

SPCR is the proportion of patients who consulted at least once during the year at a defined level of diagnostic detail (e.g. for any illness, for all respiratory illnesses, or for bronchitis), standardised for age using the European standard population.

Survival rate

Survival rate is the proportion of persons in a specified group alive at the beginning of a time interval who survive to the end of the interval. It is often studied using life table methods. See also **Relative survival**.